FUNCTIONAL

REHABILITATION IN

ORTHOPAEDICS

Trudy Sandler Goldstein, PT
Founder and Director
Quality Educational Seminars for Therapists
Burlington, Massachusetts

Senior Therapist
Arlington Orthopedic and Sports Physical Therapy
Arlington, Massachusetts

Formerly, Clinical Supervisor
New England Rehabilitation Hospital
Woburn, Massachusetts

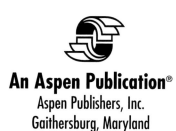

An Aspen Publication®
Aspen Publishers, Inc.
Gaithersburg, Maryland
1995

Library of Congress Cataloging-in-Publications Data

Goldstein, Trudy Sandler.
Functional rehabilitation in orthopaedics/Trudy Sandler
Goldstein.
p.   cm.
Includes bibliographical references and index.
ISBN 0-8342-0556-4
1. Physically handicapped—Rehabilitation. 2. Orthopedics.
I. Title.
[DNLM: 1. Disabled—rehabilitation.
WB 320 G624f 1995]
RD797.G65 1995
617.3—dc20
DNLM/DLC
for Library of Congress

94-27529
CIP

Aspen Publishers, Inc., grants permission for photocopying for limited
personal or internal use. This consent does not extend to other kinds
of copying, such as copying for general distribution, for advertising or
promotional purposes, for creating new collective works, or for resale.
For information, address Aspen Publishers, Inc., Permissions
Department, 200 Orchard Ridge Drive, Suite 200,
Gaithersburg, Maryland 20878.

The authors have made every effort to ensure the accuracy of the information
herein, particularly with regard to drug selection and dose. However, appropriate information sources should be consulted, especially for new or unfa-
miliar drugs or procedures. It is the responsibility of every practitioner to
evaluate the appropriateness of a particular opinion in the context of actual
clinical situations and with due consideration to new developments. Authors,
editors, and the publisher cannot be held responsible for any typographical or
other errors found in this book.

Editorial Services: Bonnie S. Lawhorn

Library of Congress Catalog Card Number: 94-27529
ISBN: 0-8342-0556-4

Printed in the United States of America

1 2 3 4 5

This book is dedicated
with love
to my family—my husband *Alan*
and my daughters *Jamie* and *Elyse.*
They have given me the support and love
to pursue my dreams.

Contents _____

Contributor

Beverly Biondi, PT
Sausalito, California

Illustrations by

Mary Fantasia Nuovo, BFA
Woburn, Massachusetts

Preface

Function is definitely the buzzword of the 1990s. Although function is addressed by the two major rehabilitative disciplines, occupational therapy and physical therapy, no one seems to work on restoring anything but the most basic functional abilities to patients with musculoskeletal disorders. Although this population represents an enormous portion of our patient caseload, little effort is spent on guiding these patients back to independence. It is assumed that they will somehow find their own way back to an independent life style. Interestingly, this same assumption is not made for the so-called more challenging patients: the neurologically involved, athletic, or industrial patient.

I have written this book to provide the rehabilitation specialist (including the physical therapist, occupational therapist, assistant, and student) with a logical treatment plan to restore function in both the ordinary patient with musculoskeletal dysfunction and the other patient populations. This highly skilled treatment plan involves the combined use of a correctional program and actual or modified functional activities.

When available, I have tried to include the actual motions and muscles needed to perform different functional activities, so that the reader understands which structures are being stressed during various functional tasks. This allows the clinician to individualize the program for each patient by appropriately modifying the activities. I have also recommended adjustments to the program that should be considered for patients with specific musculoskeletal injuries. Because of its importance, an entire chapter is devoted to the restoration of function in the geriatric population in both community and long-term care settings.

As a result of the need to prove the efficacy of our treatments, Chapter 13 deals with the topics of assessing functional level and measuring true change in functional status. To promote clinical use of functional assessment, I have included samples of actual assessment forms along with information about how to obtain them from the copyright holders. Only when therapists begin to measure functional ability accurately will we know for certain that our treatments are in fact beneficial.

Even though this program just seems to make sense on an intuitive level, I have tried to present a rationale in Chapter 4 for why function is lost in the first place and how it can best be restored on the basis of the dynamic theory of movement. This chapter deals with the complexity and interconnectedness that defines the human body and human motion. I believe this theory goes a long way toward explaining why simply restoring normal strength or range of motion does not necessarily translate into improved movement patterns. I hope the reader finds the concepts presented in this chapter as fascinating as I do.

As I lecture around the country, I find that there is always great interest in the different types of functional exercise and adaptive equipment currently available. I have therefore written two chapters (14 and 15) describing some of the functional uses of various pieces of equipment as well as whom to contact for trial use or purchase. (Although many pieces of equipment were by necessity omitted from the discussion, the reader will have a place to start in exploring equipment options.)

I hope that, by reading this book, the clinician will understand the importance of initiating a functional restoration program for all patients regardless of current ability level. Functional assessment should be a part of all evaluations and the functional program should be started in the first treatment session as a matter of course and not as an afterthought. Without the luxury of time, functional restoration can no longer be saved for the end of a rehabilitation program as a "skill to be polished." I hope this book causes the clinician to rethink traditional treatment plans and to make functional rehabilitation a treatment philosophy and goal for all patients.

Acknowledgments _____

Writing a book is an extremely time-consuming and difficult labor of love. I would like to thank the many people whose contributions made this book possible. Special thanks go to Beverly Biondi, PT, who wrote the chapter on lumbar stabilization, and to Mary Nuovo, who once again magically transformed my stick figures into illustrations. Additional thanks go to my brother-in-law, Louis Goldstein, PhD, who introduced me to the world of dynamic systems, chaos, and complexity. Because of him, I can no longer look at cloud formations, traffic jams, or my patients' movement patterns in the way I once did. Chapter 4, on movement science, is dedicated to him. I would also like to thank my husband Alan for taking many of the photographs for this text and Hyman Sandler, Lillian Sandler, Ruth-Ellen Sandler, Jamie Goldstein, and Elyse Goldstein for agreeing to be my models. In addition, I would like to thank my sister Ruth-Ellen Sandler and my coworker Mary Rojo, PT, for reading and providing valuable comments on portions of the manuscript. Special thanks also go to my parents for their love, support, and unfailing encouragement. Last but not least, I would like to express my gratitude to Loretta Stock of Aspen Publishers. Her voice across the miles was both a comfort and an inspiration and made the work involved in writing this text a pleasure.

1

Introduction to Functional Rehabilitation

The major reason why patients come to rehabilitative therapy is to return to a pain-free, active life style. They want to be as they were, to function as they did before. Until recently, rehabilitation therapists have specialized in restoring function without clearly identifying it, assessing it, or training it. In addition, the majority of the work done in this area has involved neurologically impaired patients or elite orthopaedic patients (ie, athletes and injured workers). The knowledge gained from functionally retraining these patients must now be shared with ordinary orthopaedic patients and must become a part of all rehabilitation programs.

TRADITIONAL ROLES OF PHYSICAL THERAPY AND OCCUPATIONAL THERAPY

Occupational therapy has always been the medical discipline most concerned with the restoration of function of patients. The occupational therapist (OT) teaches patients activities of daily living (ADLs), such as dressing, eating, and grooming, and creates splints and adaptive equipment for patients requiring additional stabilization or support to care for themselves. The occupational therapy department is home to the adaptive kitchen and bathroom, where patients learn to make meals and to bathe independently. In addition, the OT has a strong psychological background and helps patients overcome mental and emotional roadblocks to independence.

Physical therapy has historically been more concerned with correcting musculoskeletal dysfunction. The physical therapist (PT) instructs patients in strengthening and flexibility exercises, teaches proper body mechanics and transfers, corrects posture and gait deviations, and uses physical modalities such as ultrasound or electrical stimulation to decrease pain or promote muscle activity.

These two sister professions overlap in many areas of expertise. Both grew out of the horror of the World Wars to help heal injured soldiers and return them to purposeful lives as civilians. Today, both continue that work in restoring mobility skills and function to patients who have become disabled. Yet neither profession has been exceptional in defining function, measuring it, and specifically retraining it.

CLINICAL SETTINGS

Therapists treat patients in a variety of therapeutic settings: the acute care hospital, the rehabilitation hospital, the skilled nursing facility, the outpatient practice, and the community or

1

home care setting. To provide treatment efficiently and not duplicate services, health care facilities and insurance companies sometimes create policies to divide the patient into upper and lower body parts. OTs tend to treat the upper body parts, and PTs tend to treat the spine, pelvis, and lower extremities. In addition, OTs generally concentrate on the ability to plan and carry out activities, while PTs focus on specific musculoskeletal problems. Although therapists do not like dividing the patient up into an assemblage of arms, legs, and central processing unit, this method provides quality treatment for the most part and maintains peace between OTs and PTs. This health care delivery system is far from perfect, though, and the patient sometimes gets lost in the cracks.

Take the hypothetical case of Mrs. Richards, a 77-year-old widow who lives alone in a second-story apartment in the suburbs of Boston. Before her husband died 14 months ago, she had been extremely active. She went for daily mile walks, drove to church on Sundays, did her own shopping, loved to garden, and generally enjoyed life. When her husband became ill, she stayed at home to care for him. Six months after his death, she slipped outside on the sidewalk and cut her knee. She stopped going out unless she needed to shop or bank. Three months later, she fell at night while going to the bathroom. She tired easily. Just before her accident, Mrs. Richards' right shoulder began bothering her again, a flare-up of an old bursitis injury. She found it exceedingly difficult to carry things. Because she could no longer reach into her cupboard, she climbed a small stool to get a can of soup. Unfortunately, she lost her balance and fell, fracturing her right hip. Thus began her adventure into the medical system and her transformation from Mrs. Richards the person to Mrs. Richards the hip fracture patient.

The Acute Care Hospital

The first stop on her journey found Mrs. Richards in the acute care hospital. After examination, she underwent surgery for placement of a compression screw and plate into her right hip. Physical therapy focused on strengthening, range of motion (ROM), and basic mobility skills such as bed-to-chair transfers, ambulating to the toilet, rolling in bed, etc. Occupational therapy worked on dressing and toileting skills. Neither her PT nor her OT performed an in-depth functional assessment. They both concurred that she required moderate assistance in basic ADL skills and needed additional therapy to be able to function independently at home.

Five days after surgery, Mrs. Richards was medically stable and ready for discharge. The therapists referred her to a local rehabilitation hospital with her status as follows:

- prior to admission, patient independent
- sutures in, healing well
- strength right hip is 2/5
- passive ROM right hip: flexion 80°; abduction 20°; rotations 10°
- strength and ROM of all other extremities within functional limits
- bed mobility requires minimal assistance
- bathing and dressing of upper body independent, requires assist for lower body
- ambulation with a walker partial weight bearing, requires minimal assistance for 30 ft

Both physical and occupational therapy helped Mrs. Richards on her road to recovery. Yet assumptions were made that haunted Mrs. Richards as she continued her journey. Although the strength and ROM of her affected limb were measured with accuracy, her other limbs were vaguely categorized as "functional." If her right shoulder had possessed functional ROM in the first place, Mrs. Richards would never have needed to climb onto the stool to reach into the cupboard. Now that her ROM has been measured and determined to be "functional," one of her underlying physical problems does not officially exist in the medical record.

The Rehabilitation Hospital

Cooperation abounds in the rehabilitation hospital as patients, therapists, nurses, doctors, and social workers effectively communicate patient problems and abilities at team meetings and work together to create solutions. In this setting, functional independence is the optimal goal for all patients. However, neurological patients (patients with stroke, spinal cord injury, head injury, etc.) always seem to have priority in functional skills training. Patients with orthopaedic problems (fractures, total joint arthroplasties, etc.) receive minimal instruction in functional activities. The major emphasis is restoration of normal strength and flexibility, reduction of pain and edema, and return of basic mobility skills such as walking and transfers. It is assumed that when the musculoskeletal problem is healed, the patient will be able to resume prior activity levels without specific training.

Mrs. Richards was admitted to a rehabilitation hospital 6 days following the intertrochanteric fracture of her right hip. After additional evaluation, her OT determined that she needed a long-handled shoe horn and dressing stick to be independent in basic ADLs. Her PT began strengthening exercises and gait training with a walker. Fifteen days later at discharge, Mrs. Richards could:

- dress herself from a seated position
- toilet independently with a raised toilet seat and grab bar
- transfer on and off a tub seat
- ambulate safely with a walker for 100 ft
- climb a full flight of stairs with a railing and a cane

Her discharge plan included receiving lunch from Meals-on-Wheels and additional physical therapy at home through the local Visiting Nurse Association (VNA). The plan seemed logical and feasible, but what about the questions of her functional abilities that were not asked or answered? What about the functional treatments that were not given? A more detailed functional assessment might have shown the following:

- Mrs. Richards can sponge bathe independently in bed and can perform a tub transfer fully dressed.

But she cannot take a shower or a bath without moderate assistance.
- She can groom herself independently from a wheelchair.

But she cannot stand at the bathroom sink to wash up, brush her teeth, comb her hair, or put on make-up. (She was unable to practice these bathroom activities in the standing position because the nurses were short staffed and were unable to supervise her.)
- She can stand at a counter and make herself a sandwich.

But she cannot carry the sandwich to the kitchen table while managing the walker at the same time.
- She can reach most of the items on her kitchen counter.

But she cannot reach into the cupboards because of a painful shoulder. (Mrs. Richards never had the opportunity to use the occupational therapy kitchen because it was overbooked with high-priority neurological patients.)
- She can get onto the floor easily. (As a matter of fact, that is exactly what frightens her the most about going home.)

But she cannot get onto the floor in a safe and controlled manner, nor can she get up.

In this day of diagnosis-related groups (DRGs), Mrs. Richards was deemed ready for discharge from a rehabilitation hospital, but was she? Because her therapists did not perform an accurate measurement of her functional ability, they were unaware of the degree of her functional impairment. Although the reality of modern medicine dictates a limited number of rehabilitation days for this orthopaedic injury, Medicare guidelines never intended Mrs. Richards to return home with the inability to perform such basic ADL skills. Both her OT and her PT failed to provide her with adequate functional retraining.

Interestingly, had Mrs. Richards suffered the same fracture in the 1970s, she would not be a candidate for discharge because patients and therapists had more time to work on functional retraining after restoring sufficient strength and ROM to the affected limbs. At that time, patients with hip fractures had to make their own beds, prepare a meal in the kitchen, walk independently on all surfaces for 1000 ft, and negotiate stairs independently before returning home alone.

The Skilled Nursing Facility

Because more patients are being discharged from acute and rehabilitation settings without first achieving functional independence, there has been a large increase in the number of orthopaedic patients admitted to skilled nursing facilities instead of simply returning home. Fitzgerald et al[1] describe a 60% increase in nursing facility admissions for hip fracture patients since the implementation of the prospective payment system. In addition, there has also been a 200% increase in long-term placement at these facilities. The major correlating factor is the patient's ability to ambulate.

Therapists in this setting now need to perform full rehabilitation programs. Yet these facilities often do not have the necessary equipment or staffing to accomplish this goal. Many do not even provide in-house occupational therapy services. Time and personnel constraints often force the PT to neglect the functional retraining program.

If Mrs. Richards had been discharged to this setting, she would probably only have received standard physical therapy consisting of therapeutic exercise, modalities, and gait training. To get home, she would have required additional training, a bridge between institution life and home life. She would have needed a functional rehabilitation program. Otherwise, she might have been doomed to become another statistic in the study of Fitzgerald et al.[1]

The Outpatient Practice

As health care moves away from inpatient hospital stays, outpatient rehabilitation services grow at an astounding rate. Patients can access outpatient therapy in acute and rehabilitation hospitals, satellite centers of major hospitals, or privately owned clinics. Doctors routinely order continued outpatient occupational and physical therapy services for their neurologically impaired patients. They occasionally order continued outpatient physical therapy for their orthopaedic patients. Many PTs at these facilities work on traditional physical therapy goals of restoring strength, ROM, transfers, and gait but fail to properly address functional problems such as bathing, meal preparation, or community ambulation. If Mrs. Richards had been discharged to this setting, she would probably not have received an in-depth functional assessment. After restoration of her strength, ROM, and gait to a "functional level," Mrs. Richards would have been left to discover her way back to her prior independent status on her own.

Interestingly, these same therapists take great pains to restore their athletic and industrial patients to prior levels of function. A PT would never discharge an athlete from physical therapy until that athlete showed sufficient strength and ROM for sport as well as the capacity to run, throw, jump, etc. In other words, the athlete would need to demonstrate the necessary functional ability to safely resume the rigors of sports before being discharged. The same holds true for the injured worker, who must demonstrate the ability to properly lift, reach, type, and the like before being allowed to return to work. Why are these standards of care not equally applied to all patients?

The Home Care Setting

Community agencies such as VNAs provide physical therapy and occupational therapy services for the patient confined to home. Although unable to access the high-technology machines of standard physical therapy and occupational therapy practices, these therapists successfully restore the musculoskeletal as well as the functional problems of their clients. Nowhere in the medical community does functional restoration take on such importance. Simulation is unnecessary because the patient's home provides the functional obstacles: shelves to reach, ovens to open, sinks to wash, tables to dust, stairs to climb, and so on. Yet even here, some orthopaedic patients never reach full functional independence before their benefits expire. The problem lies mainly in the therapist's failure to assess, document, and address functional impairments in a way acceptable to insurance companies.

Mrs. Richards finds herself home at last, but a prisoner of her second-floor apartment. She is terrified of attempting the stairs by herself. She is entitled to home physical therapy but not to occupational therapy (as a result of Medicare's guidelines about duplication of services). She and her new PT work on both traditional physical therapy goals and functional restoration. Through a combination of exercise and the actual performance of functional activities, such as making breakfast, climbing the stairs, and washing a sink, Mrs. Richards begins to return to her prior level of activity. When Mrs. Richards' abilities "look OK," she is discharged from physical therapy. She officially leaves the medical realm and the role of patient behind and becomes a "person" once again. Although she can manage her self-care adequately in the home, she is afraid to walk downstairs or outdoors alone, she still cannot reach into the cupboards (no one ever assessed her shoulder, because she was a hip patient), and she has not driven her car since her fall. In spite of months of therapy, Mrs. Richards remains disabled.

FUNCTIONAL REHABILITATION FOR THE ORTHOPAEDIC PATIENT

Functional rehabilitation can no longer be a goal only for the neurologically impaired. Although the patient with neurological insult may have obvious perceptual problems, motor planning deficits, and weakness, the orthopaedic patient may have subtle but similar problems to overcome. All therapists have witnessed the patient who regains normal strength and motion but still remains nonfunctional. The assumption

that the patient can simply figure out how to return to the prior level of function without the skills of a rehabilitation specialist is simply not true in many cases.

THE ORTHOPAEDIC FUNCTIONAL PROGRAM

Functional restoration must begin immediately upon the patient's entering the medical system. The patient no longer has the luxury of time to regain strength and ROM first and then work on polishing skills such as function. Initial and follow-up evaluations must now include a functional component (see Chapter 13 on measuring function). In every clinical setting, therapists must work to restore functional limitations at the same time that they are working on more traditional therapy goals.

A Total-Body Approach

Since functional ability depends on the proper interaction of all the body parts and the brain, functional restoration requires treatment of the whole person, not just the injured portion. The entire focus of therapy can no longer be to simply regain normal strength, ROM, and gait but must include the restoration of balance, proprioception, coordination, and agility. Depending on the patient, this might mean working on quadriceps strengthening by vertical jumping (a highly skilled, total-body activity) in addition to exercising on isokinetic equipment.

Functional activities must also be done in an efficient and safe manner. Even if an activity is "functional" (ie, the patient can accomplish the task), the therapist may still need to correct the technique to make the activity less painful or easier to perform. Proper body mechanics, postures, and joint interactions must be emphasized over substituted motions to prevent future injury and to promote efficiency. Compensatory motions must be saved as last resorts because they often cause more problems than they solve.

For example, a woman with severely osteoarthritic knees is having difficulty climbing stairs. To accomplish the task independently, she flexes her trunk forward and uses both arms on the railing to pull herself up. If she continues in this fashion, she is likely to injure her back or upper extremities. Further analysis shows that she has only minimal ankle motion and Poor-plus (2+/5) strength of her ankle plantar flexors. Improving her ankle motion and strength allows her to negotiate stairs with much greater ease, alleviating the need for the compensatory trunk flexion. Even though she still needs to use one railing, stair climbing has become much easier and safer. After total-body analysis of the task and correction of the problem, she is operating on a higher functional level than before.

An Activity-Oriented Approach

Before being discharged from therapy, the patient must demonstrate the ability to safely perform the functional tasks necessary to return home. These tasks can easily be incorporated into standard strengthening and flexibility programs even in the acute care hospital. The activity of rising from a chair (sit-to-stand transfer) is an excellent way to promote closed-chain knee strengthening in a functional manner. In addition, the patient may need to simulate some activities in the clinic (eg, chopping pieces of Theraputty™ to simulate chopping vegetables). The patient must practice these types of activities often enough so that they can be performed easily and with confidence. This ability to perform tasks automatically is a major goal of functional restoration.

Because a therapist cannot anticipate every functional need for each patient, the patient must learn to apply general motor planning skills to each specific functional situation that arises in his or her particular life style. Although it sounds difficult, this is what humans do all the time when faced with a new situation. Take for example a girl learning to throw a small rubber ball. After instruction and plenty of practice, the girl learns to throw the ball with correct form and accuracy. If she now wishes to throw a football or a javelin, only minor corrections need be made in the established motor plan to successfully complete the new task.

A Realistic Approach

What level of functional restoration does a patient truly require? Therapists cannot always teach patients to be safe while performing all functional activities. By definition, some functional activities, such as rock climbing, are inherently unsafe. Neither can therapists simply restore patients to their prior functional status. This could spell disaster for the patient who had been falling for 6 months prior to fracturing a wrist. Each patient is a unique individual with separate and different needs and functions. The therapist and patient must define the risks and rewards of desired functional goals and must work together to restore important functional activities as safely as possible.

THE CHALLENGE FACING THE REHABILITATION SPECIALIST

Many health professionals claim the role of rehabilitation specialist: PTs, OTs, chiropractors, recreational therapists, hand therapists, work-hardening therapists, physiatrists, athletic trainers, human factors engineers, and so on. Each profession offers the patient a slightly different way of restoring function by either changing the patient or changing the environment. At present, there is little common terminology and few common methods for defining functional loss or returning a patient to normal function. The word *function* itself has been so abused in medical documentation that it has been rendered almost meaningless. The challenge facing all these professions concerns the ability to:

- better identify functional impairment
- measure it simply but accurately
- determine the underlying physical and/or neurological cause
- correct the physical and/or neurological cause
- restore functional capacity

The following chapters present a rational plan to restore function based on current and new scientific principles. Because research on function is only now blossoming, it is hoped that this book will serve as an introduction to this fascinating and changing field.

REFERENCE

1. Fitzgerald JF, Moore PS, Dittus RS. The care of elderly patients with hip fracture: changes since implementation of the prospective payment system. *N Engl J Med.* 1988;319:1392–1397.

2

Disability Models: Defining Terminology

In trying to restore the functional capacity of their patients, rehabilitation specialists have haphazardly established systems of evaluating and restoring function within the precepts of their own specialties. Many different terms abound: *functional capacity, functional disability, functional ambulation, functional range of motion, functional strength, functional impairments, handicap,* and so forth. The meanings of these words are unclear across and within disciplines. The concept of restoring function is inherently obvious to therapists, patients, doctors, and insurance carriers, yet the field of functional rehabilitation lacks a standard means of defining function and disability that is acceptable to all health professionals. Without standard terminology, it is difficult to assess function or dysfunction, plan treatment, and obtain outcome data as to the efficacy of the chosen treatment.

Many therapists and physicians remain unaware that classification systems in the field of function and disability exist. They continue to use vague terms as best they can to describe their evaluation and treatment procedures. This chapter introduces a classification system or taxonomy based on a theoretical model of disablement proposed by Dr. Philip Wood of Manchester, England, a consultant to the World Health Organization (WHO). By the use of standard terminology and avoidance of ambiguous labels, communication between and within disciplines should be enhanced, thereby improving patient care.

INTERNATIONAL CLASSIFICATION OF IMPAIRMENTS, DISABILITIES, AND HANDICAPS

In 1990, WHO, a specialized public health agency of the United Nations, published the *International Classification of Impairments, Disabilities, and Handicaps: A Manual of Classification Relating to the Consequences of Disease*[1] (hereinafter abbreviated ICIDH). This model, based on the work of Dr. Wood, remains the only international and interdisciplinary standard of functional terminology usable by all medical professionals, including both clinicians and researchers. Many investigators argue that, although flawed, the ICIDH represents the best taxonomy or classification of impairment and disability presently available that fosters communication among disciplines.[2-4]

The Disablement Process

Jette, a research physical therapist in Massachusetts, describes disablement as an overall process rather than a specific component of a disability model.[5] As defined by Webster's, a process is a phenomenon marked by gradual changes leading toward a particular result. Wood's model identifies four components of this disablement process that are intimately intertwined. In its simplest scenario, disease or disorder leads to impairment, which causes the person to become disabled and perhaps society to label that person as handicapped. In reality, many other factors influence this uncertain chain of events: social support systems, mental and emotional states, age, income, environmental surroundings, and the like.

Disease or Disorder ⇨ Impairment ⇨ Disability ⇨ Handicap

Disease and Disorder

Disease represents any pathological process associated with a characteristic and identifiable set of symptoms and signs.[1] The disease process is considered the stimulus for resultant impairments. For example, rheumatoid arthritis would be considered a disease that can cause the physical impairment of joint destruction. In Western society, physicians are considered the most qualified medical personnel to identify pathological processes or, in other words, to render diagnoses of disease states.

Disorder refers to other stimuli that may lead to disability. They can be acute, chronic, or congenital. They encompass traumatic and repetitive trauma injuries, congenital malformations, movement dysfunctions, and postural syndromes.[6–8] Doctors may identify these physical disorders as well. Many other rehabilitation professionals, however, are sufficiently knowledgeable and better trained to recognize and determine many of these injuries or syndromes.

Impairment

WHO defines impairment as any loss or abnormality of psychological, physiological, or anatomical structure or function within a specific organ or system of the body.[1] For the pur-

poses of this book, the discussion will focus mainly on physical impairments. (This is not to underestimate the importance of psychological impairments. In many studies, depression and other psychological issues were the major factors correlated with disability and handicap.[9,10]) Physical impairments often affect three body systems that therapists treat: the cardiopulmonary system, the musculoskeletal system, and the neuromuscular system.

Impairments can be temporary or permanent. They encompass the loss of anatomical parts, as in below-knee amputation or, less drastically, a meniscectomy, as well as muscle atrophy or loss of motor control (Table 2–1). Furthermore, they are intimately associated with functional limitations.

According to WHO, functional limitations, such as the inability to lift 20 lb or to reach above shoulder height, are used to describe the limits of function possible and can be measured by the clinician. Functional limitations are identified by variations from an ideal norm. The presence of functional limitations indicates the coexisting presence of impairments but not necessarily the presence of disabilities. Examples of functional limitations and the impairments they help define are shown in Table 2–2.

Table 2–1 Impairments of Different Body Systems

Body System	Physical Impairments
Cardiopulmonary	Diminished chest expansion
	Decreased forced expiratory volume (FEV_1)
	Varicose veins
	Myocardial infarction
	Pleural effusion
Musculoskeletal	Lateral ankle sprain
	Lumbar disc herniation
	Fascial restriction
	Weakness
	Decreased range of motion (ROM)
Neuromuscular	Rigidity
	Tremor
	Faulty motor planning
	Faulty balance
	Decreased coordination

Table 2–2 Measurable Functional Limitations To Define Impairments

Disease/Disorder	Impairment	Functional Limitations	Norm or Ideal
Cerebrovascular accident (CVA)	Glenohumeral subluxation Restricted shoulder range of motion (ROM)	Inability to comb hair Inability to put on make-up	Ability to groom self Stable glenohumeral joint
Osteoarthritis of the tibiofemoral joint	Decreased joint space 3+/5 quadriceps strength	Inability to kneel Inability to climb stairs	Ability to kneel Ability to climb full flight of stairs
Chronic obstructive pulmonary disease	Dyspnea on exertion Shortness of breath	Inability to walk 30 ft	Ability to walk 1 mi
Parkinson's disease	Rigidity	Inability to roll in bed Inability to get out of bed Ambulation velocity 97 ft/min	Full bed and transfer mobility Ambulation velocity 262 ft/min
Traumatic injury	Lateral ankle sprain	Inability to run or jump Inability to play basketball	Ability to run and jump Ability to play sports
Anterolateral impingement syndrome of hip[11]	Short hip external rotators and hamstrings Posterior pelvic tilt Excessive hip external rotation	Inability to bear weight on hip	Ability to load hip in a pain-free fashion Ability to walk

To explain further, a therapist may measure with a stopwatch the ambulation velocity of a patient with Parkinson's disease in a clinic and report that the patient can walk at a speed of 97 ft/min. Because the ideal velocity for community ambulation is 262 ft/min,[12] this patient has a functional limitation in walking. The therapist must determine the corresponding impairment (ie, rigidity) that is contributing to this limitation of ambulation function. Should this functional limitation lead to a walking disability (which is at present uncertain), the therapist will know which impairment (rigidity) to address to correct the problem (see the discussion of disability later in this chapter).

With proper assessment tools (see Chapter 13), therapists and doctors can determine functional limitations in everyday activities such as walking, running, lifting, and carrying. In fact, many physical therapists contend that physical impairment and functional limitations are well within the abilities and practice acts of physical therapists to classify (or diagnose), measure, and consequently treat.[2,13,14] Guccione, a clinical and research physical therapist, defines this area of rehabilitation expertise (ie, impairment

and functional limitation) as within the physical therapy domain[13] (Figure 2–1). Although Guccione proposed this concept of physical therapy domain based on a slightly different theoretical model of disablement (that of Nagi[15]), the idea of establishing an area of physical therapy expertise in relation to the disablement process holds true for WHO's model as well. By establishing a domain of physical therapy, Guccione's modified model can help therapists plan and direct treatment. This model defines the realm of physical therapy in relation to function and disability. Guccione logically contends that therapists should limit their treatments to only those impairments that are related to the patient's functional limitations and that can also be remedied by physical therapy intervention.[13] If the problem cannot be alleviated with physical therapy, the therapist must refer the patient to other health workers, such as psychologists, social workers, physicians, and so forth.

Other disciplines may wish to change the name of the domain to include themselves (ie, domain of chiropractic, domain of occupational therapy, domain of work hardening, etc.) by defining their own scopes of expertise. For

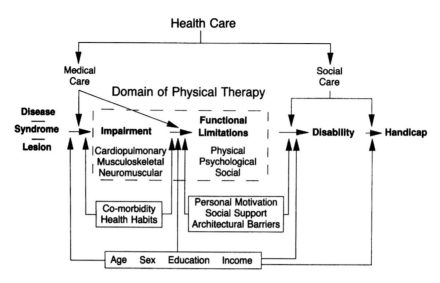

Figure 2–1. Working expansion of Nagi's[15] model of the process of disablement to account for the influence of service delivery and personal factors. *Source:* Reprinted from *Physical Therapy,* Vol. 71, No. 7, p. 502, with permission of the American Physical Therapy Association, © 1991.

example, the domain of occupational therapy may include more of the psychological aspects of functional limitations since occupational therapists have more training in this area than physical therapists. Most of these domains will overlap in some way because most of the rehabilitative disciplines share clinical skills and knowledge.

Disability

Disability is defined as any restriction or lack of ability to perform an activity in the manner or within the range considered normal for a human being.[1] Disability occurs at the person level (rather than the organ level, as in a sprained ankle). It is the patient's perception of his or her own level of ability. Jette[16] subdivides disability into four domains:

1. physical disability
2. mental disability
3. emotional disability
4. and social disability

According to WHO, disabilities may be permanent or temporary, reversible or irreversible, and progressive or regressive in nature. Other

definitions of disability, such as that of the American Academy of Orthopaedic Surgeons (AAOS), purport that disability is a permanent occurrence.

Unlike functional limitations that describe impairments, disabilities are not measures of ideals but of what occurs. If, in the example given above, the patient ambulates independently and safely and is able to carry out all normal tasks despite the functional limitation of ambulating at 97/262ths of the ideal norm, then that patient does not have a walking disability. Table 2–3 depicts two patients with similar functional limitations resulting in totally different abilities.

Therefore, not all impairments necessarily lead to disabilities or even to the same disabilities for every person. Take for example a patient with supraspinatus tendinitis who has resultant weakness and restricted range of motion in shoulder abduction (musculoskeletal impairments). She cannot reach overhead or carry any loads (functional limitations). If the tendinitis affects her dominant side, she will probably be disabled (physically, emotionally, and socially) in her everyday living such that her ability to go shopping, play sports, carry her infant child, or work as an accountant will be compromised. If

Table 2–3 Functional Limitations and Level of Disability

Disease/Disorder	Physical Impairment	Functional Limitation	Disability
Below-knee amputation	Loss of lower limb	Cane-assisted gait Slow ambulation velocity Gait deviations	None: shops Walks outside daily Attends church Visits friends
Rheumatoid arthritis	Total knee replacement	Cane-assisted gait Slow ambulation velocity Gait deviations	Unable to shop Walks indoors mostly Does not attend church Rarely sees friends

the tendinitis affects her nondominant side, she may be perfectly able to lead an independent life with only minor disruption. In other words, she would function within normal limits.

In addition, many other factors influence the progression of impairment to disability:

- environment
- economic sufficiency
- social support system
- general health
- mental fortitude
- age
- quality of medical care

These other factors can turn seemingly insignificant impairments into major disabilities. A two-step entryway into an office building may be an inconvenience for a worker with a torn meniscus who is on crutches and a complete barrier to a worker with multiple sclerosis who is in a wheelchair. The inability to afford medical care can accelerate the sequelae of disease and lead to an otherwise preventable onset of disability. In addition, the desire to achieve a goal or perform a task cannot be overstated. The old adage "Where there's a will, there's a way" holds especially true in discussions concerning disability. Of course, the opposite is equally true: Many studies indicate that the level of disability is clearly associated with the level of motivation.

Handicap

WHO defines handicap as a disadvantage for a given individual, resulting from an impairment or disability, that limits or prevents the fulfillment of a role that is normal (depending on age, sex, and social and cultural factors) for that individual.[1] Handicap occurs at a social level. A person may be considered handicapped if a task that can no longer be performed is valued by the society in which that person lives. In other words, the level of a person's handicap has little to do with the person's self-perception of ability (disability) but is determined by society. Although a paraplegic may care for himself independently, work a 40-hour week, compete in the Boston Marathon, drive a car, and coach a basketball team, our bipedal society will still label him handicapped as a result of his inability to walk. By the same token, a rock climber with plantar fasciitis may consider herself disabled because she cannot pursue an important activity in her life, but she would not be considered handicapped in American society.

Utilization of ICIDH Codes

By use of the ICIDH codes, a patient's functional status may be reduced to a simple standardized format that all medical disciplines can understand. The codes are not substitutes for each clinician's specialized notes but are a way to easily communicate the patient's functional status in numeric format. For a complete listing of ICIDH codes, the reader is referred to the ICIDH manual.[1]

The rehabilitation specialist looks up the following ICIDH types of codes in the manual:

- **I,** the impairment code, which best describes the skeletal problem facing the patient
- **D,** the disability codes, which reflect problems in functional performance or activity
- **H,** the (six) handicap codes

Although determining the proper impairment and disability codes is straightforward, the clinician may find choosing the level of handicap confusing.[4]

For example, Ms Ellen Slater is a 58-year-old woman who has just undergone total knee arthroplasty of her right leg for osteoarthritis of her knee of 10 years' duration. She is presently restricted in most areas of function. Her codes may appear as follows:

- **Diagnosis code:**   V43.6 (ICD-9 code for total knee replacement)
- **Impairment code:** 71.67 (restriction or loss of movement in one knee)
- **Disability codes:**   33.0 (bathing disability associated with transfer difficulty)
  - 35.1 (clothing disability for lower part of body)
  - 36.1 (footwear disability)
  - 40 (walking disability)
  - 41 (traversing disability: negotiation of discontinuous terrain)
  - 42 (climbing stairs disability)
  - 43 (running disability)
  - 46.1 (difficulty getting in and out of chairs)
  - 47.0 (difficulty in transfer in and out of a car)
  - 48 (lifting disability)
  - 50.0 (procuring sustenance, eg, food shopping)
  - 50.1 (transporting sustenance, eg, getting food home)

- 51.4 (manual cleaning)
- 55 (kneeling disability)
- 56 (crouching disability)
- **Handicap codes:**   1.0 (orientation—fully independent)
  - 2.5 (physical independence—short-interval dependence)
  - 3.3 (mobility—reduced mobility)
  - 4.2 (occupation—curtailed occupation)
  - 5.2 (social integration—restricted participation)
  - 6.0 (economic sufficiency—normal/disability insurance)

After Ms Slater undergoes extensive physical therapy and occupational therapy for 6 weeks in both acute and rehabilitation settings, her level of disability and handicap have improved. This change would be reflected in ICIDH code form as follows:

- **Diagnosis code:**   V43.6
- **Impairment code:** 71.67
- **Disability codes:**   40 (walking disability)
  - 41 (traversing disability)
  - 42 (climbing stairs disability)
  - 43 (running disability)
  - 55 (kneeling disability)
  - 56 (crouching disability)
- **Handicap codes:**   1.0 (orientation—fully independent)
  - 2.1 (physical independence—aided independence, eg, cane)
  - 3.2 (mobility—impaired mobility, eg, takes longer)
  - 4.2 (occupation—curtailed occupation)

5.2 (social integration—restricted participation)

6.0 (economic sufficiency—normal/disability insurance)

Clinical and Research Rationale for Using ICIDH

The WHO disability model helps the clinician identify the problem areas that need to be corrected for the patient to become better or functional. According to this classification system, the patient's disabilities are the outcomes of the present impairments. The impairments are understood to be the underlying cause. By correction of the impairments, the disability may be best corrected.[17] Therefore, the therapist must be able to differentiate between the impairments and the resulting disabilities on evaluation. The ICIDH provides a clear method of separating impairments from disabilities that all will understand.

If the clinician corrects the impairment but the patient's disability remains unchanged, the therapist can conclude that the impairment alone was not responsible for the disability. Two possibilities remain: (1) One of the mitigating factors outside the clinician's domain of expertise is influencing the patient's level of ability and requires a referral to another discipline (eg, social service, psychology, nutritionist, etc.), or (2) other impairments must be identified and addressed.

Take for example the above case of Ms Slater's continuing disabilities. The initial assumption was that there existed one underlying impairment (impairment code 71.67, restriction or loss of movement in one knee). In fact, there were many impairments observed on evaluation: strength deficits, diminished motor control, kyphotic posture, and so forth. Restoration of adequate strength and proprioceptive input in addition to proper musculoskeletal alignment in the whole body may be needed to correct the disabilities fully.

Researchers can also benefit from using a disability model. Linking impairments to subsequent disabilities can form the basis of much needed clinical research into the efficacy of treatments that have been standard in the profession for years.

Problems with ICIDH

The ICIDH classification system is not perfect for rehabilitation professionals. The following summary of some of the problems inherent in this system may help explain why the ICIDH has not been widely accepted by physical therapists, occupational therapists, and other health professionals.

The Bias toward Disease or Pathology

From a rehabilitation point of view, the ICIDH is disease biased. Because the WHO manual was written for the purpose of classifying the sequelae of disease states, the ICIDH is understandably prejudiced toward diseases. Little emphasis is placed on other stimuli (eg, disorders), such as improper posture, traumatic insult, body mechanics, movement dysfunctions, footwear, and repetitive trauma, that cause many physical impairments with resultant disabilities.

The Definition of Functional Limitation

Functional limitations are considered diagnostic indicators of impairment only. In the WHO model, their presence helps confirm or deny a suspected physical impairment. A functional assessment would be a tool similar to a radiograph or strength test. The functional limitation helps describe the impairment, but the functional limitation is not understood to be the bridge that links impairment to disability.

The Lack of Codes for Many Impairments

The manual does not provide codes for many common impairments, leaving the therapist with an incomplete assessment. This could lead a medical colleague or insurance carrier to conclude falsely that only one impairment exists when in fact many are present that simply have no corresponding ICIDH codes. The therapist can and must complement the ICIDH with evaluation and treatment notes documenting all found impairments or functional limitations.

The Connotation of the Term Disability

The word *disability* carries a stigma in American society. Webster's defines disability as the condition of being disabled, the inability to pursue an occupation because of physical or mental impairment, the lack of legal qualification to do something, and a nonlegal disqualification, restriction, or disadvantage. Already discussions and contests have been held to coin new, less-threatening terminology. Words and phrases such as *differently abled* or *physically challenged* are presently considered more politically correct. Therapists may find it difficult to accept WHO's definition of disability as a disturbance that occurs at the person level rather than as a label given by society (WHO's definition of handicap).

The Compensation and Legal Issues Associated with the Term Disability

The compensation and legal issues surrounding disability may make it even harder for therapists and doctors to use this term properly. The American Medical Association (AMA) and the AAOS define disability as a temporary or permanent injury for which the patient should or should not be compensated.[18,(p2)] Insurance carriers and lawyers desire precise determinations (in actual percentages) of the patient's loss of function to determine medical coverage and monetary compensation. Physicians reluctantly attempt to provide this information using an array of state, insurance, and AMA rating guides, but the task is often impossible in complex cases. Therefore, the AMA has recommended that physicians restrict their evaluations to impairment, which the AMA defines as "an alteration of an individual's health status that is *assessed by medical means*" rather than disability, which the AMA defines as "an alteration of an individual's capacity to meet personal, social, or occupational demands *assessed by nonmedical means.*"[18(p2)]

PROMOTING COMMUNICATION WITH THE ICIDH TAXONOMY

Because the ICIDH is not perfect for the practices of physical therapy and occupational therapy, clinicians from both disciplines have proposed modifying the codes to suit rehabilitation needs.[13,19] In addition, other models of disablement have been proposed to reflect more accurately the work done by physical therapists. For more information about these models and classification systems, the reader is referred to the works listed at the end of this chapter. Jette[2] cautions physical therapists not to accept any classification scheme as dogma while the profession is still evolving and growing. This is sound advice. No taxonomy can be accepted at present as the sole theoretical basis for functional rehabilitation. The door must be left open for alternatives to be considered in the future.

Although arbitrary, the choice to use the ICIDH terminology in this book should help promote communication among medical providers and medical insurance carriers. It is a well-known taxonomy with printed manuals that are easily accessed. Vague terms such as *functional strength* must disappear from clinical documentation and be replaced with the more standard terms *impairment, functional limitation,* and *disability.* Clinicians should only identify the patient's impairments and functional limitations and leave the patient to determine what he or she can or cannot do (ie, identify the disability level; see Chapter 4 on assessing function). The labeling of handicap will be left to society and will not be addressed further in this book.

From a documentation standpoint, the ICIDH coding system remains seriously flawed and cannot be recommended for clinical use. It is hoped that WHO will amend the codes (especially impairment and handicap) in the future to allow greater usage by health care providers. Until then, the reader is referred to Chapter 13 for more information about alternative methods of documenting function.

REFERENCES

1. World Health Organization (WHO). *International Classification of Impairments, Disabilities, and Handicaps: A Manual of Classification Relating to the Consequences of Disease.* Geneva, Switzerland: WHO; 1980.

2. Jette AM. Diagnosis and classification by physical therapists: a special communication. *Phys Ther.* 1989;69: 967–969.

3. Noyes FR, Mooar LA, Barber SB. The assessment of work-related activities and limitations in knee disorders. *Am J Sports Med.* 1991;19:178–188.

4. Wagstaff S. The use of the *International Classification of Impairments, Disabilities, and Handicaps* in rehabilitation. *Physiotherapy.* 1982;68:233–234.

5. Jette AM. Disability assessment in clinical practice (course notes). Presented at the American Physical Therapy Association Annual Conference; June 1991; Boston, Mass.

6. Wood P, Badley E. The epidemiology of disablement. In: Goodwill C, Chamberlain MA, eds. *Rehabilitation of the Physically Disabled Adult.* London, England: University Press; 1988: 6–23.

7. Harris BA, Dyrek DA. A model of orthopaedic dysfunction for clinical decision making in physical therapy practice. *Phys Ther.* 1989; 69:548–553.

8. Sahrmann SA. Diagnosis and treatment of movement system imbalances associated with musculoskeletal pain syndromes of the low back (course notes). Washington University School of Medicine; 1990. Presented at the Massachusetts Chapter of the American Physical Therapy Association Annual Conference; October 1992; Danvers, Mass.

9. Deveraux E, Carlson M. The role of occupational therapy in the management of depression. *Am J Occup Ther.* 1992;46:175–180.

10. Salaffi F, Cavaliere F, Nolli M, et al. Analysis of disability in knee osteoarthritis. Relationship with age and psychological variables but not with radiographic score. *J Rheum.* 1991;18:1581–1585.

11. Sahrmann SA, Woolsey N. Lower extremity imbalance syndromes (course notes). Washington University School of Medicine; 1990. Presented at the Massachusetts Chapter of the American Physical Therapy Association Annual Conference; October 1992; Danvers, Mass.

12. Robinett CS, Vondran MA. Functional ambulation velocity and distance requirements in rural and urban communities. *Phys Ther.* 1988;68:1371–1373.

13. Guccione AA. Physical therapy diagnosis and the relationship between impairments and function. *Phys Ther.* 1991;71:499–504.

14. Sahrmann SA. Diagnosis by the physical therapist—a prerequisite for treatment: a special communication. *Phys Ther.* 1988;68:1703–1706.

15. Nagi SZ. *Disability and Rehabilitation: Legal, Clinical and Self Concepts Measurement.* Columbus, Ohio: Ohio State University Press; 1969.

16. Jette AM. Functional disability and rehabilitation of the aged. *Top Geriatr Rehabil.* 1986;1:1–7.

17. Schenkman M, Butler RB. A model for multisystem evaluation treatment of individuals with Parkinson's disease. *Phys Ther.* 1989;69:932–943.

18. American Medical Association. *AMA Guides to the Evaluation of Permanent Impairment.* Chicago, Ill: American Medical Association, 1988.

19. Fisher A. Functional measures, part 1: what is function, what should we measure, and how should we measure it? *Am J Occup Ther.* 1992;46:183–185.

ADDITIONAL READING

Granger CV, Gresham GE, eds. *Functional Assessment in Rehabilitation Medicine.* Baltimore, Md: Williams & Wilkins; 1984.

Kessler HK. *Disability—Determination and Evaluation.* Philadelphia, Pa: Lea & Febiger; 1970.

McBride DE. *Disability Evaluation and Principles of Treatment of Compensable Injuries.* Philadelphia, Pa: Lippincott; 1963.

3

Types of Function

The simple word *function* is easily understood but hard to define. Function, in rehabilitation terms, is what humans do or how humans act. In restoring a patient's function, the clinician is attempting to have the patient do what he or she did before, whatever that may have been. The function being restored should be meaningful to the clinician, the patient, and the insurance carrier. Nobody wishes to pay for an unnecessary medical service. At present in the United States, the rehabilitation specialist and patient determine together the necessity of a treatment goal, but the true power lies with the medical insurance carrier, which determines whether the treatment is reimbursable. Because of lack of clarity in medical documentation, the insurance companies are often at odds with the medical providers in determining whether treatments are necessary and therefore reimbursable. To define function clearly for all parties concerned, this chapter reviews the presently accepted divisions of human function:

- basic or personal activities of daily living (ADLs)
- instrumental activities of daily living (IADLs)
- work activities
- sports/recreational activities

Future chapters refer to these categories of function. The use of common terminology should allow clearer communication between the providers of medical care and the ones who pay the bills, so that justification for rehabilitation treatments will be self-evident.

BASIC ADLs

The restoration of basic ADL skills has always been a major goal of occupational therapy. The emphasis on self-care activities has beneficial effects on the patient's self-perception and dignity as well as in reducing the physical and financial burdens of the caretaker and of society. Basic or personal ADLs consist of the following activities:

- bed activities (moving in bed, managing pillows and blankets, reaching for objects, sitting up, etc.)
- hygiene activities (brushing teeth, bathing, showering, washing up, toileting, combing hair, shaving, putting on make-up, etc.)
- eating activities (using utensils, managing a glass or cup, cutting meat, etc.)
- dressing activities (putting on undergarments, shirts, slacks, skirts, socks, pantyhose, shoes [tying laces], etc.)

- transfer activities (bed-to-chair, sit-to-stand from chair and toilet, into a car, etc.)
- walking activities (walking on level surfaces and uneven surfaces, negotiating curbs and stairs, opening doors, walking and carrying items, etc.)

These basic activities form the keystone of most inpatient occupational therapy programs. The occupational therapist (OT) initially assists the patient bedside with these tasks and may prescribe devices, such as long-handled shoe horns or elastic laces, so that the patient can achieve independence. The patient progresses by successfully performing some actual tasks in the occupational therapy kitchen and bathroom in the hospital setting or in the patient's kitchen and bathroom at home. For the patient with severe stroke or spinal cord injury, months may be needed to accomplish these tasks. Some patients never regain these abilities.

Physical therapy has consistently addressed some of these basic self-care tasks as well, but from a different perspective. The physical therapist (PT) views these functions as mobility issues:

- bed mobility (rolling from side to side, scooting, supine-to-sit, etc.)
- transfer mobility (bed-to-chair, wheelchair-to-stand, floor-to-stand, etc.)
- walking mobility (distance, velocity, assistive devices, weight bearing, gait deviations, stair climbing, etc.)

The PT works on restoring the patient's neuromuscular pathways, strength, and cardiovascular endurance (ie, impairments) so that the patient can accomplish the needed tasks. This is usually done in a controlled environment. Bed mobility is often performed on mats and plinths, while gait training is initially done on level hospital corridors. The patient achieves a higher level of mobility skills, but this does not immediately translate into a higher level of functional ability. Because of the different objectives of these two disciplines, the PT and OT are often at odds during team meetings. The OT might report that a patient is functionally ambulating with a walker for 50 ft, whereas the PT reports that the patient is ambulating 35 ft with a cane and assistance. Both are accurate in their observations. The OT wonders at the PT's purpose in introducing an ambulation device that makes the patient unsteady and therefore unable to operate in the real world (where assistance may not be available). The PT wonders why the OT is limiting the patient to life-long dependence on a bulky piece of equipment by reporting the patient independent in ambulation (which will in all probability terminate medical coverage). The PT is trying to maximize mobility skills, and the OT is trying to maximize independent function skills. The perfect answer lies somewhere in between, as the patient must work with newly regained mobility skills to achieve true function in a more realistic environment.

In an outpatient setting, many orthopaedically injured people lose the ability to perform some basic ADL tasks or lose their proficiency or prior skill level. They will display measurable functional limitations. A patient with trochanteric bursitis of the hip may ambulate with decreased velocity, a patient with patellar tracking problems may find squatting painful, and a patient with low back dysfunction may have difficulty brushing his or her teeth. In this healthy setting, the clinician must assist the patient in returning to both high-skill levels (working or playing sports) and basic self-care levels.

The necessity of restoring these basic human functions is generally obvious to all concerned: the patient, the clinician, and the medical insurance company. Documentation deficiencies, such as failure to identify the impairment(s) and to measure the functional limitations, can cause reimbursement problems for the health care provider (see Chapter 13 on measuring function).

IADL

IADLs could also be called advanced ADLs. To live in the community (rather than an institution), a person must be able to perform some of

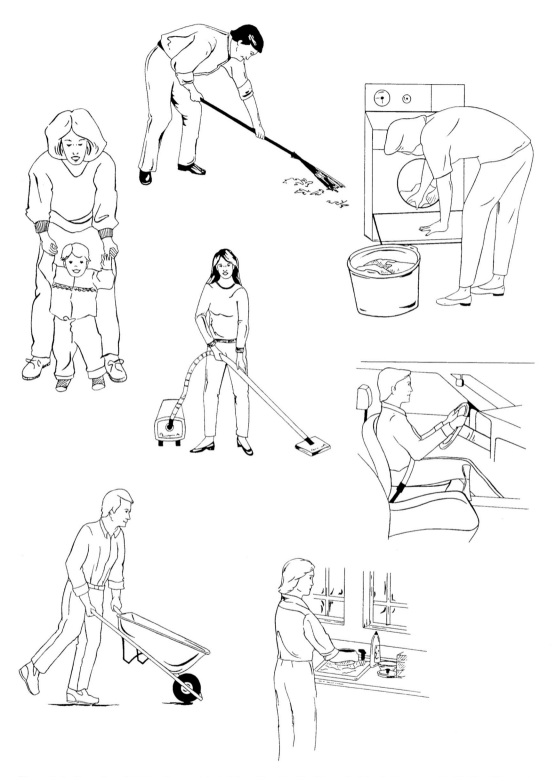

Figure 3–1. Examples of IADLs. *Source:* Adapted from *Your Healthy Upper Body* by L. Demers p. 16, 28, 29, with permission of Ergonomics Plus, © 1991.

these functional tasks (see Figure 3–1). Once again, occupational therapy is the discipline that historically has addressed these issues in both physical and cognitive domains. IADLs consist of the following:

- meal preparation—Cutting vegetables, carrying milk, cracking eggs, turning on the oven, stirring, measuring ingredients, etc.
- light housework—Dusting, washing dishes, mopping floors, cleaning sinks, etc.
- check writing—Manipulating a pen, adding and subtracting, reading a bill, etc.
- local shopping—Pushing a wagon, carrying grocery bags, reaching shelves, walking, getting money out of a pocket or purse, etc.
- having sex—Getting in and out of positions, manipulating clothing, etc.
- driving a car—Getting in and out of car, adjusting mirrors, turning the wheel, understanding traffic rules, reaching the pedals, etc.
- gardening—Kneeling, raking, digging, watering, etc.
- communicating—Using writing tools, using the telephone, etc.

IADLs also include the ability to engage in hobbies, shovel snow, go to church, take public transportation, go to the movies, and so forth. The ability to perform these activities correlates with the patient's perception of quality of life. In general, this higher level of function requires greater cognitive as well as physical skills. The patient must be able to conceptualize traffic rules, money, recipes, etc. in addition to being able physically to complete the tasks.

In settings where occupational therapy is not available, physical therapy can and must work on IADLs. Often times an orthopaedic patient is unable to perform these high-level functions because of a physical impairment that can easily be treated by physical therapy. Simulations for many of the activities can be created in the physical therapy clinic, or the patient can perform the actual tasks at home.

WORK ACTIVITIES

The activities required to perform a job are as varied as the number of occupations themselves. In spite of that, experts in the field of industrial rehabilitation have compiled a generalized list of physical demands that a worker may need to perform:

- lifting
- carrying
- stooping
- pushing
- pulling
- reaching
- kneeling
- manipulating
- climbing
- sitting
- standing
- walking

Although orthopaedic PTs have commonly treated the injured worker in the acute and chronic stages, combined treatment by occupational therapy and physical therapy is now common in work-hardening centers. In these facilities, emphasis is placed on returning to work rather than returning to normal.

Work conditioning, as defined by the American Physical Therapy Association, is a work-relevant, intensive, goal-oriented treatment program specifically designed to restore an individual's systemic, neuromuscular function (strength, endurance, movement, flexibility, and motor control). Many orthopaedic physical therapy clinics use this cost-effective program to help return the majority of injured workers to their jobs. As the acute symptoms subside, the worker begins an exercise program specifically designed to address the physical impairments and functional limitations that are preventing him or her from performing job-related tasks. In addition, the worker begins aerobic training and some simulated job tasks using proper body mechanics and posture.[1]

The more physically and psychologically involved workers require the comprehensive program of work hardening. In 1989, specific national guidelines were created by the Commission on Accreditation of Rehabilitation Facilities (CARF), precisely defining work-hardening programs. Briefly, work hardening involves a multidisciplinary approach including physical and occupational therapy, vocational counseling, and psychology. The program lasts 4 to 8 hours daily and often uses circuit training, consisting of work simulators for precise retraining, as well as a cardiovascular fitness program for improving general health.[2]

SPORT AND RECREATIONAL ACTIVITIES

The restoration of skills needed for sports and recreation has traditionally fallen within the domain of the certified athletic trainer (ATC) and more recently in the domain of the orthopaedic PT. The skills needed are sport specific and player position specific and generally involve total-body abilities. A partial list of some sport-specific activities follows:

- walking—Forward, retro, sideways, on a level surface, etc.
- jogging—Forward, retro, on grass, on a track, on hills, in water, etc.
- sprinting—Forward, retro, on grass, on a track, on a basketball court, etc.
- cutting—Large circles, small circles, figure 8s, crossovers, etc.
- jumping—Vertical, forward, retro, side to side, on a level surface, from a height, etc.
- throwing—Underhand, overhand, two handed (basketball), with different types of balls, etc.
- catching—Two-handed, one-handed, with different sizes and weights of balls, etc.
- batting—Baseball bat, tennis racquet, field hockey stick, golf club, etc.
- swimming—Crawl stroke, breast stroke, backstroke, whip kick, flutter kick, etc.

The ATC or PT not only attempts to restore the athlete's previous ability but tries to achieve a higher level of functioning and conditioning. The field of sports medicine has evolved from the days of steamy training rooms equipped with little but whirlpools, hot packs, white tape, and bottles of liniment oils to being the premier provider of quality rehabilitation. Innovations in rehabilitation began here, and sports medicine continues to break new ground in the restoration of function. As it became obvious that simply restoring strength and range of motion was insufficient to allow an athlete to return to the sport safely, sports clinicians began to identify more areas that required intervention. These pioneers in functional rehabilitation determined that the athlete also needed:

- initial protective immobilization, including rest, ice, compression, and elevation (RICE) to reduce edema and promote healing
- proprioceptive retraining (neuromuscular re-education) to restore the normal kinesiologic input to the nervous system by the joint mechanoreceptors
- both open- and closed-chain exercise to promote total-body functioning
- specific exercise to promote function per the specific adaptation to implied demands (SAID) principle
- muscular speed and power
- plyometrics, the combination of strength and speed that allows for fast acceleration (explosive-reactive type motion) and also deceleration
- agility
- cardiovascular endurance[3]

These concepts should be applied to all functional retraining programs. Many of these treatment ideals have already been adopted by work-hardening programs. Some even label the injured worker an industrial athlete. This book introduces the concept of defining all our high-level patients as community athletes and treating them as such.

REFERENCES

1. Darphin LE, Smith RL, Green EJ. Work conditioning and work hardening. *Orthop Phys Ther Clin.* 1992;1(1): 105–124.

2. Twelves JW. Physical therapy in industry. *Clin Manage.* 1990;10:14–19.

3. Harrelson GL. Introduction to rehabilitation. In: Andrews JR, Harrelson GL, eds. *Physical Rehabilitation of the Injured Athlete.* Philadelphia, Pa: WB Saunders; 1991.

4

Movement Science

The belief that the higher centers of the brain exert control of motor function over the lower centers of the brain has influenced rehabilitation strategies until the present. The majority of neurological reeducation for patients with stroke or brain injury has consisted of inhibiting lower brain reflexes and facilitating normal movement using sensory pathways. The treatment philosophies of Rood,[1] Brunnstrom,[2] Bobath,[3] and Knott and Voss[4] developed as a way to influence the hierarchic structure of the central nervous system (CNS) to promote normal movement.

Because orthopaedic patients do not have damage to the CNS, treatment strategies have focused on correcting musculoskeletal impairments such as strength and range of motion. Perhaps this is just as well. New theories of motor control are replacing the old ones. The new theories of motor learning and skill acquisition are based on different assumptions of how the nervous system is organized. Higher centers do not control lower centers. All the components of the nervous system, from cerebral cortex to pressure receptors, influence each other. These new theories help explain how function can be so adversely affected by a seemingly minor insult to the musculoskeletal system.

NONLINEAR SYSTEMS AND COMPLEXITY

Because they are easier to learn and understand, linear systems are taught in most basic sciences (eg, chemical equations that remain in perfect equilibrium, geometric equations that determine circumference, physics equations that determine velocity, etc.). In each of these linear systems, the whole is exactly equal to the sum of its parts. Breaking a linear system down into its component parts (or reducing it) helps us understand that system better. If all systems in the known universe were linear, everything from the origin of life to New England's weather would be predictable and equally easy to understand. This is not the case.

Although many phenomena can be explained in linear terms, other systems that are more complex, such as the human body, cannot be so easily understood. Simply reducing a human to an assemblage of tissues and cells does not explain how that entity develops the capacity to think and move. Mapping the brain to determine control centers cannot explain awareness or consciousness; neither can it explain skill acquisition and motor control.

The whole is almost always equal to a good deal more than the sum of its parts. One nonlinear phenomenon known as "chaos" declares a simple but profound message: Everything is connected, often with incredible sensitivity. In a well-studied complex system, the weather, scientists believe that the flap of a butterfly's wings in Texas can change the course of a hurricane in Haiti.[5] Similarly, an ingrown toenail can change a patient's ability to push-off, thereby altering an entire gait pattern and perhaps even interfering with the performance of functional activities.

Such is the real world, full of interacting agents and systems. In this nonlinear world, order emerges out of apparent randomness. Complex systems of all kinds (physical, chemical, biological, etc.) organize themselves spontaneously. Atoms merge to become molecules, single-celled organisms evolve to become multicellular entities, animals organize themselves into societies, and so on. These complex systems are not static phenomena but rather are always changing and adapting to their environment. They are dynamic systems. Under new circumstances or conditions, molecules split and become something different, organisms mutate, and societies rise and fall.

This nonlinear science is named "complexity." Investigators of complexity study the "emergence" of order and chaos in complex systems. Complexity helps explain the possible origins of life and the workings of the brain.[6] Instead of reducing a system into its component parts, complexity looks to the larger picture for understanding. In that sense, a person is not a brain and a bunch of limbs with a connecting torso but a person interacting with an environment. The mind and body are not separate but one. Although complexity is far from understood, movement scientists are already trying to understand how patterns of movement result from underlying control of dynamic systems. For those clinicians frustrated with the limitations imposed by assuming that learning and movement are exclusively controlled by higher centers, the theories of complexity offer a small window of understanding into how we humans function in the real world. These theories help explain why some patients lose functional capacity and how they can best restore it.

For the purposes of this book, further discussion of nonlinear dynamics is limited to a basic introduction of the complex system of human movement (motor control) and skill acquisition (motor learning). The reader is referred to the texts and articles on nonlinear systems listed at the end of this chapter for a truly eye-opening view of the universe.

THE DYNAMIC PATTERN THEORY OF MOTOR CONTROL

The dynamic pattern theory (DPT) was derived from synergetics, a nonlinear physical theory of self-organization and pattern formation.[6] Instead of breaking down the system of movement coordination into smaller and smaller parts (until a microscopic level is reached), DPT attempts to discover laws of coordination that can be observed by the clinician.[7] Because the study of complex systems (in this case, human movement) applies to the macroscopic (rather than the microscopic) world, it is usable by clinicians and not just researchers.

Transition of Movement Patterns

Many patterns exist in the real world: cloud formations, a flock of geese in flight, or the physical states of matter (solid, liquid, and gas). Unless the environment changes, these patterns maintain their form or, in other words, remain stable. A change in prevailing conditions, however, may destabilize the pattern and cause a new pattern to emerge. For example, if water is placed in a freezer, the drop in temperature causes the molecules in the liquid to transition into a crystalline structure (ice). To destabilize the liquid pattern of water, the system needs to be exposed to a change in temperature. Temperature is therefore considered the property in the environment that controls the physical state of water, and it is called the control parameter.

Animals also act or move in patterns. In general, there are many possible movement patterns available to an entity wishing to accomplish a specified goal. Take for example a horse wishing to cross a field to graze on a greener pasture. With no time constraints, the horse begins to walk in the desired direction. If the horse gets hungry, it may break into a trot to get to the pasture sooner. If it is really hungry, the trot will turn into a gallop. DPT helps explain why a horse switches from the movement pattern of trotting to galloping when it wishes to increase its speed. The horse does not think, "Now I will gallop." This change in pattern occurs spontaneously, not by some conscious choice but as a result of a control parameter (in this case, a critical velocity) causing the system to transition to a new pattern of coordination.[7]

A similar phenomenon perhaps occurs when a patient who has been using a walker is asked to walk normally while holding the therapist's arm for support. The gait pattern remains slow and uneven with a majority of the time spent in two-legged support. The pattern does not return to normal until the therapist requests that the patient walk as quickly as possible. The increase in velocity (without the fear of falling) helps the patient transition to a different walking pattern (one hopes a more normal one). The therapist does not have to instruct the patient to push off on the toes at the end of the stance phase or to take larger steps (in fact, sometimes too much verbal cueing causes a more confused and uncoordinated gait pattern to emerge). The only instruction usually needed is "go faster."

The spontaneous change in a movement pattern is believed to be caused by a loss of the initial pattern's stability. It is assumed to result from the self-organization of the neural networks. The pattern is neither imposed nor commanded but results from the interaction of all the neural networks, including both the CNS and the peripheral nervous system.[7]

Available Movement Patterns

If a person or a horse can change between coordinated movement patterns in response to a need or environmental demand, it presupposes that the movement patterns exist in memory somewhere in the neural network. They could be instinctive or learned patterns. It is probably important to note that these movement patterns are not "hard-wired" or unchangeable, reflex-like movements.[8] They are "available" to the being if and when needed. Depending on the being's physical state (degree of strength, height, flexibility, etc.), mental desires (go fast, be safe, etc.), and the environment (flat and even surfaces, many obstacles, etc.), movement patterns are switched on or off to accomplish functional tasks. This means, of course, that there is no single correct movement pattern for all humans for all functional tasks under all conditions. There is no single right way to get out of a chair, walk, or lift a bundle of groceries (some ways are of course better than others). There are, however, many correct ways to perform functional activities under different prevailing conditions.

A study by Ford-Smith and VanSant[9] on movement patterns used to arise from bed further clarifies this point. They studied 93 adults ranging from 30 to 59 years of age performing the activity of daily living of getting up and out of bed. They discovered great individual variation but also some general movement patterns that related to age (see Figures 4–1 and 4–2). They concluded that the older group appeared to separate the rising task into two distinct components: coming to sitting from supine, and coming to standing from sitting. The younger group seemed to roll off the bed in one smooth movement. Is the control parameter for this activity age? Perhaps. But what if the control parameter is the ability to balance or a certain level of abdominal strength? This could also account for a switch in movement patterns. (Anyone who has had a hangover will clearly remember getting out of bed the next morning slowly and in a movement pattern similar to that of the older group. Light-headedness and unsteadiness, not age, may account for this automatic switch in movement pattern.)

In addition, a patient can be stuck in a movement pattern as a result of his or her own physical condition or the environment. The inability to switch out of the stuck movement pattern in response to needs or desires may make a patient nonfunctional. Under the current conditions (such as physical weakness or thick carpeting),

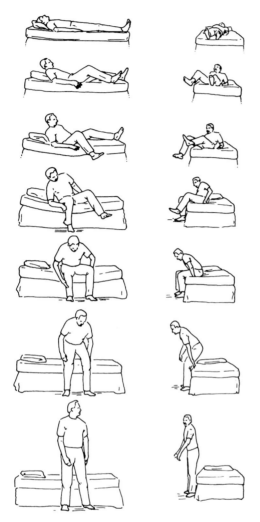

Figure 4–1. Most frequent movement patterns demonstrated by the 30- to 39-year-old subject. The subjects seems to roll off the bed in one smooth movement. *Source:* Reprinted from *Physical Therapy,* Vol. 73, No. 5, p. 305, with permission of the American Physical Therapy Association, © 1993.

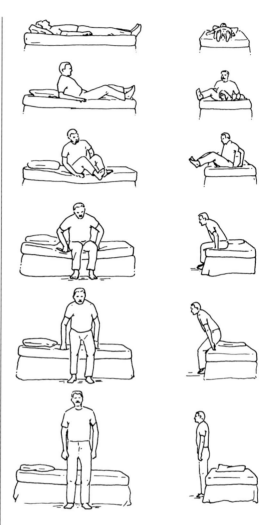

Figure 4–2. Most frequent movement patterns demonstrated by the 40- to 49-year-old and 50- to 59-year-old subject. Note that the task appears to be broken into two parts: supine-to-sit and sit-to-stand. *Source:* Reprinted from *Physical Therapy,* Vol. 73, No. 5, p. 306, with permission of the American Physical Therapy Association, © 1993.

the desired pattern change cannot occur because it is simply not available to the patient.[7,10] Physical impairments can prevent a stored, coordinated pattern from being used by the body. Environmental conditions, such as slippery floors or congested sidewalks, may also prevent the use of a particular movement type. A change or modification of the smallest prevailing physical or environmental condition can affect the entire movement pattern of a patient, the same

as a butterfly flapping its wings in Texas can affect New England's weather.

Influencing Pattern Change

If this theory proves to be true, it will help explain why a patient loses the ability to function normally in the first place. The nonfunctional patient needs to use a different movement pattern because, for some reason, perhaps a painful left knee, the original movement pattern is no longer available to the patient. The resulting antalgic gait pattern is a spontaneous pattern change that allows the patient to achieve his or her goal of walking. (The patient does not think, "Oh, I have a painful knee, so therefore I will limp.") If the pain resolves in a short while, the abnormal gait automatically disappears without the patient ever being aware of its existence. If the pain lasts for weeks or months, the new pattern might become normal to the patient (even when the pain is no longer present). In dynamic systems, this normal antalgic pattern is called an "attractor" because the system falls into the pattern easily and returns to that pattern when perturbed or interrupted.[8] Therapy may be needed to help this patient regain the original movement pattern (ie, return to function).

By finding each situation's control parameter (within the patient or the environment), the therapist can influence a change in the movement pattern. The clinician searches for the control parameter in the patient's physical abilities, mental abilities, and the surrounding environment (this is not necessarily an easy search). Improving a known impairment or changing the environment may be the catalyst needed to cause a movement pattern transition. When the critical level necessary for change is reached, the original pattern spontaneously occurs. The therapist usually exclaims, "See, that's it! You're walking normally now. Doesn't it feel better?"

Nonlinear or dynamic systems theory helps explain how and why the smallest of insults to the physical being or changes in the environment can render a patient nonfunctional. The underlying assumption is that biological organisms are complex, cooperative systems, with no one subsystem (posture, musculoskeletal, CNS, etc.) having priority for organizing the behavior of the system.[4] By changing the patient's physical characteristics through rehabilitation (ie, altering the subsystems by increasing strength, stability, balance, etc.) or by changing environmental demands (decreasing the height of a stair riser, using arm rests on chairs, inserting orthotics, etc.) original movement patterns spontaneously emerge.

MOTOR LEARNING

A motor learning or skill acquisition model developed by Carr and Shepherd[11] also rejects the neurotherapeutic theories of proprioceptive neuromuscular facilitation (PNF), neurodevelopmental technique (NDT), etc. Their model recognizes the complexity of human movement and incorporates some of the theories of nonlinear systems. A short review of their work and its relation to functional retraining and skill acquisition follows. Other motor learning models of equal importance exist in the literature but are beyond the scope of this book. For more information about motor learning (and motor control), the reader is referred to the four-part series on movement science in *Physical Therapy* listed at the end of this chapter.

Underlying Theories of Motor Control

Carr and Shepherd's[11] motor control theory is compatible with the DPT presented above and in some ways is similar. The basic premise of their motor control theory is that most skilled movements depend on preplanned patterns of neural output, which may be called motor programs (DPT calls these coordinated movement patterns). The performance of any motor task in a complex environment is governed by a predictive or anticipatory mode of control and by interrelated postural adjustments and limb movements. The role of the sensory system is to help shape ongoing movement as well as to influence future movements by updating the body's motor programs.[11,12] The sensory system therefore is not separate from the motor system but rather is an interactive part of it (this concept may seem strange to clinicians taught in the old way of sensory input and motor output).

Skill Acquisition

The behavior of all animals is directed to the accomplishment of goals. Skill is defined in terms of consistency in attaining a goal with some economy of effort. A skilled action involves achieving a goal efficiently through movement patterns shaped by the physical characteristics of the performer and configured to fit the environmental demands.[13]

Learning a skill is not a matter of copying a specific movement pattern but of learning a general strategy for solving a problem. Each environment and task situation demands a unique solution.[12] Reaching for a can of peas in a cupboard requires a slightly different movement pattern than reaching for a can of corn behind the peas. A short person with limited shoulder range of motion may need to climb on a stool to reach the can of corn, which lies only 2 small inches farther away than the can of peas.

Learning is a matter of doing or practicing. Practice involves a testing of various strategies in such a way that a person gradually selects and then optimizes the proper control strategy.[12] It is not simply a repetition of the same movement. Bernstein states, "Practice, when properly undertaken, does not consist in repeating the *means of solution* of a motor problem time after time, but in the *process of solving* this problem again and again by techniques we have changed and perfected from repetition to repetition."[14(p127)] Skill level is known to improve in proportion to the amount of practice. Practicing throughout the day is therefore much more effective than having the patient practice only while in therapy.

The Motor Relearning Program

Although originally described to assist in recovery after stroke, Carr and Shepherd's[11] motor relearning program has relevance to the non–brain injured as well. Most patients have motor programs stored in memory to help perform everyday functional activities. The therapist's job is to help the patient rediscover those motor programs. In DPT, this would be akin to making the movement patterns available again to the patient. Based on the underlying assumptions already mentioned, the investigators present the four steps of their program:

1. analysis of task
2. practice of missing components
3. practice of task
4. transference of training

Analysis of Task

The therapist observes the patient perform a task. The therapist then determines whether the performance accomplished the task (ie, met the functional goal) and was biomechanically efficient. If not, the patient's movement pattern and environment are analyzed more thoroughly to find the impairment or environmental cause that is preventing normal achievement of the task. The therapist must differentiate between the primary problem and compensatory problems that also have arisen. DPT calls this analysis the search for the control parameter (see Chapter 5 for more information about functional activity analysis).

Practice of Missing Components

Carr and Shepherd[11] advocate practicing the motor task in its entirety when at all possible. However, when the patient cannot perform the whole activity, individual components of the task may first be practiced separately. These components can consist of one or more of the following:

- an observable joint displacement (eg, knee extension)
- a muscle or muscle group (eg, the quadriceps femoris)
- a spatiotemporal relationship between muscles (the timing, sequencing, and/or rhythm of a movement)

Take for example the functional activity of getting out of a chair. After observing the patient's attempt to perform the task, the therapist concludes that weak quadriceps are contributing to the inability to arise efficiently from the chair. The therapist instructs the patient to practice the missing component of the task: knee extension. This can be done by sitting and kicking out the leg (open-chain extension) or in weight bearing by doing minisquats (closed-chain extension). After the patient regains sufficient knee extensor strength, the entire task can be practiced.

Practice of Task

Carr and Shepherd[11] point out that, in reality, practice of the missing component and practice of the actual task occur right after each other or at the same time. The therapist should constantly reevaluate the entire performance, checking especially for proper body and limb alignments that ensure that the appropriate muscles are placed at a mechanical advantage for the desired action.

During this stage the patient progresses from the cognitive phase of learning to the automatic phase of learning. The task should be made increasingly more difficult for the patient by changing the speed of the task or by changing the environmental context. In the example above of the patient learning to get out of a chair, the therapist wishes to change the difficulty of the task by altering the environment (the chair). When the patient is still too weak to accomplish the task without assistance, the therapist places two pillows on the chair (raising the seat height), so that the quadriceps have sufficient strength to perform the task without additional assistance. Progression consists of decreasing the seat height (removing the pillows) and then trying the activity out on different types of chairs and stools, including, of course, a toilet.

Transference of Training

During this phase, the patient practices the activity a sufficient number of times and in variable environmental contexts, so that the pattern of the movement becomes normal. The patient automatically uses the new pattern consistently and safely to accomplish functional goals.

The patient tries out and develops different strategies to adapt to the changing environment as well as changing behavioral goals. The patient needs to explore various movements and strategies. By trying different movement patterns and making mistakes, the patient learns to solve the functional problems present in life by discarding ineffective approaches and keeping the ones that work.

DYNAMIC MOVEMENT SCIENCE AND FUNCTIONAL REHABILITATION

The neurophysiological theories that provide the basis for PNF and NDT have been unable to explain in full the functional losses of motor control seen clinically. They represent a linear or hierarchical approach to the problem of motor control. The so-called higher centers of the brain, however, do not have enough time to properly control and inhibit the lower centers and reflexes. We would move too slowly in robotic fashion. We humans cannot think about and therefore control all our daily functions, nor can we rely solely on hard-wired reflexes that cannot adapt to change.

In addition, we initiate behaviors and actions. We do not simply react to the environment; we proact. We anticipate and predict. If we anticipate lifting a heavy load, we set our postural muscles accordingly, beforehand and without conscious thought. We do not think, "Now I am going to do this." We simply do it. We transition in and out of movement patterns to adapt to our changing environment and our changing abilities. Each movement is similar to those of our fellow humans but also uniquely our own based on our body build and other characteristics.

We are interconnected with incredible sensitivity. One system influences another. The old song line "the hip bone's connected to the knee bone" strikes a true chord. A tight Achilles tendon can manifest itself as foot pain, knee pain, or back pain, depending on the patient. Because humans are individuals with different physical and mental characteristics, each also recovers differently from injury. Some automatically regain functional ability as their injury heals, and some need help to make original motor patterns available again.

Rehabilitation specialists have always understood these ideas on some intuitive level. The statements presented here are not really new or profound. But now with greater understanding of what has in some ways always been known, therapists can better assist patients on the road to full functional recovery. New treatment strategies for restoring function, such as the ones presented in this book, will develop based on these dynamic theories of movement science. We are at the dawning of a new way to look at real patients trying to operate in the real world. It is a wonderfully complex world full of complex organisms acting in complex ways but perhaps governed by simple rules. As these complex systems and their simple rules become better understood, the entire focus of medical and rehabilitative treatment may change drastically. The treatment strategies presented in this book are an attempt to glimpse into that future.

REFERENCES

1. Rood MS. Neurophysiological mechanisms utilized in the treatment of neuromuscular dysfunction. *Am J Occup Ther.* 1956;10:220–225.

2. Brunnstrom S. *Movement Therapy in Hemiplegia.* New York, NY: Harper & Row;1970.

3. Bobath B. *Adult Hemiplegia: Evaluation and Treatment.* 2nd ed. London, England:Heinemann;1978.

4. Knott M, Voss DE. *Proprioceptive Neuromuscular Facilitation.* 2nd ed. New York, NY: Harper & Row;1968.

5. Waldrop MM. *Complexity: The Emerging Science at the Edge of Order and Chaos.* New York, NY: Simon & Schuster; 1992.

6. Haken H. *Synergetics, an Introduction: Non-Equilibrium Phase Transitions and Self-Organization in Physics, Chemistry, and Biology.* New York, NY: Springer-Verlag; 1983.

7. Scholz JP. Dynamic pattern theory—some implications for therapeutics. *Phys Ther.* 1990;70(12):827–843.

8. Kamm K, Thelen E, Jensen JL. A dynamical systems approach to motor development. *Phys Ther.* 1990; 70(12):763–775.

9. Ford-Smith CD, VanSant AF. Age differences in movement patterns used to rise from a bed in subjects in the third through fifth decades of life. *Phys Ther.* 1993; 73(5):300–307.

10. Bradley NS. Animal models offer the opportunity to acquire a new perspective on motor development. *Phys Ther.* 1990;70(12):776–787.

11. Carr JH, Shepherd RB: *A Motor Relearning Programme for Stroke.* Gaithersburg, Md: Aspen; 1987.

12. Gordon J. Assumptions underlying physical therapy intervention: theoretical and historical perspectives. In: *Movement Science Foundations for Physical Therapy in Rehabilitation.* Gaithersburg, Md: Aspen; 1987:15–17.

13. Gentile AM. Skill acquisition: action, movement, and neuromotor processes. In: Carr J, Shepherd R, eds, *Movement Science Foundations for Physical Therapy in Rehabilitation.* Gaithersburg, Md: Aspen;1987:93–154.

14. Bernstein NA. *The Coordination and Regulation of Movements.* New York, NY: Pergamon;1967.

ADDITIONAL READING

Warning: The reference materials presented here are sufficient to get an interested reader hooked on complex systems. The information is a bit radical, weird, and crazy, but that is what it is like on the frontier of a new science: wild and crazy but exciting with possibilities. The reading requires intense thought and concentration. If you get hooked, though, you can never look at the world as you did before. Suddenly complex systems are everywhere. Once your eyes are opened to the universe of complexity, you can never go back.

Gleick J. *Chaos: Making a New Science.* New York, NY: Penguin; 1987.

Movement science (part 1). *Phys Ther.* 1990;70(12): 758–872.

Movement science (part 2). *Phys Ther.* 1991;71(1):25–67.

Movement science (part 3). *Phys Ther.* 1991;71(2):123–164.

Movement science (part 4). *Phys Ther.* 1991;71(3):215–259.

5

Determining the Cause of the Disability

In the United States, the presence of disease dictates entry into the health care system, yet many functional losses are due to disorders or physical and mental impairments, not just diseases. Although the disability models discussed in Chapter 2 help the clinician understand the potential functional loss associated with disease, there is a lack of exact correlation between disease and functional ability. In addition, the severity of a disease or the number of diseases present does not necessarily determine the level of functional disability, especially in the elderly.[1,2] To treat a patient successfully, the therapist must be able to establish a relationship between physical impairment and disability. Rehabilitation specialists have not always clearly assessed and documented a patient's functional ability (or disability) while at the same time relating that functional level to the presence of physical impairments. Physical therapy has generally been more interested in evaluating the musculoskeletal impairments present, such as weakness or loss of range of motion (ROM), but has often failed to correlate them with functional loss. Occupational therapy has always evaluated function, but has often failed to correlate the patient's function with a treatable impairment, such as shoulder instability or faulty motor control.

The therapist first documents the functional losses as determined by a functional assessment or questionnaire (see Chapter 13). To determine the cause of the functional loss, the clinician must then analyze the functional activity and, through detective work, deduce the impairments or environmental constraints (control parameters) that are preventing normal movement from occurring.

FUNCTIONAL ACTIVITY ANALYSIS

No matter how simple or complex the functional activity, the therapist, in combination with a cooperative patient, can analyze it and discover which aspect or component of the activity the patient is unable to complete in an efficient, pain-free manner. The process of analysis is the same for the elderly patient having difficulty rising from a chair, the worker who cannot lift packages overhead, and the athlete who is unable to maneuver on the soccer field.

The Big Picture

The therapist must view the patient as a human being trying to interact with the environment with different degrees of success. Of paramount importance is what the patient deems to be important behavior. The basis of therapy is to emphasize the functional activities that the patient wishes to pursue (this alleviates motivational problems). After the patient determines the direction of rehabilitation, the therapist uses anatomy, biomechanics, postural alignment, and movement science to discover the component of the activity that is preventing the patient from accomplishing the behavioral goal (in dynamic movement science, this is the search for the control parameter that is preventing stored patterns from being used by the person). The big picture includes patient goals of the following type:

- I want to be able to do everything.
- I want to be able to play basketball (or any other sport).
- I want to be able to walk.
- I want to be able to hold my grandchildren.
- I want to return to work.
- I want to be able to go to the bathroom by myself.
- I want to go to church (or any other religious event).
- I want to go to the movies or a restaurant.
- I want to paint again.
- I keep losing my balance. I don't want to fall and break my hip.

Breaking It Down

After picking one goal on which to work, the therapist mentally reduces the functional activity to its major component parts. This step is simple but vital. The therapist then asks the patient questions to determine which of the major components is at fault. For example, an outpatient with knee dysfunction establishes a functional goal of grocery shopping. The major physical components of grocery shopping include the following:

- getting to and from the store (transportation)
- pushing a grocery cart
- walking up and down the aisles

- reaching onto shelves
- placing items into the cart
- standing in line
- reaching into the cart and lifting the items out onto the conveyor belt
- carrying the grocery bags into the home
- putting the items away in the home

In addition, the cognitive skills of deciding what is needed, making a shopping list, knowing the location of the store, calculating the approximate amount of money needed, understanding money management, and the like are obviously prerequisites to the instrumental activity of daily living (IADL) of going shopping.

Other IADLs have been grossly analyzed, broken down, and reported in the literature. Boblitz[3] identifies the physical demands of being able to drive a car (Table 5–1) or ride a public bus (Table 5–2). In industrial circles, similar analyses have also been performed. Ellexson[4] analyzes the job of a packer (Table 5–3). Most other work activities have been analyzed and described in the book *Selected Characteristics of Occupations Defined in the Dictionary of Occupational Titles*[5] as well as in the *Dictionary of Occupational Titles*[6] itself. Sporting activities can be broken down into major components as well. For example, the game of baseball includes the following:

- throwing a baseball
- catching a baseball
- batting
- running on dirt and grass or Astroturf
- fielding ground balls

Depending on the player's position, more time is spent performing some of the components than others.

The therapist then questions the patient as to which aspect of the activity seems to be difficult or painful. In the example above concerning the functional activity of grocery shopping, the patient may reply that the problems lie within three components: transportation, pushing the grocery cart, and carrying the grocery bags.

Table 5–1 Basic Physical Driving Tasks

Task	Evaluation Location	
	Simulator	Actual Vehicle
1. Opens/closes car door		✔
2. Transfers to/from seat		✔
3. Opens/closes front side windows		✔
4. Adjusts seat/mirrors		✔
5. Fastens/unfastens seat belt and/or harness		✔
6. Depresses/releases foot brake	✔	
7. Releases/depresses parking brake	✔	
8. Shifts gears	✔	
9. Depresses/releases clutch	✔	
10. Depresses/releases accelerator	✔	
11. Controls steering	✔	
12. Turns signals on/off	✔	
13. Turns head/body upon backing/pulling out	✔	
14. Turns head to observe road environment	✔	

Source: Reprinted from *Rehabilitation Management of Rheumatic Conditions,* Second Edition by G.E. Ehrlich, p. 209, with permission of Williams & Wilkins, © 1986.

Table 5–2 Categorical Functional Activities Required by Ambulatory Passengers in Public Bus Use

Activities	Critical Activities	Potential Operator-Assisted Activities
1. Walks two blocks to bus stop carrying 10 lb	✔	
2. Stands waiting at least 10 minutes	✔	
3. Identifies correct bus	✔	
4. Ascends front bus steps from curb	✔	
5. Ascends front bus steps from street	✔	
6. Places change in coin box/shows reduced fare card/obtains transfer		✔
7. Walks to seat while bus is stationary	*	*
8. Walks to seat while bus is moving		✔
9. Transfers to seat while bus is stationary	✔	
10. Transfers to seat while bus is moving		✔
11. Sits and maintains balance while bus is moving	✔	
12. Stands and maintains balance while bus is moving		✔
13. Stands up from seat while bus is stationary	✔	
14. Stands up from seat while bus is moving		✔
15. Pulls signal cord		✔
16. Walks to front exit while bus is stationary	*	*
17. Walks to front exit while bus is moving		✔
18. Walks to back exit while bus is stationary	*	*
19. Walks to back exit while bus is moving		✔
20. Descends front bus steps to curb	✔	
21. Descends front bus steps to street	✔	
22. Descends back bus steps to street		✔
23. Walks two blocks to destination carrying 10 lb	✔	
24. Stands waiting at least 10 minutes to transfer to another bus	*	*

*Neither critical nor potential operator-assisted activities.
Source: Reprinted from *Rehabilitation Management of Rheumatic Conditions,* Second Edition by G.E. Ehrlich, p. 227, with permission of Williams & Wilkins. © 1986.

Table 5–3 Example of an Analysis of Work Activity

Job Title: *Packer*

Essential function: packing individual cobbler cups for shipping

Steps

1. Select a box
2. Place the box on the conveyor side rack
3. Pick up one cobbler cup in each hand
4. Place the cups into the packing box
5. Repeat steps 1–2 until 36 cups are in a box
6. Place the filled box on the "sealing table"
7. Fold the short flaps of the box flap
8. Fold the long flaps of the box flap
9. Tape the long flaps of the box down using the manual taping machine
10. Place the sealed box on the pallet

Source: Reprinted from *Orthopaedic Physical Therapy Clinics of North America,* Vol. 1, No. 1, p. 17, with permission of W.B. Saunders Company, © 1992.

Each of the three tasks is then further analyzed to determine the basic problem areas. Upon further questioning, the patient states that the really difficult part of the transportation task is getting in and out of the car without hurting the knee (ie, car transfers). In addition, pushing the cart is not so hard in the beginning, but as it gets full the knee pain begins again. In other words, there is a critical mass of the cart (control parameter) that, when reached, prevents the activity from being accomplished in a pain-free, efficient manner. The entire task of lifting and carrying the grocery bags also causes increased pain in the impaired knee. Sufficient information now exists for the clinician to begin the process of determining which impairments correlate with the basic problem areas of car transfers, pushing, and carrying.

To perform a functional task analysis, the therapist must possess the qualities of an organized and logical mind in addition to excellent deductive reasoning skills. The clinician must also understand the need and importance of categorizing the patient's function to dedicate the time necessary to conduct an intensive interrogation about the patient's activities and desires in life. With time constraints only worsening, the therapist must resist the temptation to treat immediately and instead must spend the time finding out what really needs to be treated to restore function.

OBSERVATIONAL ANALYSIS

From a therapy standpoint, the clinician needs to know in which component of the movement task (such as car transfers, lifting, or carrying) the problem occurs. As mentioned in Chapter 4, Carr and Shepherd[7] theorize that at least three major components exist: joint displacement, muscle action, and/or the spatiotemporal relationships among muscles. Fisher and Yakura[8] believe that four major components of movement must be observed by the clinician. These two theories are compatible with each other and may be extensions of the same idea. Fisher and Yakura's four biomechanical descriptors of movement behavior are as follows:

1. base of support
2. alignment
3. sequence of movement
4. stability/mobility

By observing the patient performing the functional task (or one of its components) with regard to the biomechanical descriptors listed above, the therapist continues the process of analyzing the activity to discover the physical impairments or environmental constraints that are preventing normal motion and function.

Base of Support

Base of support is defined simply by Fisher and Yakura[8] as the weight-bearing structure(s). Klein-Vogelbach[9] describes the human body as a chain of links each representing a mobile body segment (ie, the head, thorax, pelvis, legs, and arms). When a person is lying down, each body segment possesses its own center of gravity and its own base of support. When the person changes the relations among the body segments and gets up, the body segments become linked by muscular activity, and the five joined body parts acquire a common center of gravity and a need for a stable base of support. In bilateral standing, the feet, ankles, knees, hips, and vertebral column all support some of the weight-bearing load. The support area or base consists of the space occupied by the feet (Figure 5–1). During a push-up, the hands, wrists, elbows, and shoulders as well as the toes and metatarsal joints bear weight. The base of support consists of the entire area from hand contact to foot contact. The therapist observes the functional task, such as a car transfer or walking, and notes the overall dimension of the base of support (eg, wide or narrow) and how it changes during the activity, from starting posture, including the movement itself, to ending posture.[7]

The therapist looks for pain patterns or movement patterns related to potential problems with the base of support as well as at the body's weight-bearing structures. Knowledge of joint anatomy and biomechanics is imperative to discover any interrelationships between an activity and the body's base of support. Does the patient hold one leg in external rotation (toe-out) to increase the base of support? Does the knee pain increase only on weight-bearing activities? If so, is the pain more on the medial (weight-bearing) compartment than on the lateral? Is there a difference during gait in the amount or quality of the pain on heel strike, when the weight-bearing forces are directed posteriorly versus midstance, when the weight-bearing forces are directed

more anteriorly? By having the patient perform variations of the activity that alter the control parameters (eg, heel walking and toe walking are variations of gait), the therapist can determine whether the base of support or the structures that support weight are causing a problem for the patient during a particular activity. This information brings the therapist one step closer to discovering the exact impairment or impairments impeding normal function.

Alignment

Alignment refers to both the relationship of the body's center of mass over the base of support and the relationships of the body segments to each other. The alignment is also observed from initial posture and throughout the movement until final posture.[8]

Importance of Alignment

The initial postural alignment of a person dictates the movement options available. The delicate interrelationships within the body are never more evident than when one is discussing the cascade of events that occurs from maintaining a forward head posture (Table 5–4). The resultant dysfunctions wind their way to the shoulder

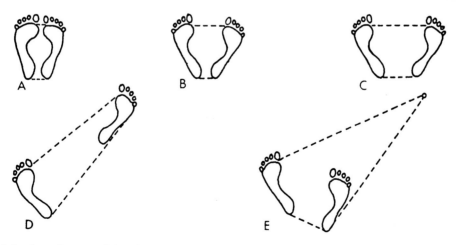

Figure 5–1. Base of support: Various foot positions in standing that provide various areas of support. The base increases in size from *A* to *D*. *E* illustrates the large area of support made possible by the use of a cane. Crutches would increase the base considerably. *Source:* Reprinted from *Therapeutic Exercise for Body Alignment and Function,* Second Edition by L. Daniels and C. Worthingham, p. 5, with permission of W.B. Saunders Company, © 1977.

Table 5–4 Postural Sequence for the Forward-Head Posture

Forward bending of the midcervical facet joints

Backward bending (extension) of the occiput atlas

Shortening of suboccipital muscles, resulting in potential impingement of the greater or lesser occipital nerves

Imbalance between the sternocleidomastoid, the levator scapula, and the trapezius

Imbalance between the anterior cervical musculature (including the suprahyoid and infrahyoid muscles) and posterior cervical extensors

Shoulder girdle protraction with internal rotation (the latissimus, subscapularis, pectoralis, and teres major being involved)

Increased thoracic kyphosis with decreased lumbar lordosis

Increased activity of the accessory respiratory muscles due to poor diaphragmatic breathing and poor expansion of the lower rib cage

Elevation of the first rib by increased scalene activity

Anterior and posterior restriction of the first rib articulations

Tendency toward thoracic outlet symptomatology

Cervical imbalance with a tendency toward degenerative joint disease from C-5 through C-7

Muscular imbalance leading to abnormal muscle firing (some muscles become facilitated with trigger points)

Joints and soft tissues maintained in shortened range lead to restriction of joint capsules and loss of proprioception

Source: Reprinted from *Myofascial Manipulation Theory and Clinical Application* by R.I. Cantu and A.J. Grodin, p. 81, Aspen Publishers, Inc. © 1992.

girdle, causing scapular protraction (round-shouldered posture) with resultant internal rotation of the humerus. The now malaligned humerus (in relation to the glenoid fossa) will impinge on the coracoacromial arch sooner during elevation activities than if the joint was optimally aligned. This will cause a different movement pattern to arise spontaneously.

Klein-Vogelbach[9] contends that pathologic posture and resulting movement lack harmony and economy. She further states that the ability for fine adjustment is reduced. With postural malalignment, strain on the passive structure increases, and inappropriate demands are made of the musculature.

Sahrmann[10] believes that the initial alignment is also an important factor in movement disorder. Her second hypothesis in her movement system balance theory is, "Ideal (optimal) postural resting alignment is a prerequisite for precise movement because faulty initial alignment does not permit maintenance of the optimal path of instantaneous center of rotation. . . . "[10(p3)] This is of course exactly what occurs in the shoulder impingement scenario described above. Sahrmann attributes the deviation from optimal postural alignment to an alteration in muscle length. In other words, Sahrmann has correlated some movement disorders with the presence of physical impairments. The postural fault must be corrected by restoring optimal muscle length to both shortened and lengthened muscles to restore the original movement pattern.

(*Author's personal note:* In doing the research for this book, somehow I knew it would all come down to my mother being right. Without any thought to movement science or access to expensive laboratory analyzing equipment, mothers throughout the ages have admonished their children to attain proper posture. So, to all mothers everywhere who pleaded with their adolescent teenagers to "Stand up straight and pull your shoulders back!", my personal salute. And to all those teenagers who ignored all those mothers go the thanks of the entire physical therapy profession for keeping us gainfully employed.)

Exploring Posture Further

After the initial obligatory check for major postural deviations, the therapist must truly explore the patient's postural alignment during functional activities and special tests. Many investigators, including Sahrmann,[10] Daniels and Worthingham,[11] Klein-Vogelbach,[9] and Kendall and McCreary,[12] have written extensively about the subject. The reader is referred to these texts for additional information about postural assessment. This in-depth, fact-finding tour of body alignment holds the key to many of the patient's movement problems and cannot be dismissed as simply poor posture. Table 5–5 lists Kendall and McCreary's[12] examples of common postural faults of the lower extremities and the resultant muscle length changes that may occur. When postural alignment can be correlated with painful movement patterns, the muscular or fascial faults can be discovered and corrected through minimal manual therapy and moderate physical exercise.

Sequence of Movement

Sequence is defined by Fisher and Yakura[8] as the order of occurrence, timing of changes, and direction of movement of the segments. They emphasize that the initiation of movement, or which body segment moves first, influences the progression of the entire movement.

A change in sequence often occurs in a patient with frozen shoulder syndrome. With loss of glenohumeral joint motion, the patient attempts to elevate the arm with the only available movement pattern present: scapular abduction, elevation, and upward rotation. As the frozen shoulder slowly resolves, the patient may continue using the pathological pattern (called reverse scapulohumeral rhythm). The patient shrugging the shoulder during the first 90° of shoulder elevation looks wrong and clues the clinician to a sequencing or coordination problem (Figure 5–2). Even if the original physical impairment of capsular dysfunction gets better, the patient does not until the secondary coordination impairment is corrected. The therapist must provide guidance with verbal, visual, and tactile cues to correct the patient's movement pattern.

Stability/Mobility

To analyze a task properly, Fisher and Yakura[8] wish to identify which of the body seg-

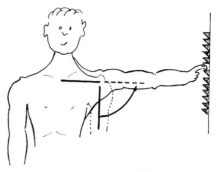

normal scapulohumeral rhythm

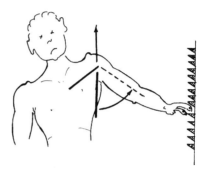

reverse scapulohumeral rhythm

Figure 5–2. (Top) Normal scapulohumeral rhythm; note the horizontal level of the clavicle. **(Bottom)** Reverse scapulohumeral rhythm; note the elevated clavicle. *Source:* Adapted from *Shoulder Pain* by R. Cailliet, with permission of F.A. Davis Company, © 1966.

ments acts as part of a postural support system (what Klein-Vogelbach[9] calls stabiles) and which serve as moving segments (what Klein-Vogelbach calls mobiles).

As mentioned previously, Klein-Vogelbach[9] describes the functional body segments as consisting of the thorax, the pelvis, the legs, the head, and the arms. The five body segments work together, with the thorax acting as the primary site of stabilization and the distal segments moving and interacting with the environment (Figure 5–3). During different activities, mobile segments act as stabile segments, and vice versa.

The thorax consists of the 12 thoracic vertebrae, ribs, and sternum. This region houses the cardiopulmonary center of the body. For body

Table 5-5 Faulty Leg, Knee, and Foot Positions: Analysis and Treatment

Postural Fault	Anatomical Position of Joints	Muscles in Shortened Position	Muscles in Lengthened Position	Treatment Procedures*
Hyperextended knee	Knee hyperextension, Ankle plantar flexion	Quadriceps, Soleus	Popliteus, Hamstrings at knee	Instruct regarding overall postural correction with emphasis on avoiding knee hyperextension. In hemiplegics, short-leg brace with right-angle stop.
Flexed knee	Knee flexion, Ankle dorsiflexion	Popliteus, Hamstrings at knee	Quadriceps, Soleus	Stretch knee flexors, if tight. Overall postural correction. Knee flexion may be secondary to hip flexor shortness. Check length of hip flexors; stretch if short.
Medially rotated femur (often associated with pronation of foot; see below)	Hip joint medial rotation	Hip medial rotators	Hip lateral rotators	Stretch hip medial rotators, if tight. Strengthen hip lateral rotators, if weak. Young children should *avoid* sitting in reverse tailor fashion ("W" position; see below for correction of any accompanying pronation).
Knock-knee (genu valgum)	Hip joint adduction, Knee joint abduction	Fascia lata, Lateral knee joint structures	Medial knee joint structures	Inner wedge on heels, if feet are pronated. Stretch fascia lata, if indicated.
Postural bowlegs	Hip joint medial rotation, Knee joint hyperextension, Foot pronation	Hip medial rotators, Quadriceps, Foot everters	Hip lateral rotators, Popliteus, Tibialis posterior and long toe flexors	Exercises for overall correction of foot, knee, and hip positions. *Avoid* knee hyperextension. Strengthen hip lateral rotators. Inner wedges on heels to correct foot pronation. Stand with feet straight ahead and about 2 inches apart. Relax the knees into an "easy" position, ie, neither stiff nor bent. Tighten the muscles which lift the arches of the feet, rolling the weight *slightly* toward the outer borders of the feet. Tighten the buttocks muscles to rotate the legs slightly outward (until kneecaps face directly forward).
Pronation	Foot eversion	Peroneals and toe extensors	Tibialis posterior and long toe flexors	Inner wedges on heels (usually 1/8 in on wide heels and 1/16 in on medium heels). Overall correction of posture of feet and knees. Exercises to strengthen the inverters. Instructions in proper standing and walking.
Supination	Foot inversion	Tibials	Peroneals	Outer wedge on heels. Exercise for peroneals.
Hammer toes and low metatarsal arch	Metatarsophalangeal joint hyperextension, Proximal interphalangeal joint flexion	Toe extensors	Lumbricals	Stretch metatarsophalangeal joints by flexion; stretch interphalangeal joints by extension. Strengthen lumbricals by metatarsophalangeal joint flexion. Metatarsal pad or bar.

*If indicated on the basis of tests for alignment and muscle length and strength tests.
Source: Reprinted from *Muscles Testing and Function*, Fourth Edition by F.P. Kendall, E.K. McCreary, and P.G. Provance. p. 108, with permission of Williams & Wilkins, © 1993.

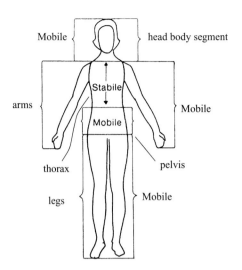

Figure 5–3. Klein-Vogelbach's functional body segments as stabiles, which remain unmoving, and mobiles, which are body segments that move around the stabiles. *Source:* Adapted from *Functional Kinetics* by S. Klein-Vogelbach, p. 80, with permission of Springer-Verlag, © 1990.

movement purposes, this area acts mainly as a stabilizing center for posture and peripheral movements. Through synergistic and antagonistic muscle activity (also called dynamic stabilization), the thorax is able to receive, absorb, and transmit all incoming movement forces.[9]

The pelvis consists of the five lumbar vertebrae, sacrum, ilium, ischium, and pubic bones. This region protects the digestive and reproductive organs of the body. For body movement purposes, this area acts to achieve a balance between the functions of the thorax and the legs. The pelvis helps control, coordinate, and transmit the forces generated by the legs to the vertebral column.[9]

The legs consist skeletally of the femurs down to the phalanges and are considered the region of locomotion. All movements of the legs influence the pelvis, too. In addition, the legs afford a mobile foundation that supports the vertebral column. By absorbing many of the weight-bearing forces, the legs contribute to the health of the spinal column.[9]

The head body segment consists of the seven cervical vertebrae and the skull. It houses and protects the brain and the major sense organs.

Perched atop the thorax, the head requires great potential mobility to properly scan the environment with eyes, ears, and nose.[9]

The arms consist of the entire shoulder girdle down to the phalanges. The arms are considered the region of manual skill and allow the body to interact with the environment with great precision. Both arms generally act independent of each other. They connect to the trunk via the shoulder girdle by embracing the thorax like a pair of tongs.[9]

PHYSICAL IMPAIRMENTS

By analyzing the task through its components and through observation, the therapist may be able to identify the physical impairments or environmental causes of functional loss. The impairments can derive from any of the body's major systems, cardiopulmonary, neuromuscular, or musculoskeletal.

In general, multiple impairments overlap, causing a confused clinical picture initially. Only some (the control parameters) may actually be the root of the observed functional loss. The areas of greatest interest are:

- flexibility
- strength/power
- balance
- coordination/motor control
- sensory input

All these base elements influence each other as the person attempts to interact with the environment.

Flexibility

Flexibility, or the amount of motion available at a given joint, has always been a major goal of both physical and occupational therapy. Flexibility refers to both the length and the elasticity of the muscles, joint ligaments, joint capsules, and other connective tissue structures. Generally measured with a goniometer, normal ROMs have been determined and are available in many texts. By measurement of joint ranges during basic functional activities, some functional ROMs have also been estimated (Table 5–6). These measures of motion should not be viewed as definitive for individual patients. Flexibility also depends on a patient's body build and anatomical structure.

The obsession with restoring normal ROM has caused a backlash of unintended but real injuries to patients. Many therapists used to crank on their patients' joints in the "no pain—no gain" era of therapy to return the motions to normal. Because this was done without regard to the particular structure preventing the motion, trauma was induced in all the tissues surrounding the joint and even in other joints. The results were horrendous. Some of this passive ranging still occurs today. A large percentage of the shoulder pain that stroke patients experience can be attributed to the unskilled passive ranging of the hemiparetic arm causing tears in the rotator cuff.

Therefore, the clinician needs to determine which structures are too short: the muscles, the joint capsule, or the fascia (connective tissue). Perhaps even more important, the clinician needs to determine which structures are too loose. Injuries and pain rarely occur at hypomobile joints; they are too stabile and secure. Most pain occurs at the hypermobile joints, where the muscles or joint capsule may be excessively long. In other words, the system gives way at its weakest or, in this case, its loosest link. Sahrmann[10] refers to this concept as the principle of relative flexibility. She contends, "The body takes the path of least resistance for motion."[10(p4)] This means that motion will occur at the loosest joint first rather than where it should occur.

A flexible patient is not necessarily a pain-free one. Take for example a 38-year-old fitness trainer with a primary complaint of left knee pain following three surgeries. She reports that she has always been a flexible person. Although she can palm the floor, she cannot simultaneously extend her knee fully. Further investigation reveals shortened hip extensors (ie, hamstrings), which are causing a posterior pelvic

Table 5–6 Estimated Joint Functional ROM

Joint	Estimated Functional ROM
Ankle*	Dorsiflexion 10°
Knee†	0°–105° with 10° of tibial rotation, abduction, and adduction
Hip‡	120° flexion, 20° abduction, 20° external rotation
Shoulder§	100° flexion, 90° abduction, 30° external rotation, 70° internal rotation
Elbow/forearm‖	30°–130° extension to flexion, 50° pronation, 50° supination

Source: Data from *Normal and Abnormal Function of the Foot* by M.L. Root et. al., Clinical Biomechanics Corp, © 1977; †*Physical Therapy*, Vol. 52, No. 1, p. 34–42, American Physical Therapy Association, © 1972; ‡*Basic Biomechanics of the Skeletal System* by V.H. Frankel and M. Nordin, p. 156, Lea & Febiger, © 1980; §*Physical Therapy*, Vol. 66, No. 12, p. 1890, American Physical Therapy Association, © 1986; ‖*The Elbow and Its Disorders* by B. Morrey, ed., p. 68, W.B. Saunders Company, © 1985.

tilt. Her major source of flexibility comes from her low back. Upon further questioning, the patient reports a long history of intermittent low back pain (interestingly, she has recently developed pain at her ischial tuberosity, the insertion of the hamstrings). A clinician can easily be fooled by such a fit patient who presents with such apparent flexibility. To restore normal low back, hip, and knee mechanics, the hip flexors need to be stretched out, and the low back needs to be stabilized.

Strength/Power

Strength is one of those terms that is commonly misused or misconstrued. It is mainly a property of the muscular system. However, the skeletal system must be intact and able to withstand the compressive and tensile forces generated by the contracting muscles or a bone fracture will occur. Strength can be considered a measurement of the tension produced by muscular contraction. Rothstein[13] writes that strength has been used to describe both the ability to move and the ability to hold, which are clearly not the same. He recommends that muscles be thought of as transducers (a device that converts energy from one system to another in a different form) and be measured in terms of power, where power = work/time.

The power (or strength) needed to accomplish functional tasks has not been measured, but is easily observed by an experienced clinician. What is not as easily observed is which muscle group is actually the weak one. Changes in muscle length (as in a stretched or shortened muscle) alter the anatomical, biochemical, and physiological properties of the muscle. Shortened muscles have decreased numbers of sarcomeres with increased sarcomere length, while lengthened muscles have increased but smaller sarcomeres (Figure 5–4). In addition, the length-tension curves are altered, with the shortened muscles showing the greatest changes.[14] Kendall and McCreary[12] have named the weak-

ness they noted in lengthened muscle stretch-weakness, but it may be more accurately called a loss of strength at a specific muscle length. Sahrmann[9] calls this positional strength.

Insufficient strength at a muscle or muscle group causes the person to compensate, or to substitute other muscles or motions. As mentioned previously in Chapter 4, this substitution is spontaneous and not under conscious thought. A person climbing the stairs with a weak gastrocnemius does not think, "Oh, I will use my quads more." Instead, an entire movement pattern emerges: foot flat on the stair, increased flexion of the hip, knee, and ankle, and increased tension produced by the quadriceps. If other system reserves are low, as often happens with the elderly, insufficient strength can contribute to major functional losses of even the most basic activities of daily living.

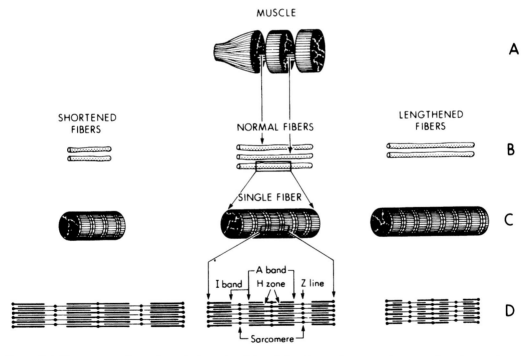

Figure 5–4. The structure of normal muscle (**center**) and the relative changes that occur when a muscle undergoes changes due to a shortened position (**left**) or lengthened position (**right**). (**A**) Skeletal muscle composed of single fibers (cells). (**B**) Single fibers. (**C**) Single fiber enlarged to show myofibrils; note decreased and increased sarcomere numbers in the shortened and lengthened fibers, respectively. (**D**) Myofibril enlarged to show contractile proteins of the sarcomere (actin and myosin myofilaments); note increased and decreased sarcomere length in the shortened and lengthened fibers, respectively. *Source:* Reprinted from *Physical Therapy*, Vol. 62, No. 12, p. 1800, with permission of the American Physical Therapy Association, © 1982.

Balance

Balance is the ability to maintain one's center of mass over one's base of support. It requires complex interactions of the sensorimotor system to constantly adjust joint position and muscular activity.[15] Balance involves both the ability to react to perturberances, such as bumping into someone, and the ability to anticipate the environment, as in walking up a grassy slope. As a complex system (see Chapter 4), balance is not solely under the control of the central nervous system (CNS) but is a dynamic function of the entire neuromotor system. Unlike balance problems in the brain-injured population, where balance deficits result mainly due to CNS insult, balance problems in the orthopaedic population show up more often in the peripheral systems. Weakness of the ankle dorsiflexors, knee extensors, and hip abductors and extensors as well as loss of sensory perception in the feet, ankles, and knees can alter the ability to balance. Diminished sensory input from vision (which occurs often in the elderly) has a profound effect on the ability to maintain balance.[16] Possible changes in gait pattern to increase the base of support would show up as:

- increased toe-out
- lack of heel strike
- increased step width
- decreased step length
- increased time in double support

The balance deficit is no less real or less dangerous in the orthopaedic patient than in the stroke population and needs to be addressed. Although many of these adjustments in gait pattern help maintain a safe and stable ability to ambulate, especially in the healthy elderly population,[17] they may also be seen as warning signs that a correctable problem exists in the balancing mechanism. Table 5–7 describes some other common balance problems in patients with musculoskeletal dysfunction.

Coordination/Motor Control

Any injury affects the person's ability to move in a pain-free, efficient manner. This complex system is addressed more fully in Chapter 4. To reiterate briefly, the control of motor performance of any being is the result of the self-organization of the entire neural net, from the CNS to the periphery. Motor control and coordination are influenced by the behavioral goals and physical characteristics of the being as well as by the surrounding environment. Problems in this system manifest themselves to the observer as movements that are labored, slow, stiff, difficult, excessive, etc.

Sensory Input

The head sits on top of the body and scans the environment with its four major sense organs. Other sense organs feel the outside world. From within the body, more information is gathered about the condition of internal organs and other tissues. Sensory information floods the neural net and allows the being to interact with itself and its environment.

Subjectively, we believe that we live in the immediate present. When discussing skill acquisition, however, Gentile[18] points out that we actually live in the immediate past as a result of neural transmission time delays. Lagging behind the real world by less than 1 second does not, at first thought, appear to be a big problem. It can be important, however, when one is interacting with a complex environment, such as driving a car in traffic. The ability to predict the environment based on sensory information helps avoid future injury.

Specialized receptor cells transmit streams of data about internal and environmental conditions via afferent nerves into the neural net. Afferent nerves have been discovered in muscle, tendon, ligaments, and joint capsules.[19–21] Although an in-depth discussion of the sensory system is not within the scope of this book, a brief review of the joint receptors is provided in Table 5–8.

The exact mechanism of function of these receptors is not completely known, despite much

Table 5–7 Common Balance Problems in Patients with Musculoskeletal Dysfunction

Ankle Problems

History

Chronic sprains

Subtalar pronation

Weakness of peroneus longus

Posture

Pronated feet associated with valgus and hyperextension at the knee

Internal rotation of hip

Balance

Sensory

Decreased static and dynamic proprioception

Static

Increased sway with eyes closed

Difficulty balancing on one leg

Perturbed balance

Sway increased on unstable surfaces, eyes closed

Inability to balance on unstable surface, eyes closed, head turning

Inability to stand 10 seconds on toes, eyes closed

Postural reactions

Good

Postural strategies

Moves to early hip strategy with unstable support

Shoulder Impingement Syndrome

History

Usually more than one episode

Has pain when reaching behind or out to side; hard to get on coat

Slow onset, but really noticed after activity such as polishing car

Painful arc

Has a desk job

Posture

Side view, head and shoulders forward

Increased lumbar lordosis and flat thoracic spine

Balance

Static

Easily perturbed

Center of balance posterior

Response to perturbations

Increased sway with unstable surface

Postural reactions

Good

Postural strategies

Uses hip strategy or steps easily

Does not stabilize trunk

Behavioral characteristics

Feels odd to be upright and aligned

Has difficulty recognizing that head is forward

Table 5–7 Common Balance Problems in Patients with Musculoskeletal Dysfunction (continued)

Chronic, Degenerative Low Back Pain

History

    Back pain for years; may have old disk injury

    Usually decreased ROM

    May or may not have radicular signs/symptoms

Posture

    Variable; usually some asymmetry in medial/lateral or anteroposterior alignment

    Military type posture or sway back not uncommon

Balance

    Static

        Center of balance backward but still in the middle in the frontal plane

        Similar to normals in stable conditions, eyes open and closed

        Some difficulty with one-footed balance on painful side, eyes open

    Response to perturbations

        Increased sway with unstable support surface

        When successfully maintains balance after perturbed by the support surface, brings center of balance forward

        Inability to stand on one leg, eyes closed (10 seconds)

    Postural reactions

        Good except poor trunk rotation with righting on one leg

    Postural strategies

        Hip strategy appears to be the basic strategy rather than ankle, particularly in mildly unstable situations

    Behavioral issues

        Feels odd when aligned properly; cannot find own neutral

Idiopathic Scoliosis

History

    May have history of motion sickness, seasickness

    May have secondary instability of the ankle (pronated feet)

    Scoliosis usually progressing or greater than 20°

Posture

    Lateral deviation of the spine with rotation; right thoracic curve most common

Balance

    Static

        Normal standing balance when stable support surface, eyes open or closed

        Center of balance often posterior and to side of concavity curve

    Response to perturbation

        Increased body sway with unstable support surface, especially tandem feet

        Inability to maintain balance when vestibulospinal pathways challenged with head turning (unstable support surface, eyes closed, head turning)

        Difficulty with one-legged balance, either leg, eyes closed

    Postural reactions

        Slow to respond to protect; may indicate does not know which way falling

        Mixed results regarding proprioception: increased sensitivity to vibration or decreased joint position sense

    Strategy

        May move earlier into a hip strategy when perturbation still mild, especially with medial/lateral perturbation

Source: Reprinted from *Orthopaedic Physical Therapy Clinics of North America,* Vol. 1, No. 2, pp. 228–229, with permission of W.B. Saunders Company, © 1992.

Table 5–8 Basic Joint Receptors

Receptor Type	Receptor Location	Detects
Free nerve endings	Joint surfaces Joint capsules	Joint pain
Golgi type	Ligaments about the joint capsules	Change of joint rotation Rate of movement Static joint position
Pacinian	Near tendons and joints	Vibration Pressure Rate of joint movement
Ruffini's endings	Joint capsules	Fast change of direction Joint position Intraarticular pressure change

Source: Data from *Textbook of Medical Physiology,* Fifth Edition by A.C. Guyton, pp. 649–652, W.B. Saunders Company, © 1976; *Scientific Bases of Human Movement,* Third Edition by B.A. Gowitzke and M. Milner, pp. 282–286, Williams & Wilkins, © 1988.

study. As part of the peripheral neural net, the input from these receptors, along with the muscle and cutaneous receptors, helps the being modulate its activity while interacting with the environment. In addition, the proprioceptors probably play an adaptive role, updating motor patterns so that movements can be corrected afterward, making the next attempt better.[6] Injury to the musculoskeletal system can cause delays in the afferent transmissions of these proprioceptors. This can cause difficulties in kinesthetic awareness and balance[22] and can cause further injury.

The special senses' importance in movement should not be overlooked. The influence of vision on movement has been studied extensively and found to be extremely important. Vision helps shape ongoing movement in an ever-changing environment.[7] Together with the otoliths, vision helps maintain postural orientation and the perception of uprightedness.[16]

ENVIRONMENTAL CONSTRAINTS

Environmental obstacles often prevent desired actions from occurring. A small river stops an otherwise fully abled person from crossing to the other side, especially if that person cannot swim or does not wish to get wet. A mountain stops all but the rock climbers. No one can jump across the Grand Canyon.

The person unable to cross the river does not necessarily have a physical impairment that is preventing the task from being completed. The river itself may simply be too wide to swim across for the average abilities of the human being. In other words, most humans are not made to swim across a mile-wide river (it could be similarly argued that humans are not made to sit in chairs in front of computer terminals for 8 hours a day). If the desire or behavioral goal is great enough, human ingenuity can devise ways to alter the environment to allow the task to be accomplished. To cross the hypothetical river, a bridge or a boat can be built. The therapist must evaluate the environmental context in which the patient operates to determine whether the environment can be altered to fit the needs of the patient.

Static Environment

A static environment is one that is stationary or nonmoving. Examples of a static environment are a flight of stairs, an empty hallway, and a quiet therapy gym. It is relatively easy for humans to scan a static environment and interact within it. The more consistent the environment (chairs of the same height, level floors, etc.), the easier it is to plan movements. Variability in the environment (grassy slopes, cluttered rooms, etc.) makes it harder to motor plan.

Occupational therapists and physical therapists have always performed home visits to evaluate the static environment of the patient's residence. After observing the patient behave within his or her own home, the clinician completes an assessment of the physical layout (Exhibit 5–1) and recommends needed structural changes. The most common recommendations usually decrease the amount of variability in the environment and can include removing scatter rugs, eliminating unnecessary clutter, and securing electrical cords.

Exhibit 5–1 Home Visit Check-List

Therapist: _____

Date: _____

Name: _____

Address: _____

Diagnosis and disability: _____

Number of persons living with patient: _____ Adult: _____ Children: _____

I. Arrival:

  A. Car transfer: _____

  B. Pathway: Length: _____ Surface: _____

  C. *Entrance to home:*

    1. number of stairs: _____ 2. height of stairs_____

    3. is there a handrail: _____ left _____ right _____ (facing house)

    4. doorway width: _____

    5. are there other entrances that might be used: _____

      describe: _____

    6. is construction of a ramp feasible: _____

    7. *Additional Comments:*

II. Interior:

  A. *First floor*—number of rooms: _____

  B. *Bedrooms:*

    1. location _____

    2. width of doorway: _____ 3. is there a doorsill:_____

    4. rug elevation: _____ 5. height of bed: _____

    6. is bed suitable for attachment of: side rails: _____

                          trapeze bar: _____

    7. can furniture be arranged more conveniently: _____

      describe: _____

    8. can patient reach closets: _____ bureaus:_____

    9. is there room for wheelchair to maneuver: _____

    10. is there room for additional furniture: _____ (eg, commode, seat, etc.)

    11. *Additional Comments:*

  C. *Bathroom:*

    1. location _____

    2. width or door: _____ 3. is there a doorsill:_____

    4. type of bathtub—roll rim: _____ square rim: _____ wide square rim: _____

    5. height of tub: _____ 6. height of toilet seat:_____

    7. can wheelchair get close to sink: _____ toilet: _____ bathtub: _____

continues

8. is tub enclosed by—shower curtain: _____ sliding doors: _____

9. is there a separate shower stall: _____

10. is bathroom on same floor as: bedroom: _____ living room: _____ kitchen: _____

11. is it feasible to install handrails on: tub: _____ walls: _____ toilet: _____

12. *Additional Comments:*

D. *Kitchen:*

1. location: _____

2. width of doorways: _____ 3. is there a doorsill:_____

4. is there room for movement of wheelchair: _____

5. are cupboards within reach: _____

6. can patient use kitchen utilities: _____ (range, sink, refrigerator)

7. is rearrangement of furniture feasible: _____

8. *Additional Comments:*

E. *Other Rooms:*

1. width of doors: _____ 2. are there doorsills:_____

3. are light switches in easy reach: _____

4. would furniture arrangement be feasible: _____

5. is telephone conveniently located: _____ type:_____

6. if needed, is there suitable space for parallel bars: _____

F. *Stairways:*

1. Handrail: right: _____ left: _____

2. height of risers: _____ 3. width of steps:_____

4. *Additional Comments:*

G. *Functional Activities of Patient:*

1. can patient enter and leave home independently: _____ if not, what assistance is needed:_____

   _____

2. responsibilities of patient at home: (homemaker, etc.) _____

3. which transfer activities is patient unable to perform independently:

   bed to chair: _____ chair to bed:_____

   toilet: _____ bathtub: _____

   shower: _____ automobile: _____

III. Additional Comments:

Source: University of Connecticut School of Allied Health, Storrs, Connecticut, unpublished course notes.

Another common environmental evaluation performed by therapists and human factor engineers (ergonomists) is an assessment of the workplace. For office workers, the chair and desk (workstation) need to fit the worker. The chair should fit so that proper body alignment of all body segments can be maintained for the desired type of seated position: reclined, upright, or forward. Although many older texts on proper seating recognize only the upright seated position as optimal, the other positions may better fit individual patients' needs and situations (see Chapter 6 for more information about chair design and seating). Other areas to explore include the space (distances between areas), the equipment, the lighting, noise, odors, and the like.[3] Many texts have been written on work-site analysis; these same principles apply to all environmental analyses that the clinician might need to perform.

After assessing the static environment, the therapist needs to determine whether the environment is preventing desired behaviors from occurring. Is a poorly fitting chair the cause of a neck and shoulder problem? Is a toilet height so low that the patient cannot get up from it in a safe, efficient manner? Is the carpeting so shaggy that the patient cannot safely walk on it? In other words, is the river too wide for this particular patient to get across? Is a bridge needed?

Dynamic Environment

A dynamic environment describes the moving world in which we live. The environment can move in a consistent fashion (eg, a conveyor belt, an escalator, etc.) or, more commonly, in a variable fashion (eg, a crowded shopping mall). When a person contacts a dynamic environment, the senses must scan the moving objects and predict their future path while the body moves to avoid contact and achieve its behavioral objective. The motor planning involved is identical for the holiday shopper picking her way through the crowd or a football running back picking his way through potential tacklers.

The dynamic environment can be a frightening place for the injured patient. Unable to use previous movement patterns as a result of physi-

cal impairment, the patient can become paralyzed with fear while attempting to negotiate through dynamic surroundings. Witness the patient who works on gait pattern for an entire therapy session but, upon leaving the clinic, begins limping again. The therapist has to be aware that the patient's home or the clinic is a relatively stationary, safe milieu. For functional rehabilitation, the therapist must shape the environment in a progressively dynamic manner until the patient regains the ability to interact safely and with confidence in the real world.

REFERENCES

1. Jette AM. Functional disability and rehabilitation of the aged. *Top Geriatr Rehabil.* 1986;1:1–7.
2. Rhode Island Health Services Research, Inc. *Profiles from the Health Statistics Center.* RI: Rhode Island Health Services Research; 1977. Series 4(1).
3. Boblitz MH. Transportation evaluation, counseling, and training. In: *Rehabilitation Management of Rheumatic Conditions.* 2nd ed. Baltimore, Md: Williams & Wilkins;1986:206–231.
4. Ellexson MT. Analyzing an industry job analysis for treatment, prevention, and placement. *Orthop Phys Ther Clin.* 1992;1(1):15–21.
5. US Department of Labor, Employment and Training Administration. *Selected Characteristics of Occupations Defined in the Dictionary of Occupational Titles.* Washington, DC: Government Printing Office;1981.
6. US Department of Labor, Employment and Training Administration. *Dictionary of Occupational Titles,* 4th ed. Indianapolis, Ind:J IST Works;1991.
7. Carr JH, Shepherd RB. *Movement Science: Foundations for Physical Therapy in Rehabilitation.* Gaithersburg, Md: Aspen; 1987.
8. Fisher B, Yakura J. Movement analysis: a different perspective. *Orthop Phys Ther Clin.* 1993;2(1):1–24.
9. Klein-Vogelbach S. *Functional Kinetics.* Berlin, Germany: Springer-Verlag; 1990.
10. Sahrmann S. Diagnosis and treatment of muscle imbalances associated with regional pain syndromes. (Course notes, 1990). Presented at the Massachusetts Chapter of the American Physical Therapy Association Annual Meeting, Danvers, Mass; 1992.
11. Daniels L, Worthingham C. *Therapeutic Exercise for Body Alignment and Function,* 2nd ed. Philadelphia, Pa: Saunders;1977.
12. Kendall FP, McCreary EK. *Muscles: Testing and Function,* 3rd ed. Baltimore, Md: Williams & Wilkins;1983.
13. Rothstein J. Muscle biology—clinical considerations. *Phys Ther.* 1982;62:1824–1827.

14. Grossman MR, Sahrmann SA, Rose SJ. Review of length-associated change in muscle—experimental evidence and clinical implications. *Phys Ther.* 1982;62(12): 1799–1807.

15. Ivenson BD, Gossman MR, Shaddeau SA, Turner ME. Balance performance, force production, and activity levels in noninstitutionalized men 60 to 90 years of age. *Phys Ther.* 1990;70(6):348–355.

16. Byl NN. Spatial orientation to gravity and implications for balance training. *Orthop Phys Ther Clin.* 1992;1(2): 207–242.

17. Winter DA, Patia AE, Frank JS, Wait SE. Biomechanical walking pattern changes in the fit and healthy elderly. *Phys Ther.* 1990;70(6):340–347.

18. Gentile AM. Skill acquisition: action, movement, and neuromotor processes. In: Carr JH, Shepherd RB, eds. *Movement Science: Foundations for Physical Therapy in Rehabilitation.* Gaithersburg, Md: Aspen;1987,101–102.

19. Gowitzke BA, Milner M. *Scientific Bases of Human Movement,* 3rd ed. Baltimore, Md: Williams & Wilkins; 1988.

20. Schulz RA, Miller DC, Kerr CS, et al. Mechanoreceptors in human cruciate ligaments. *J Bone Joint Surg Am.* 1984;66:1072–1076.

21. Kennedy JC, Alexander IJ, Hayes KC. Nerve supply of the human knee and its functional importance. *Am J Sports Med.* 1982;10:329–335.

22. Garn SN, Newton RA. Kinesthetic awareness in subjects with multiple ankle sprains. *Phys Ther.* 1988; 68(11):1667–1671.

6

Functional Exercise Progression

After analyzing functional tasks and determining some physical impairments and environmental constraints, the clinician must create an individual rehabilitation program to restore the patient's ability to function. The exercise portion of the program must be specific to correct the physical impairment(s) suspected of blocking the patient's ability to function and at the same time must protect injured structures that are healing. In keeping with Carr and Shepherd's[1] motor learning program, it must be done in conjunction with a functional task. The exercise can even be the actual functional task in a modified form, so that the patient can complete it. Then the patient needs to practice the functional activity, exploring different movement strategies (ie, making mistakes) until the optimal way is discovered or found again. Only when the patient has full confidence in this new found ability will return to activity be efficient and automatic.

ELIMINATING THE BARRIERS TO FUNCTION

Assuming that the patient wishes to be independent in function (behavioral goals), the two major roadblocks (control parameters) mentioned above are physical impairments and envi-

ronmental constraints. The therapist has a choice of improving the patient's physical capabilities or improving the physical surroundings. Usually the therapist does a little of both.

Correcting the Physical Impairments

Chapter 5 describes in detail the observations of patient performance that need to be made to determine which physical impairments require improvements. Many of the categories overlap in real life. Treatments for correcting these areas will be as specific as possible, but they will overlap as well. For the purposes of this book, rehabilitation of physical impairments will center on the following combined areas:

- postural alignment and base of support
- flexibility and mobility
- strength and dynamic stability
- sensory input
- sequence of movement and coordination/motor control

Each of these combination impairment categories influences and is influenced by the others. Attempting to correct one of the five areas may simultaneously correct other areas or cause new problems to emerge. Therefore, the therapist must constantly observe and evaluate the patient's abilities because they will change from treatment to treatment and perhaps from moment to moment.

Postural Alignment and Base of Support

After identifying suspected malalignments or deviations from the standard base of support, the therapist asks the patient to voluntarily correct the faults. The patient usually needs verbal and tactile cues to assist in overcoming a habitually "normal" pose. Therefore, the clinician needs to demonstrate the corrections by mimicking the patient's posture and then showing the more optimal alignment. With access to video equipment, the therapist can also point out to the patient the exact problematic alignments. With the help of a full-length mirror, the patient begins attempting to correct the problem. At first the patient may complain that this new alignment feels awkward or of feeling as if he or she is leaning forward or backward. The therapist assures the patient that this is a normal reaction to the correction but encourages the patient to maintain the correction for as long as possible. Although the patient will revert to the habitual pose, he or she is instructed to become more aware of the abnormalities and to correct them when able throughout the day. Soon the more optimal alignment will feel better, and the habitual pose will begin to feel awkward.

Figure 6–1 illustrates a common deviation from optimal two-legged standing. The patient unconsciously assumes a pose of overweighting the right lower extremity while externally rotating the left hip. In effect, the patient has increased the base of support through the increased space occupied by the left foot. This posture is often seen in people who studied ballet in their youth or in someone with a painful left lower extremity. Often one-legged balance is a major issue with this patient and needs to be addressed. When this patient attempts to stand on one leg (Figure 6–2), pelvic or hip rotation or trunk lean may occur to compensate for the lack of muscular strength needed to stabilize the leg and pelvis body segments.

The postural correction exercise is simply to attempt optimal alignment while balancing on the left foot. The patient begins to balance on one leg while using a mirror for visual feedback and, if needed, a surface to touch, such as a table or wall. The exercise progresses by first removing the additional support of the upper extremities for balance. Then the patient tries to stand in optimal alignment for increasing amounts of time, up to 1 minute for adults. The last part of the exercise involves removing the mirror for visual feedback while the patient maintains the posture through proprioceptive input.

If voluntary intervention is insufficient to correct the malalignment, the therapist can work the soft tissues (muscle, capsule, fascia, etc.) to stretch out shortened structures while strengthening any weakened muscles that may be contributing to the inability to hold a more optimal posture. The patient is not allowed to sacrifice one body segment for another (unless compensation is the only way remaining to return the patient to function).

Flexibility and Mobility

After any injury to the musculoskeletal system, problems with flexibility and range of motion (ROM) commonly occur. Loss of motion also accompanies movement disorders and hypokinetics or decreased activity (eg, couch potato syndrome).

Internal restrictions of joint mobility can include muscle shortening, insufficient muscle strength, and tightening of the connective tissue (joint capsule and fascia). Appropriate modalities, such as hydrocollator packs and ultrasound, help prepare the soft tissues for manual work. Passive stretch, massage, and hold-relax techniques work well on shortened muscles. Joint mobilization (gentle passive oscillations or stretch to the joint capsule) and myofascial release (slow stretch to the myofascia) can be effective in improving connective tissue mobility, although controversy still exists as to the efficacy of both manual treatments.[2] For more detailed information about these techniques, the reader is referred to the manuals listed at the end of this chapter.

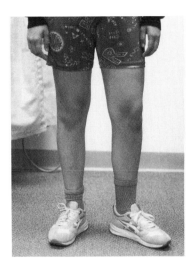

Figure 6–1   Faulty habitual two-legged posture. Note excessive weight bearing on the right lower extremity and excessive hip external rotation of the left lower extremity. The toed-out posture of the left foot increases the base of support. This posture is commonly seen in dancers and persons with painful left lower extremities. Over time this posture can cause shortening of the left hip external rotators, with abnormal forces crossing the anterior hip joint and the patellofemoral joint.

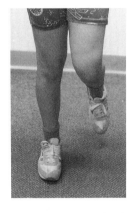

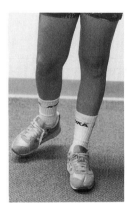

A   **B**

Figure 6–2   One-legged standing accentuating the faulty posture. Normally, the positive Trendelenburg action of the gluteus medius maintains pelvic alignment while the hip lines up with the knee over the smaller base of support. (**A**) When the patient with faulty alignment tries to stand on the right foot, excessive hip internal rotation becomes evident. (**B**) When she attempts to stand on the left foot, the shortened external rotators pull the pelvis into rotation. By looking into a mirror, the patient attempts to correct the malalignments for increasing amounts of time up to 1 minute.

In whatever manner ROM is achieved, the patient must begin using the new motion immediately through active exercise or functional activity. Although the patient will appear weak in the new ROM, working into end range ensures that less of a rebound effect will occur. Often the patient reports pain when performing eccentric work in the new range at the glenohumeral joint and hesitates to exercise. This is probably due to the inability of the rotator cuff to stabilize the humeral head in the glenoid in this increased range.[3] The therapist must encourage the patient to power the limb, as if pushing against a great resistance, through the end of range and back again. By cocontracting the agonist and antagonist, the pinching sensation does not materialize. Within about 10 repetitions, the patient attempts again to concentrically and eccentrically control the limb (without benefit of cocontraction). If pain free, the patient continues actively using the limb in the greater range. If the pain persists, the patient may need specific exercises to increase humeral head stability (see below).

Sometimes it is necessary to restore flexibility without the benefit of modalities or manual techniques. The therapist may not wish to introduce a machine upon which a patient may become dependent. Alternatively, the therapist may want the patient to take greater responsibility for getting better and not rely on therapy for the cure. In any event, the patient can be taught to increase ROM through self-stretching as well as through strengthening of the antagonist.

Strength and Dynamic Stability

Strengthening programs generally pose no problems for experienced physical therapists and occupational therapists. Although improved strength can increase the likelihood of functional gains, strength is but one component needed for independent function.[4] Many research articles have been written on the various types of strength training and have compared differing protocols. It is beyond the scope of this book to cover in any detail what has already been written, and the reader is referred to some of the exercise texts and articles listed at the chapter's end for more information. With all the controversy abounding as to the best exercise to teach, however, a brief review of the different exercise types and their application to functional restoration is provided.

For the exercise to be functional, it must be specific to the patient's needs. No strengthening exercise program in and of itself is wrong or outdated, but any exercise can be wrong for a given patient. Understanding the benefits of closed-chain exercising does not necessitate abandoning all open-chain work. It is the therapist's job to create a varied exercise program that the patient finds challenging and fun but *do*able. The only wrong exercise is one that fails to protect an injured part or one that the patient finds boring.

Active and resistive exercise provides the mainstay of the strengthening program. Resistance can be provided by free weights, elastic tubing, water paddles, or machinery (eg, Nautilus equipment, stationary bike, Stairclimber, Cybex, etc.) or by using the patient's own body weight. Depending on the patient's injuries and abilities, the exercise can be isometric, isotonic, isokinetic, or any combination of the three.

Isotonic strengthening exercises include two phases: concentric (muscle shortening) contractions and eccentric (muscle lengthening) contractions.[5] Both types of contractions are needed for most functional activities, depending on the circumstances. Concentric strength is required for lifting grocery bags out of a car, climbing up a hill, getting out of bed, etc. Eccentric strength is needed for descending stairs, restraining a child from running into the street, decelerating the shoulder during ball throwing, and so forth.

Strengthening exercise can also be classified as open chain or closed chain. This terminology refers to the concept of Steindler[6] that people are made up of segmental links in a kinetic chain. Whenever the most distal link is bearing weight, such as the foot during the stance phase or the hands during a push-up, the kinetic chain is considered closed. Whenever the most distal link is free and not bearing weight, such as the foot during the swing phase or the hand when throwing a ball, the kinetic chain is considered open (Figure 6–3). The muscle groups fire in different patterns to move the body and limbs, depending on whether the chain is open or closed. Functionally, people use both types of activities with great frequency, so that both types of exercise should be performed.

Plyometrics, or stretch-strengthening, tries to use the myotatic stretch reflex to produce a more powerful contraction. It consists of an eccentric contraction to decelerate a movement followed quickly by a concentric contraction. This occurs naturally in many high-skill activities, such as sprinting. According to Voight, "the goal of plyometric training is to decrease the time required between the yielding eccentric muscle contraction and the initiation of the overcoming concentric contraction, thereby allowing the muscle to produce maximum strength in the

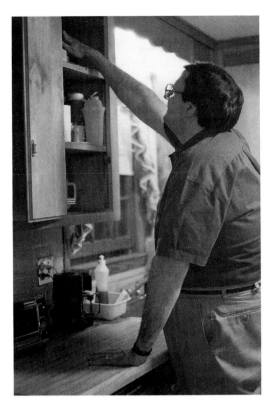

Figure 6–3 Examples of open-chain and closed-chain elbow extension. A man reaches for a serving plate in a high cupboard, which requires that he extend his right elbow while his hand is not bearing weight (open chain). For added reach and support, he pushes down on the counter with his left hand by extending his elbow (closed chain).

shortest possible time."[7(p 244)] Although used primarily in sports training, which requires both strength and speed, low-level plyometrics should be used for strengthening all patients for everyday activities (Figure 6–4). The accelerations and decelerations needed for daily living are commonplace. Failure to retrain this ability is one of the reasons why some patients never return to their prior level of function. Contrast the carefree manner in which an uninjured person bounds down a flight of stairs with the painstakingly slow and laborious style of someone with a sprained ankle. Life is full of starts and stops, and the ability to maneuver quickly is essential for someone trying to walk along a crowded sidewalk or quickly cross a street to avoid being hit by a car.

When determining the progression of a strengthening program, the therapist must balance intensity with safety. In general, an exercise is contraindicated if it causes an increase in the patient's symptoms (eg, pain or swelling) or if abnormal movement patterns emerge. The therapist can adjust the following variables to change the intensity or purpose of the exercise:

- resistance
- speed
- distance/direction
- number of repetitions
- number of sets

Although strength gains are related to functional improvements, it is not known exactly how much strength is needed to perform functional activities. Some therapists argue that the strength required to move the body or its limbs is not quite as important as the strength needed to stabilize the body or limbs. Bernstein[8] wrote that the body has difficulty managing the multiple links (degrees of freedom) that compose it. The key to coordinated movement is control or stabilization of the excessive motion available to the body. Many others agree.[9–13] The success of the patellofemoral and lumbar stabilization programs lies in increasing the strength of the body's stabilizing musculature to curtail harmful, excessive motion (see Chapter 9). The stabilizers are initially trained through submaximal isometric contractions. Small-range isotonic exercises are then superimposed on the system. As the patient gains the ability to stabilize the joint in question, the isotonic range progresses to full, and resistance can be added. Table 6–1 shows a dynamic stabilization protocol for diminished rotator cuff control of the humeral head. This program could be implemented for the person who has shoulder pain on eccentric lowering of the arm.

Sensory Input

As mentioned previously, the sensory system is an integral part of the neural net controlling movement patterns. The type and quality of movement patterns available to a person are dependent in part on the information provided

A   **B**

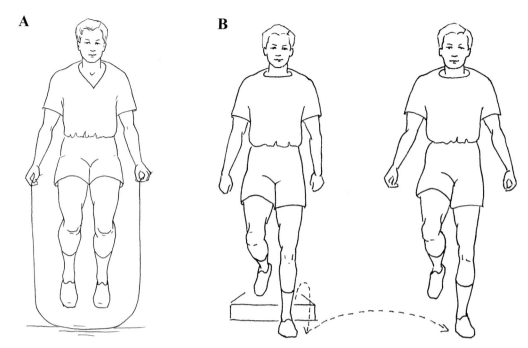

Figure 6–4 Examples of plyometric training. (**A**) Low level. Bilateral slight vertical leaps (**B**) High level. One-legged box jumping with side cut.

Table 6–1 Humeral Head Stabilizing Exercises

Submaximal Isometrics
    Abduction at 30° and 60°
    Surpraspinatus at 30° and 60° (empty can position or scaption)
    ER at 0° shoulder abduction
    IR at 0° shoulder abduction
    Biceps isometrics

Short Arc Isotonics
    Abduction: from 30°–90° of motion
    Supraspinatus: from 30°–90° of motion
    Flexion: from 30°–90° of motion
    ER at 30° (shoulder abduction) with towel roll with tubing
    IR at 30° (shoulder abduction) with towel roll with tubing
    Biceps isotonics tubing at 35°–40° flexion (shoulder)
    D_2 flexion RS at 30°, 60°, 90°, and 120°

Rotator Cuff Dynamic Stabilizing Sets*
    Arm elevation from 0°–60° isometric hold 2 seconds (2 points in range)
    Arm elevation from 60°–120° isometric hold 2 seconds (2 points in range)
    Supraspinatus from 0°–60° isometric hold 2 seconds (2 points in range)
    Supraspinatus from 0°–90° isometric hold 2 seconds (2 points in range)
    D_2 flex UE, RS, and SRH at 0°, 60°, 120°, and 160°
    Tubing D_2 flex with isometric holds

Abbreviations: ER, external rotation; IR, internal rotation; D_2, proprioceptive neuromuscular facilitation pattern for upper extremity (UE); RS, rhythmic stabilization; SRH, slow reversal hold.
*Begin with no weight program to 1 lb, then gradually increase.
Source: Reprinted from *Orthopaedic Physical Therapy Clinics of North America,* Vol. 1, No. 2, p. 344, with permission of W.B. Saunders Company, © 1992.

about the being itself as well as about the world outside. Enhancing sensory input can increase the person's awareness of the self in relation to the environment. Too much input can create an information overload, however, causing uncoordinated movements to occur. The key to restoring function is for the therapist to provide the minimal amount of cues that allows the patient to successfully complete an activity.

The special senses, especially vision and touch, assist in regulating movements. A baseball outfielder backpeddles or in some other way alters course to catch a fly ball while tracking its trajectory. The ability to feel at the soles of the feet provides a person with needed information to maintain balance. The therapist can use the patient's senses to augment the functional program. Focusing attention on a particular sense causes immediate results. Therefore, using a mirror (vision) helps a patient better understand and correct body alignment. Keeping a night light on prevents some elderly persons from falling. Improving tactile input at the feet by changing the shoe shank to a more flexible type allows a person with peripheral neuropathy to feel the floor better and remain upright. Using surface electromyography (EMG) over selected muscle groups assists the person by visually providing feedback in feeling a desired contraction or in quieting an unwanted contraction.

In addition, the importance of the special senses in scanning the real world for dangers (smelling smoke, tasting spoiled food, hearing a fire alarm, etc.) is often forgotten in the environmentally controlled world of rehabilitation. The clinician must impress upon the patient the importance of wearing prescription glasses while performing activities of daily living (ADLs), especially at night when going to the bathroom. Hearing aids are equally valuable in evaluating the environment for approaching people, animals, cars, and so forth. More information about tips for making persons with visual and auditory impairments safer can be obtained from the following organizations:

American Foundation for the Blind
15 West 16th Street
New York, NY 10011
(212) 620-2000

National Association of the Deaf
814 Thayer Avenue
Silver Spring, MD 20910
(301) 587-1788

The body's ability to tune into itself, providing sensory information about internal conditions, is called proprioception. The mechanoreceptors and nociceptors within the musculoskeletal system (see Table 5–8) monitor joint alignment, the rate of joint movement, deep pressure at joint surfaces, muscle tension, and even intraarticular pressure. This information flows into the neural net and helps shape movement patterns.

Because proprioception is not perceived completely on the conscious level, it has been difficult to measure. Other systems tend to reflect proprioceptive input. For example, the reflex inhibition commonly seen at the quadriceps femoris may be caused by the detection of increased intraarticular pressure (swelling) in the knee by the Ruffini receptors.[14] The therapist will perhaps observe quadriceps atrophy or loss of medial glide of the patella. The patient may only be aware of knee pain or a vague feeling of instability. Another example is the patient who is unaware of the posture of excessive external hip rotation. Both patients require input from the visual sense to augment diminished proprioceptive input. The actual act of performing one-legged balance in front of a mirror to correct alignment simultaneously retrains the proprioceptors.

Proprioceptive retraining involves joint movements (preferably performed actively) that change speed and direction and are done in both weight-bearing and non–weight-bearing postures. This activates the different mechanoreceptors discussed in Chapter 5 and summarized in Table 5–8. Tactile input can increase the patient's ability to sense internal conditions. Placing cuff weights on a patient's ankles and wrists or even weighting an assistive ambulation device provides additional feedback that allows for increased motor control. There is even evidence to support the hypothesis that Neoprene sleeves, athletic tape, and even McConnell tape at a joint provide minimal physical support but great proprioceptive input.[15] The patient can indirectly monitor whether proprioception is being improved by visually assessing postural corrections, watching greater EMG output displays, or feeling less pain.

The proprioceptors of any joint that has undergone direct or indirect trauma should be retrained on the assumption (which is difficult to prove but is seen often clinically) that the afferent input has been altered in some way. Examples of different types of proprioceptive activities for both upper and lower extremities are provided in Table 6–2.

Sequence of Movement and Coordination/ Motor Control

Oftentimes the therapist will observe a problem with the quality of the patient's movement, which can appear jerky or painful. Although there may be an underlying reason for such a movement pattern to emerge, the therapist cannot change it (eg, meniscectomy) or perhaps cannot find it as yet. By altering some of the movement characteristics, a more coordinated movement pattern may develop. The therapist can change:

- the speed of movement

- the joint ROM

- the initial postural alignment

- the sequence of muscle activation

Increasing the speed of an activity often requires less precise control and can be easier to perform (but too much speed can literally get out of control, causing more damage). To protect the integrity of the joints, the patient should exercise in midrange, avoiding the ends of available motion. Alignment differences and sequence of muscle activation differences may enable a smoother motion to emerge in either open-chain or closed-chain exercise (circumstances will dictate which exercise is preferred for each patient).

For example, a patient with a tibial plateau fracture comes to therapy 6 weeks after the injury. After working on the most obvious physical impairments first, such as loss of motion, weakness, and swelling, the therapist notes a loss of overall quality of motor control (this may be a vague impression that the person simply does not appear to be moving normally). When the therapist places the patient prone and requests knee flexion, the patient responds with a slow, laborious effort. The patient's cautious compliance is a protective reaction to an anticipated pain that may or may not come. The therapist acknowledges the patient's apprehension and places a towel under the thigh just above the patella to prevent patella compression and a pillow under the lower leg and ankle to prevent full knee extension. The therapist again asks the patient to flex the knee in a pain-free range. When the patient realizes that the motion is possible without pain, the speed of the exercise is increased with emphasis on quickness of reversal

Table 6–2 Examples of Proprioception Exercises (Exercises Progress from Bilateral to Unilateral)

Training Level	Lower Extremities	Upper Extremities
Basic	Rocking chair with feet on floor Sitting with feet on wobble board Ambulation with cuff weights	Rhythmic stabilization in quadruped position or sitting with hands on a table Isometrics in different positions
Intermediate	Supported standing on a wobble board Ambulation on even surfaces Ambulation in different directions	Rocking in quadruped position Wall or table push-ups Table wobble board
Advanced	Unsupported standing on wobble board Plyometrics (leaps, hops, Fitter*, etc.) Beginning sport skills	Floor push-ups Plyometrics (plyoball, Fitter*, etc.) Beginning sport skills

*See Chapter 14, Functional Exercise Equipment, for more information concerning Fitters.

of motion from flexion to extension and vice versa. Through this type of motion retraining, the therapist may note increased knee ROM and a more pain-free gait (even though those areas were not specifically addressed through passive stretching or gait training). The change in motor control has influenced other impairments in a positive manner.

Sometimes pain-free motion does not occur because a muscle or muscle group is recruited at the wrong time. This can result from the dominance of a secondary mover (gastrocnemius) over the primary mover (hamstrings) or an imbalance within the same muscle group (eg, medial versus lateral hamstrings).[9] If the sequence of muscle activation is altered, normal motion returns. The therapist can restore muscle balance through verbal cueing or with the help of surface EMG to augment proprioceptive input.

Protecting Injured Structures

The clinician designs the rehabilitation program to correct physical impairments while protecting injured structures while they heal. If no force is placed upon an injured site, it weakens. If too much force acts on an injured area, it breaks down further. The therapist must act in partnership with the patient to create an exercise program that is just right. Common injuries requiring protection include:

- bone fracture
- total joint arthoplasty
- muscle strain or tear
- ligament sprain or rupture
- capsule or labrum tear
- meniscal tear
- anterior cruciate ligament reconstructions
- any wound or surgery

Protection may include limited weight bearing, submaximal exercise, avoidance of end ROM, and the like. Protecting one area may stress another area more. Limiting the weight bearing at the right ankle by use of crutches increases the weight bearing of the other three

limbs. Other body systems may also require protection. Patients with history of cardiovascular disease, balance disorders, Alzheimer's disease, or Parkinson's disease require special modifications to the functional rehabilitation program to reduce the risk of further injury.

Improving the Environment

A patient may lose the ability to function when a musculoskeletal injury combines with a hostile environment. The static environment may pose an insurmountable physical barrier, such as a mountain, or may be too dynamically complex, such as a crowded airport terminal, for the patient to interact with it safely.

The Static Environment

Not all barriers to normal function reside within the patient. Many result from natural or artificial environmental designs. Temporary or permanent alterations of the surroundings can help a patient function independently. The physical characteristics of the environment can be changed to accommodate many of the patient's current limitations. The growing field of ergonomics has much to offer in making the environment fit people rather than forcing people to fit the environment.

Chairs, including desk chairs, wheelchairs, lounge chairs, dining room chairs, and so forth, can be adjusted for improved body alignment and ease of use. A person should be able to sit with the feet flat on the floor or on foot rests and with the thighs and back supported comfortably. An adjustable seat tilt is recommended to allow the preferred seat position of reclined, upright, or forward.[16] Figure 6–5 illustrates an adjustable chair design for office work.

In addition to postural support, adding or changing the chair's dimensions alters the biomechanical forces necessary for ADLs. A chair with arm rests and/or a raised seat height requires less force production across the lower extremity joints and is therefore easier for a patient to get in and out of. Patients with weight-bearing restrictions at the hip should therefore have raised toilet seats to prevent excessive

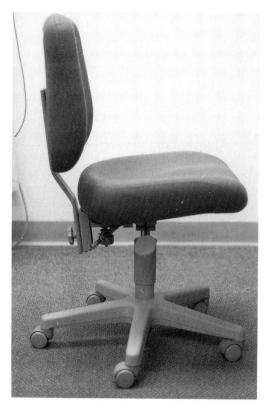

Figure 6–5 Adjustable chair design for office work. The worker should be able to adjust the seat height, tilt, or slope as well as the back rest height and angle to the seat. Care should be taken to ensure that the seat possesses sufficient depth and width for the worker. The need for arm rests, a swivel chair, and casters also should be assessed.[16]

force production at the joint (in addition, patients with total hip arthoplasties may need the additional seat height to prevent the artificial joints from dislocating).

Many other aspects of the environment may need to be evaluated for their postural and biomechanical effects on function. For some patients, an inch height difference in a stair or curb may spell disaster. Using a foam doughnut to relieve pressure on a metatarsal head can alleviate pain and cause independent ambulation to return. Other areas to look at include the following:

- doors (heaviness, type of door knob, etc.)
- walking surface (uneven, slippery, carpeted, grassy, etc.)

- stairs (riser height, railings, carpeted, etc.)
- bathtubs (shower doors, grab bars, bath mats, etc.)
- footwear (flexible shank, heel height, materials, etc.)
- kitchens (cupboard heights, refrigerator/ freezer set-up, stove controls, etc.)
- laundry (top loading, location of controls, types of laundry baskets, etc.)
- living area (chair types, clutter, remote controls, etc.)
- transportation (automatic transmission, seat adjustments, etc.)

This list could go on and on and on. In addition to the home area, patients need evaluations of the many environments in which they interact, such as work, recreational, social, and sports environments. Each environment can be altered to benefit the patient temporarily during healing and rehabilitation or as a compensation for a permanent disability (see Chapter 15 for more information about adaptive equipment).

The static environment can also be altered to challenge the patient instead of to protect the patient. Therapists are perhaps guilty of overprotecting their charges. Therapy gyms are often wide open areas of perfectly carpeted space for ambulation activities. Stairs have rough treads in contrast colors with railings on both sides. Often clinicians will clear away obstacles in the patient's path or will open doors for the patient. Although courteous and safe, these actions do not force the patient to create solutions for environmental problems that occur in everyday living. Navigating through and around static objects should begin with the first treatment session. As the patient's abilities improve, the therapist must introduce progressively more clutter into the usually perfect therapeutic environment.

The Dynamic Environment

Oftentimes the environment is not static but a moving blur of people and machinery. Examples of interacting with a dynamic environment include walking on the deck of a ship, running a track race, or holding a squirming toddler. Interacting with a dynamic environment places higher demands on the neural net. To step safely onto an escalator, a person must visually track the moving stairs, predict their path, and move accordingly to step on one without falling. In other words, the person must now time his or her movements to match the environment. Obviously, a dynamic environment is more complex and difficult to move about in safely because of the temporal constraints placed on the person. It is no longer good enough to be able to walk from point A to point B; one now has to be able to walk fast enough to avoid being hit by an oncoming car.

Clinically many patients have difficulties interacting within a complex environment. Anyone with a vision problem will find it hard to scan the moving objects. Other people may not be able to move quickly enough without loss of balance. Some are overwhelmed by the movement swirling around them and become paralyzed with fear. The therapist must address the issue by creating progressively more complex dynamic problems for the patient to solve. One such example is a therapeutic game called bumper cars (see Exhibit 11–2 in Chapter 11). It simulates the act of walking through a crowded mall or on a sidewalk in a progressively more difficult fashion.

Providing a New Environment

What if the world possessed such different physical features and properties that our bodies moved in strange new patterns? It would be like setting foot on another planet. The now familiar bounding gait of the astronauts on the moon emerged as a more efficient gait pattern than Earth-normal ambulation. With the loss of any meaningful gravitational pull at all, astronauts in orbiting shuttles devise new ways of transporting themselves throughout the spacecraft and performing the ADLs of eating, grooming, and toileting (sometimes these alterations from Earth normal require adaptive equipment). Although the astronauts and their movement abilities do not change after blasting into space, the

environment they occupy differs so drastically from conditions on Earth that new movement strategies are required to function.

A similar world can be found on Earth. The aquatic environment offers to therapists and patients alike a new environment with wonderfully different properties for recreational or rehabilitational purposes. Because of the different characteristics of water, patients find that some movements that are impossible to accomplish on dry land can be performed easily in water. The converse is true as well. Although aquatic therapy has been around for thousands of years, its benefits have recently been rediscovered and refined by clinicians. Many books and articles have been written on aquatic rehabilitation, and the reader is referred to them for more information. Presented here is a brief review of the unique properties of this environment and its implications in functional rehabilitation.

Hydrostatic Pressure

Water molecules apply a force or pressure on the surface of an object immersed in water. The pressure is applied equally in all directions but changes depending on the depth of the object (Pascal's law). When exercises are performed underwater, this pressure may be used to control or reduce swelling.[17] Caution should be observed in the patient with cardiopulmonary dysfunction, however, because hydrostatic pressure also resists chest expansion.[18]

Buoyancy

Buoyancy results from the differences in hydrostatic pressure at different depths causing an upward thrust. This thrust is equal to the weight of the water displaced (Archimedes' principle of buoyancy) and acts in the opposite direction of the force of gravity. The therapist can use buoyancy to unload the joints. There is approximately a 90% apparent weight loss in shoulder-depth water.[19] In addition, buoyancy (like its counterpart gravity) can be used to progress an exercise program. Buoyancy increases as a limb nears the surface or as the limb is lengthened (by lengthening the lever arm, the moment of buoyancy increases). Therefore, an arm moving into abduction will be assisted by buoyancy, especially as it nears the surface. Flexing the elbow, or shortening the lever arm, will diminish the buoyant effect (Figure 6–6). Adding floats at the wrists increases the effect of buoyancy by moving the center of buoyancy of the limb distally.[17] Buoyancy-resisted exercises are movements that directly oppose the upward thrust of buoyancy and are similar to isokinetic exercise.[20] Exercises that move toward the bottom of the water, such as shoulder adduction or leg squats, must overcome the force of buoyancy through muscular action.

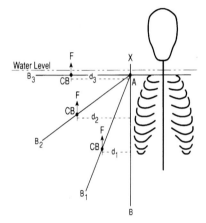

Effect of buoyancy increasing on abduction.

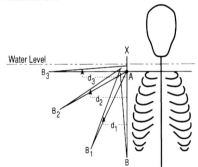

A weaker effect due to bending the elbow.

Figure 6–6 Turning effect of buoyancy. A lever (A–B) is submerged in water. *F,* force of buoyance; *d,* distance from vertical; *x,* point about which the turning effect is exerted. *Source:* Reprinted from *Sports Medicine Update,* Vol. 7, No. 2, p. 6, with permission of HEALTHSOUTH Rehabilitation Corporation, © 1992.

Viscosity

Viscosity is the resistance of fluid flow.[18] It is the friction that occurs between individual molecules as they attempt to move by each other.[20] Because water has greater viscosity than air, there is more resistance when one is moving through water than through air. As a body moves through water, the pressure is increased in front of the body and decreased behind it. Water rushes to the area of reduced pressure, causing turbulence or eddies that tend to drag the body backward. The faster the movement, the greater the turbulence and the larger the drag force or resistance to movement.[17] The shape of an object also affects turbulence, with streamlined shapes causing less eddies. Exercises and equipment can therefore be designed to create more or less turbulence, making the exercise harder or easier to perform in water.[20]

It is interesting to note that air also possesses the property of viscosity. The new exercise of chuting, or running while wearing a parachute, utilizes the same principles discussed above. The increased drag of the parachute causes greater resistance to running.

Aquatic Functional Program

The rehabilitation specialist can use the water environment to make the performance of functional activities easier, more challenging, or simply different for the patient. The buoyant properties of water can compensate for many physical limitations, such as weakness or limited weight bearing, that interfere with the patient's ability to function on dry land. Activities such as sit-to-stand transfers, squats, lifting, and slow walking are generally easier to do in water. If the depth of the water is lowered, the activities become progressively harder to perform. The water can also be used to make activities more difficult. Walking briskly through waist-high water eliminates 50% of the weight-bearing forces, but requires greater muscular force production to overcome the increased turbulence (resistance).

Many pieces of rehabilitation equipment have been developed for aquatic therapy, from webbed gloves and kickboards to underwater treadmills and stairclimbers (see Chapter 14 for more information about aquatic equipment). Pushing a kickboard through the water (Figure 6–7) can prepare a patient for other dry-land pushing activities, such as pushing a grocery cart or pushing open a heavy door. Sports activities, such as swinging a tennis racquet, sprinting, or doing plyometrics, can be done in the pool as well.

Finally, the pool environment can be used to allow new movement patterns to emerge as the patient attempts to solve problems under different circumstances. By interacting in this water world, new ways of moving become available to the patient. Some of these movement solutions may carry over onto dry land.

Water Worries

Although exercising in water benefits many patients, there are some inherent dangers to this otherwise fun and exciting treatment medium. Before instituting an aquatic program, the clinician needs to look into the following safety issues:

* the patient's fear of water
* the patient's cardiopulmonary history and status
* life-saving equipment
* water safety certification (including first aid and cardiopulmonary resuscitation)
* water temperature
* infection control

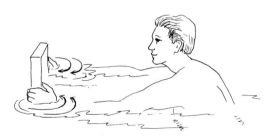

Figure 6–7 Simulating functional activities in the water. Pushing a kickboard through the water forces the patient to overcome the increased turbulence (arrows) and drag. This is similar to the dry-land activity of pushing a grocery cart or pushing open a heavy door.

For more information about these safety issues, the reader is referred to the references listed at the end of this chapter.

MODIFYING THE FUNCTIONAL TASK

Although the rehabilitation specialist must be aware of the patient's physical impairments and constraining elements in the environment, the most important portion of the functional retraining program is to have the patient exercise by performing the actual functional task(s). Obviously if the patient could already perform functional activities in a pain-free manner, he or she would not need therapy. Therefore, the clinician must create an environment in which the disabled patient can attempt to solve functional problems. Based on past motor performance and through trial and error, the patient tries to do various activities. If the therapist is clever enough, the environment can be modified in such a way that the activity can be accomplished with moderate difficulty but independently. Verbal cues should initially be limited to "Try to figure this out for yourself" or "Just try it." As the therapist observes the patient's attempts, a small amount of advice can be offered.

If the patient has access to a pool, the functional activities can be started in the aquatic environment (see above). Many patients can become water free before they can become functionally independent on land. Because pool therapy is frequently unavailable, however, the clinician generally must make do with the real world. This is simpler than one might think. The therapist assesses which tasks pose a problem for the patient through functional activity analysis (Chapter 5) and identifies the problem areas so that the patient can begin working on them. If needed, the rehabilitation specialist provides environmental modifications that increase the available movement patterns for the patient. As the patient becomes proficient at accomplishing the modified task, the therapist changes the task to challenge the patient to solve a progressively more difficult motor problem. Depending on the circumstances, the therapist can devote 2 minutes or the entire treatment session to the functional part of the program (the patient is also exercising in a traditional manner to correct the physical impairments present).

For example, an outpatient complains that he has pain driving his car. This prevents him from socializing and doing errands. After task analysis, the therapist and patient conclude that the really painful part of driving is getting in and out of the car (especially getting out). Low back pain begins when the patient attempts to move the left leg over the door sill onto the street (hip flexion and abduction). At this point the therapist has two choices: to teach the patient a new way to get out of the car, or to help the patient return to his normal way of getting out of the car. Initially the clinician might teach the patient to protect his low back by:

- carefully turning his entire body until it faces the car door
- sliding to the edge of the seat
- using the arms for additional support
- performing a sit-to-stand transfer

Only if the patient's pain is severe enough, however, will he continue to perform this biomechanically safe transfer because it requires so much additional time.

To be able to get out of a car as he did before, the patient must begin practicing the missing functional task in the clinic or at home (see Figure 7–22). The patient first flexes his left hip in increasing increments of range (in either sitting or standing position). Then he attempts hip abduction and external rotation, also in increasing increments of range. Next he combines the two motions as he would in the real task, exploring his body's limitations and figuring out how to get the job done within those limitations. As the movement pattern normalizes the physical limitations begin to change, and as the physical limitations change new movement patterns will emerge. The therapist can alter the criteria for successful task completion by adding barriers of various heights for him to lift his leg over (simulating the door sill of the car). Success is determined by pain-free accomplishment of the task in an efficient manner. (The traditional exercise part of the program might include lower extremity strengthening as well as a lumbar stabilization program.)

RETURN TO FUNCTIONAL ACTIVITY

Training one specific task at a time can be counterproductive because it fails to teach the patient how to solve generalized problems in life. The therapist cannot be with the patient as each new situation arises. The patient needs to learn general motor patterns that can be altered to fit each unique problem. This means that the patient must be allowed to try new movement approaches when alone as well as when in therapy. The patient needs to take some calculated risks, make mistakes, and finally come to an efficient solution to functional problems that occur. The therapist, family, or institution may have a policy preventing the patient from doing these types of things when alone. This is ostensibly to protect the patient from making a movement error that would cause further physical injury. Therein lies the Catch-22: The patient cannot engage the environment risk free to learn how to be independent, and the patient can never learn to be independent without trying alternative movement strategies in different and sometimes unsafe environments.

Nowhere is this absurd scenario more evident than in a rehabilitation hospital. There the patients spend 3 hours a day learning ambulation, transfers, and functional independence only to be confined to wheelchairs to get from therapy to therapy or even to the bathroom. Because of liability issues, many patients must even learn to get washed and dressed from a wheelchair. The few patients who try to be independent are usually admonished by well-meaning staff. Although filling out incident reports in triplicate is not pleasant, the staff (or family) must allow a competent patient the right to make mistakes and perhaps in the process to get better (maybe some sort of release from liability form could be signed by the patient to protect everyone's rights).

Patients who live at home can be encouraged to try out activities and report back to the clinician as to the success or problems of their attempts. The risks and benefits must be explained in detail to them. Depending on the patient's abilities, this can be a short walk or jog around the block or an attempt at rollerblading. It can even be as protected an activity as rising from a chair independently with a sturdy table placed strategically in front of the patient in case of balance loss. Whatever the activity, the more the patient practices it and corrects performance errors, the more the movement will become spontaneous or automatic. Only when a movement is automatic will a patient actually use it in everyday life. The problem with most rehabilitation programs is that the therapist believes that the patient will perform an activity at home if that patient has successfully performed the activity in therapy. Doing an activity once or twice, or even 10 times, is not nearly enough practice to make an activity automatic and safe. Both the patient and the clinician need to understand that therapy is only the beginning. The patient must take the information learned in therapy and tailor it to suit his or her own needs and ways. There are too many patients held prisoner at home because of fear of doing an activity that they supposedly can perform independently.

REFERENCES

1. Carr JH, Shepherd RB. *Movement Science: Foundations for Physical Therapy in Rehabilitation.* Gaithersburg, Md: Aspen; 1987.

2. DiFabio RP. Efficacy of manual therapy. *Phys Ther.* 1992;72(12):853–864.

3. Wilk KE, Arrigo C. An integrated approach to upper extremity exercises. *Orthop Phys Ther Clin.* 1992;1(2):337–360.

4. Judge JO. Resistance training. *Top Geriatr Rehabil.* 1993;8(3):38–50.

5. Albert M. *Eccentric Muscle Training in Sports and Orthopaedics.* New York, NY: Churchill Livingstone; 1991.

6. Steindler A. *Kinesiology of the Human Body under Normal and Pathological Conditions.* Springfield, Ill: Thomas; 1973.

7. Voight ML. Stretch-strengthening: an introduction to plyometrics. *Orthop Phys Ther Clin.* 1992;1(2):243–252.

8. Bernstein NA. *The Coordination and Regulation of Movements.* New York, NY: Pergamon; 1967.

9. Sahrmann S. Diagnosis and treatment of muscle imbalances associated with regional pain syndromes (course notes, 1990. Presented at the Massachusetts Chapter of the American Physical Therapy Association Annual Conference, Danvers, Mass; 1992.

10. Klein-Vogelbach S. *Functional Kinetics.* Berlin, Germany: Springer-Verlag; 1990.

11. McConnell J. Patellofemoral syndromes (course notes). Marina del Ray, Calif: The McConnel Institute; 1991.

12. Irion JM. Use of the gym ball in rehabilitation of spinal dysfunction. *Orthop Phys Ther Clin.* 1992;1(2):375–398.

13. Jull GA, Richardson CA. The muscular protection of the lumbar spine (course notes). 1992 National Orthopaedic Symposium of the Canadian Physiotherapy Association, Toronto, Ontario, Canada; 1991.

14. Gowitzke BA, Milner M. *Scientific Bases of Human Movement.* 3rd ed. Baltimore, Md: Williams & Wilkins; 1988.

15. Worrell T, et al. Effects of patella taping on patella position and perceived pain. *J Med Sci Sports Exerc.* 1993; 25(9):989–992.

16. Benner E. Have a seat? Ergonomics for seated occupations. *Orthop Phys Ther Pract.* 1994;7(2):9–12.

17. Fawcett CW. Principles of aquatic rehab: a new look at hydrotherapy. *Sports Med Update.* 1992;7:6–9.

18. Johns KM. Aquatic therapy: therapeutic treatment for today's patient. *Phys Ther Prod.* 1993;4(3):24–25.

19. Sova R. *Aquatics: The Complete Reference Guide for Aquatic Fitness Professionals.* Boston, Mass: Jones & Bartlett; 1992.

20. Thein LA, McNamara CA. Aquatic exercise in rehabilitation and training. *Orthop Phys Ther Clin.* 1992;1(2): 191–206.

ADDITIONAL READING

Aquatics

Aquatic Physical Therapy. *Orthop Phys Ther Clin.* 1994; 3(2):83–260.

Aquatic rehabilitation. *Sports Med Update.* 1992;7(2):4–30.

Duffield MH. *Exercise in Water.* 2nd ed. London, England: Balliere Tindall; 1976.

Hydrotherapy. *Clin Manage.* 1991;11(1):14–37.

McWaters G. Aquatic rehabilitation. In Andrews JR, Harrelson GL, eds. *Physical Rehabilitation of the Injured Athlete.* Philadelphia, Pa: Saunders; 1991:473–503.

Mobilization Techniques

Kaltenborn FM. *Manual Mobilization of the Extremity Joints.* 4th ed. Oslo, Norway: Olaf Norlis Bokhandel; 1989.

Cantu RI, Grodin AJ. *Myofascial Manipulation Theory and Clinical Application.* Gaithersburg, Md: Aspen; 1992.

Maitland GD. *Peripheral Manipulation.* 2nd ed. London, England: Butterworth; 1977.

Manheim CJ, Lavett DK. *The Myofascial Release Manual.* Thorofare, NJ: Slack; 1989.

Manual therapy. *Phys Ther.* 1992;72(12):839–936.

Mennell JM. *Joint Pain.* Boston, Mass: Little, Brown; 1964.

Strengthening Exercises

Albert M. *Eccentric Muscle Training in Sports and Orthopaedics.* New York, NY: Churchill Livingstone; 1991.

Andrews JR, Harrelson GL. *Physical Rehabilitation of the Injured Athlete.* Philadelphia, Pa: Saunders; 1991.

Daniels L, Worthingham C. *Therapeutic Exercise.* Philadelphia, Pa: Saunders; 1977.

Gould JA. *Orthopaedic and Sports Physical Therapy.* St Louis, Mo: Mosby; 1990.

Kendall F, MacCreary EK, Provance P. *Muscles: Testing and Function.* 4th ed. Baltimore, Md: Williams & Wilkins; 1993.

Kisner C, Colby LA. *Therapeutic Exercise: Foundations and Techniques.* 2nd ed. Philadelphia, Pa: Davis; 1990.

Smythe R. *Plyometrics.* Portland, Ore: Speed City; 1987.

Timm KE. Exercise technologies. *Orthop Phys Ther Clin North Am.* 1992;1(2):191–407.

7

Functional Exercises for the Lower Extremities

As a unit, the lower extremities function mainly to provide a means of transportation for the body. They are the first part to contact the ground during walking, and they act to absorb the impact of the ground reaction forces that travel up to the other body segments. The legs require sufficient strength to propel a person forward and to decelerate or control all ambulatory and postural movements.

GENERAL FUNCTIONAL PROGRAM

When designing the functional program versus a standard exercise program, the therapist addresses the barriers to function previously mentioned in Chapter 6 (postural alignment and base of support, flexibility and mobility, strength and dynamic stability, sensory input, and sequence of movement and coordination/ motor control) through correctional exercises (phase I) and goal-oriented activities (phases II and III).

For the program to work, the interrelationships of the lower extremities with themselves as well as with the other body segments must first be considered. In other words, the patient must learn to align the lower body segments properly before initiating functional activities.

Although some malalignments may be caused by skeletal deformity, a surprising number can be corrected through voluntary control of the muscular system. The therapist should keep a special watch on the long muscles of the legs that cross two joints:

- gastrocnemius
- hamstrings
- rectus femoris
- sartorius
- tensor fascia lata (TFL) together with the iliotibial band (ITB)

These commonly can shorten and dominate over or substitute for the primary movers. In addition, the therapist must keep a close eye on the patient's hip rotations and their relation to patella tracking. Distally, the therapist observes the ankle/foot complex, looking for any faulty motions or posture (eg, foot pronation) that could cause compensations farther up the kinetic chain.

The patient begins the lower extremity functional program simply by attempting the following locomotor activities (phase I) at the proper ability level (basic through to advanced):

- standing
- gait

- chair-to-stand transfers
- floor-to-stand transfers
- stair climbing

As mentioned previously, the therapist makes sure that the patient is properly aligned and is using a properly sequenced motor plan. The therapist changes the environmental conditions either to assist or to challenge the patient's abilities. For some high-level patients, such as athletes, many of the exercises in the phase I or beginning locomotor program will be easy to perform. The clinician must know by evaluation or by trial and error at what level the patient should enter the program. Generally, the easy activities can be used as a quick warm-up for such a patient. By the same token, a severely debilitated patient in a nursing home setting might find even the easiest activities in the phase I program quite challenging. Many times, this type of patient may have to begin the lower extremity program by performing closed-chain ankle and foot exercises in a sitting position before progressing to simple standing (this is especially true if the patient does not have full weight-bearing orders). Although the nursing home patient might never reach the athlete's level of function, it is hoped that the program will begin to restore meaningful functional ability to both people.

By itself, the lower extremity phase I program is essentially a fine closed-chain exercise regimen. To improve functional capacity, however, the patient cannot spend all cerebral effort on exercise, but must concentrate instead on accomplishing functional tasks or goals. Therefore, the patient simultaneously engages in a total body program (phase II), which begins to integrate the lower extremity segments back into the rest of the person. Examples of phase II integration types of activities are:

- lifting
- carrying
- pushing or pulling
- squatting or crouching
- sport tasks

As mentioned in Chapter 6, functional ability cannot be achieved only by attending therapy. The patient must practice the functional tasks in phases I and II at home or in a hospital room. They are the building blocks that can cause new or old motor patterns to emerge. The patient must then incorporate these movement patterns into true functional activities (phase III). A true functional activity is an action taken by a person to achieve a behavioral goal (the goal must be the patient's, not the therapist's). These are the functional activities previously listed in Chapter 3 and include basic activities of daily living (ADLs), instrumental ADLs (IADLs), work activities, and sports/recreational activities. The patient must practice solving real problems in the real world, first under supervision and then alone. This level of interaction in the real world involves an element of risk that the patient must choose to undertake. The potential danger is further injury and incapacitation. The potential benefit is return to independent function.

Standing

The activity of standing is necessary for many functional tasks and is a prerequisite for ambulation. The patient must be able to maintain balance under various circumstances. The lower extremities must be strong enough to support the entire body weight and flexible enough that the pelvic and thoracic segments do not have to move unnecessarily. When the patient practices the standing program, the therapist acts to ensure that the patient's trunk remains erect, the iliac crests remain even, the hips remain in neutral rotation, and the patellae remain centrally tracked. If any deviations occur or if the patient reports pain, the therapist must alter the environment so that the task can be performed correctly.

Phase I: Beginning Locomotor Activities

The clinician can create the surroundings to fit the patient's needs by varying the following conditions:

- patient's base of support (wide versus narrow)

- sensory input (visual, tactile, and proprioceptive)
- floor surface (even versus uneven, smooth versus textured, etc.)
- environment (static versus dynamic)

The easiest conditions in which to maintain standing exist when the patient is in bilateral standing (ie, wide base of support), with eyes open (visual input), near a supporting structure such as a wall or table (tactile input available from the hands), on a low-pile carpet (even, textured surface), and in a quiet room (static environment). In this position, the patient should be able to shift weight from leg to leg and slightly forward and backward without loss of balance or increase in symptoms. The patient progresses by being able to maintain balance with a change in some of the parameters, such as standing on one leg (ie, narrow base of support) with eyes closed (no visual input) and in an open space (no tactile input from the hands) but remaining on a low-pile carpet in a quiet room (Figure 7–1).

The clinician may need to increase the patient's tactile input from the soles of the feet or decrease the input if weight bearing causes pain. This can be accomplished by altering the floor surface (carpet, linoleum, cement, etc.) or the patient's footwear (barefoot, sneakers, pumps, orthotics, etc.). In addition, the patient needs to assume various postures even while stationary. The standing program therefore must include strengthening exercises of ankle heel-offs and toe-offs, knee squats, and upper extremity and trunk movements (Figures 7–2 through 7–4). These exercises are precursors to activities such as standing on tip-toes to reach for an item on a high shelf or crouching low to pick up something from the floor. These exercises will of course also increase the patient's strength in a functional pattern so that other tasks, such as walking or stair climbing, will be affected in a positive manner.

As the patient improves, the therapist must also change the environment to a more dynamic one, as might be encountered when trying to stand on the deck of a ship or on wet sand. The

Basic Standing Balance

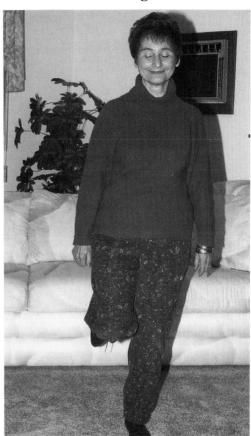

Figure 7–1 Phase I: basic standing balance. The easiest conditions in which to maintain standing exist when the patient stands on two feet near a supporting structure, on a level surface, with eyes open, and in a quiet room. Standing can be made more difficult by changing some of the conditions, such as standing on only one foot in an open space, on a level surface, with eyes closed, and in a quiet room (shown above). Other conditions could be altered instead to challenge the patient's standing ability.

clinician can provide a solid but unstable surface by using a wobble board, a biomechanical ankle platform system (BAPS) board, or Ethafoam™ roller. The progression from easy to harder remains the same, with the patient first practicing in bilateral standing near a supporting structure, then trying unilateral standing, and eventually progressing toward an open space. For safety reasons, the patient with even the slightest limitation should perform the

Standing Ankle Exercises

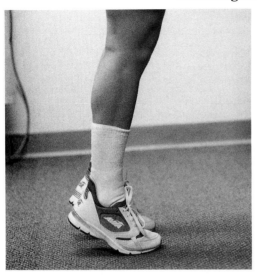 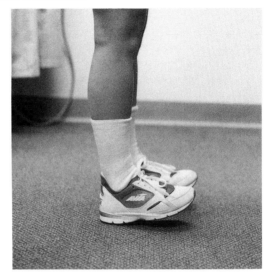

Figure 7–2 Phase I: standing ankle exercises. (**A**) Having the patient perform heel-offs (plantar flexion) decreases the base of support while simultaneously strengthening the gastrocnemius and soleus muscles. (**B**) Toe-offs (dorsiflexion) are generally more difficult, especially for elderly patients, because they also decrease the base of support while causing a posterior postural sway. The therapist can alter the difficulty by allowing a supporting structure, such as a doorjamb, to be positioned nearby. For safety reasons, these types of exercises should be performed with eyes open.

Standing Minisquats

A   B   C

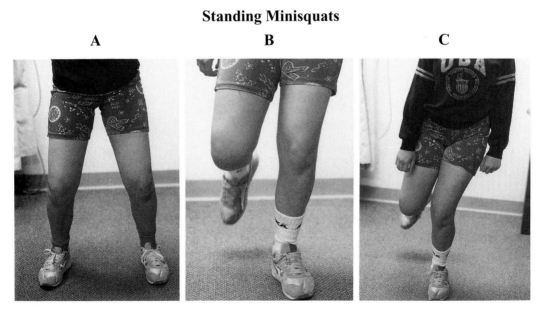

Figure 7–3 Phase I: standing minisquats. This exercise is a precursor for crouching, getting up from a chair, or negotiating stairs. The therapist needs to ensure that proper patella tracking is occurring with the hips in neutral rotation by instructing the patient to keep the knee over the second toe of the foot. The program progresses by going from a two-legged squat (**A**) to a one-legged squat (**B**). Once again, a supporting structure nearby affects the difficulty of the activity. The person in (**C**) demonstrates incorrect technique, with valgus forces being generated at the knee as a result of excessive hip internal rotation. This can cause patellofemoral pain.

Standing with Upper Extremity and Trunk Movements

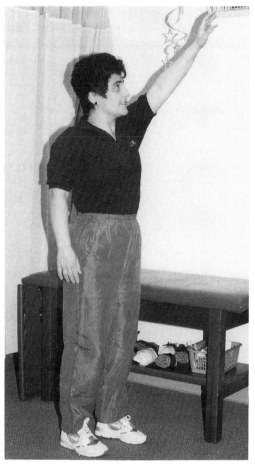
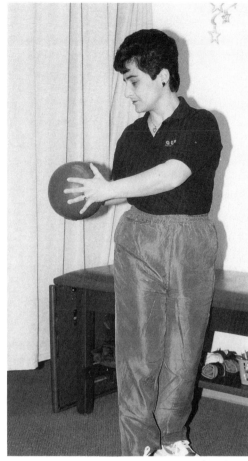

A   **B**

Figure 7–4 Phase I: standing with upper extremity and trunk movements. The patient also needs to be able to maintain standing balance while the upper extremities (**A**) or trunk (**B**) are in motion. This exercise causes the lower extremities to assume their role as postural stabilizers. The patient can alter the width of the base of support to change the difficulty of this activity.

program on the unstable surface with eyes open (Figure 7–5).

Phase II: Beginning Integration Program

With the foundation built through standard exercises and the phase I program, the patient needs to integrate the formerly dysfunctional lower extremities back into the body as a whole. The patient needs to forget which is the bad leg, the sprained ankle, or the fractured hip and has to begin doing things again with the entire body. Phase II of the functional rehabilitation program involves beginning activities common to many types of function. While automatically maintaining balance on both feet, the patient concentrates on accomplishing different objectives. Examples of these types of activities are:

- squatting or crouching
- throwing or catching a ball (Figure 7–6)
- lifting an object
- reaching overhead for an item
- hitting a foam ball with a paddle

Standing on an Unstable Surface

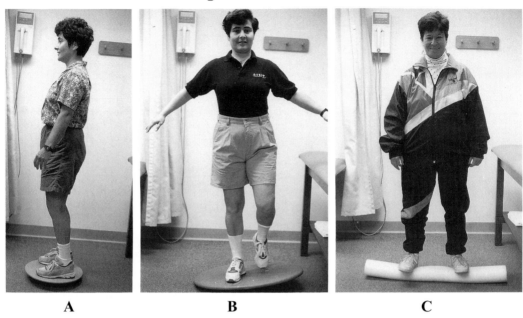

| A | B | C |

Figure 7–5 Phase I: standing on an unstable surface. A more dynamic environment is created when the patient tries to maintain standing balance on a firm but unstable surface, such as a wobble board (**A**), BAPS board (**B**), or Ethafoam™ roller (**C**). Proper joint alignments must be maintained. Patients of all levels should perform these activities with their eyes open for safety reasons. Supporting structures should be used as needed, especially with the elderly. Photo **A** is courtesy of Spri Performance Systems, Deerfield, Illinois.

The list could include as many exercises as there are real-life activities. Each is a further progression of the phase I standing program. Crouching and lifting involve performing a more difficult squat. Throwing or catching a ball or reaching overhead requires the legs to assume their stabilizing role while the upper extremities perform a separate task. Hitting a foam ball with a paddle requires trunk rotation and upper extremity motion. All these activities cause the patient to preset postural and balance mechanisms automatically, recalling movement patterns from prior experience. With greater abilities present, the old patterns once again become available to the patient.

Phase II activities follow immediately on the heels of the phase I program. If possible, the patient begins these activities in the same treatment session as the phase I exercises. Neither the therapist nor the patient possesses the luxury of time to begin these activities after successfully completing an exercise and/or phase I program. They must be done practically simultaneously, each one flowing effortlessly into the other.

The phase II program is usually different and fun for a patient who is used to "just exercising." Games, sports, and other functional activities challenge the patient's ability to maintain standing posture under changing circumstances. Because the patient's mind is engaged in winning, scoring, or catching, the physical impairments that have so strongly commanded the patient's attention are deemphasized. The patient is slowly becoming a person again.

Phase III: Solving Functional Problems

The last phase of the functional rehabilitation program involves returning to everyday function. Simply learning to do some activities in therapy 3 to 6 hours a week does not guarantee that the patient will carry the movement pat-

Integration of the Lower Extremities into the Whole Body

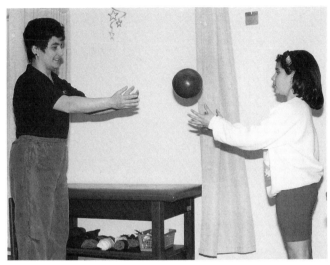

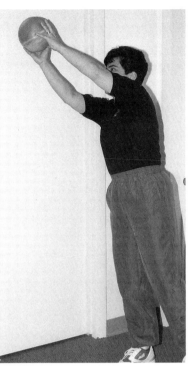

A   **B**

Figure 7–6 Phase II: beginning integration of the lower extremities into the body as a whole. Fun activities, such as throwing and catching a ball (**A**), require the patient to stop focusing on maintaining balance and instead to concentrate on the ball. As balance is maintained automatically, the activity can be made more difficult by throwing the ball away from the patient (**B**) so that she must reach for it without losing her balance. A plyoball (or weighted ball) requires more strength and stability from the lower extremities as well as from the whole body to maintain upright posture.

terns over into real life. The patient must be instructed to try the standing program in some protected way independent of the clinician. This provides the patient with the opportunity to create solutions to life's problems independent of the clinician's professional recommendations. By backing off, the therapist forces the patient to take action that will accomplish the patient's behavioral goals in a safe fashion. The patient must understand that making mistakes is not only OK but necessary for learning to occur. (On the other hand, falling from a standing position can have dire consequences.)

This might involve standing by the bathroom sink to perform hygiene or grooming. A spouse at home or a nurse in the hospital could judiciously place a chair nearby in case the patient fatigues and needs to sit down. Only by performing the standing task of grooming day in and day out will the patient develop the most efficient means of doing it. Circumstances are always changing. Even in the most mundane functional tasks such as grooming, new problems arise that are similar to the ones of yesterday but ever so slightly different. This of course requires unique solutions, similar to the ones of yesterday perhaps but ever so slightly different. If the brush has been moved from the right side of the sink to the left, the standing postural alignment will need to differ a tiny bit to accommodate the change.

Other standing activities that can be practiced first under supervision and then independently could include any of the following:

- waiting in line in a grocery store
- standing to get dressed
- standing to prepare meals
- standing to putt or drive a golf ball

Once again, the list is endless and dependent on the patient's personal desires. The rehabilitation specialist's instructions change from "Pour yourself a glass of milk here in the occupational therapy kitchen" to "Go home and try to make yourself a snack. Report back to me on Friday with any problems you might have encountered." For an institutionalized patient, the therapist might request that the patient try to get dressed alone in the standing position.

After successfully interacting with the environment, the patient should gain confidence in his or her own ability to stand safely while doing things. Without conscious thought, the patient begins to do other activities from the standing position automatically and without major effort. Standing function has been restored.

Gait

As Perry[1] succinctly reports, walking is basically a means of traveling from one place to another to reach a position in time and space to do something else of greater importance. Therefore, walking should only require minimal amounts of energy while providing the rest of the body with a smooth ride to the desired destination.

Gait has been studied thoroughly from many viewpoints and has been written about extensively in the literature. Perry[1] gives six functional descriptors of gait: weight acceptance, trunk glide, push, balance-assist, pick-up, and reach. These correlate with the more commonly used temporal descriptors of gait (Table 7–1). Appendix A at the end of this book concisely reviews Perry's analyses of the many events that occur during the gait cycle. She describes five major points as having the greatest significance for normal walking:

1. Beginning to balance on one limb causes a definite valgus thrust on the weight-bearing knee.

Table 7–1 Comparison of Perry's Functional Descriptors of Gait Phases with the More Common Temporal Descriptors

Functional Descriptors of Gait	Temporal (Classic) Descriptors of Gait
Weight acceptance	Heel strike (early stance)
Trunk glide	Midstance
Push	Push-off (late stance)
Balance-assist	Push-off (late stance)
Pick-up	Early swing
Reach	Late swing

Source: Data from *Principles of Lower-Extremity Bracing* by J. Perry and H. Hislop, eds., p. 14–15, American Physical Therapy Association, © 1967.

2. As the pelvis rotates and tilts, the weight-bearing hip goes through adduction, internal rotation, and extension during the stance (or reach) phase.
3. The plantar flexors (with help from the hip extensors) prevent the knee from buckling during weight acceptance and trunk glide (stance phase). The quadriceps are less important but useful when present.
4. The body weight can advance in front of the foot only if approximately 10° of ankle dorsiflexion is available. If not present, a strong hyperextension force will exist at the knee and the hip must be able to support weight in flexion.
5. During the initial swing phase, any toe drag is due to lack of pick-up activity by the hip and knee flexors. Later during the reach phase, toe drag is caused by lack of dorsiflexion.

The gait pattern described by Perry differs when a person maneuvers around an object or backs up to a toilet. In addition, an increase in velocity changes the pattern to that of a jog or a sprint. Each of these ambulatory patterns has unique characteristics that may need to be retrained for the patient to become functional again.

When the patient practices the gait program, the therapist acts to ensure that no obvious gait deviations are occurring that could interfere with economic, pain-free locomotion. Some commonly observed gait deviations are:

- circumducted gait
- abducted or waddle gait
- shortened step length
- increased step width
- increased double support
- decreased push-off
- decreased pelvic rotation
- decreased trunk rotation
- increased foot pronation or supination
- decreased tempo or fluidity of motion

Phase I: Beginning Locomotor Activities

Aside from the many gait deviations mentioned above, the clinician works first to ensure that the lower limb segments from foot to pelvis are properly aligned. The therapist adjusts the following variables in the functional program to assist the patient's return to normal walking or running:

- *Size of step:* Increasing the step size causes increased weight bearing and requires increased balancing ability on the stance leg. Many patients reduce their normal step size when injured for protection.
- *Resistance:* Increasing the resistance by using surgical tubing, a sled, or a parachute (see Chapter 14) requires increased muscle tension both to move and stabilize the lower extremity joints and also causes greater joint reaction forces.
- *Surface:* Changing from a level surface to a sloped surface or from flat to uneven terrain requires greater balancing ability and accommodations by the foot and leg to absorb increased forces. Most people need the ability to walk on different types of surfaces.
- *Velocity:* Increasing the velocity requires greater muscle tension both to move and to stabilize the lower extremity joints and also causes increased joint reaction forces. The ability to accelerate and decelerate on demand is essential for safety in everyday life and for all sports and work activities.
- *Environment:* Changing the environment from static to dynamic forces the patient to

begin scanning and anticipating the surroundings. With the additional ability to change velocity on demand, the patient progresses from merely walking to maneuvering.

The phase I gait program consists of some of the locomotor activities required to interact with the patient's environment at home, in the nursing home, on the athletic field, or at work. As such, it includes the following activities (Figures 7–7 through 7–15):

- forward walking (or jogging or running)
- sidestepping
- backward walking or retrowalking
- crossover or Carioca stepping
- circular and figure-of-eight walking
- shuttle walking
- plyometrics
- treadmill walking

Many of these functional rehabilitation techniques are already commonly used by therapists for high-level athletes with great success. Yet they are not commonly used in the rehabilitation of the geriatric patient with hip fracture or arthritis or, for that matter, in the rehabilitation of a working mother with knee pain. With creativity, the rehabilitation specialist can create a program that delivers benefits similar to those of an athletic workout but without similar risks for reinjury. For more information about a high-level phase I gait program than is provided here, the reader is referred to the books on improving athletic performance listed at the end of this chapter.

Phase II: Beginning Integration Program

The patient must also reintegrate the injured lower extremity back into the whole person. The phase II integration program assists in accomplishing this goal by having the patient concentrate on basic functional activities while automatically using gait patterns to travel. The following examples of phase II activities should be initiated simultaneously with phase I exercises, even

Forward Locomotion

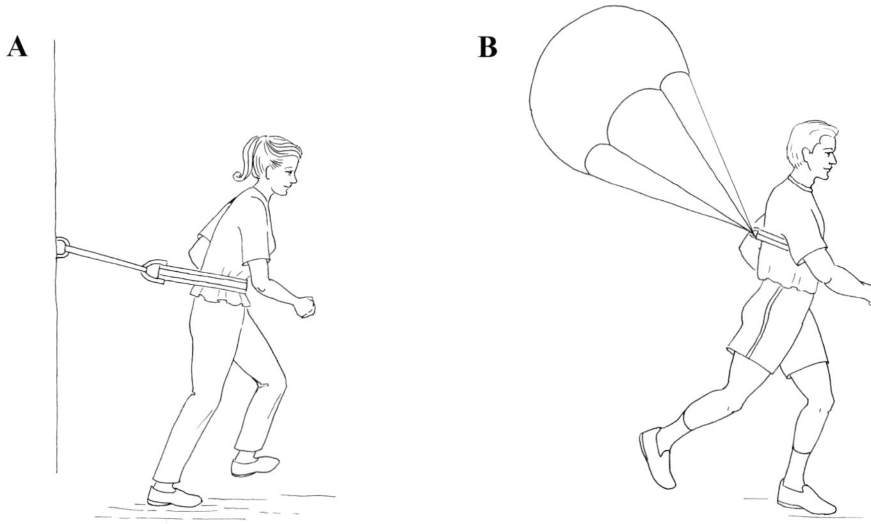

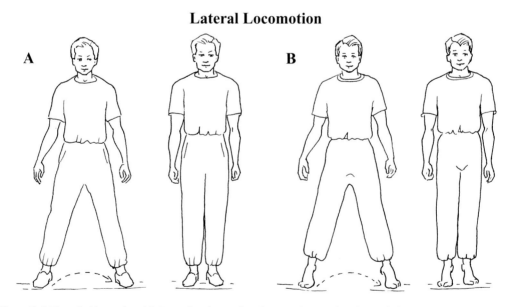

Figure 7–7 Phase I: forward walking or running. The program progresses from walking (or running) with a normal gait pattern in an open space to negotiating uneven terrain. If desired, the clinician can request that the patient alter the tempo or velocity of the walk (or run) to as fast as possible or slower than normal. During running, the knee extensors absorb the impact loads while the ankle plantar flexors provide propulsion.[2] Resistance can be achieved through the use of surgical tubing (**A**) for the low-level midlevel patient or with a sled or parachute for the high-level athlete (**B**). When the resistance is removed, the patient usually walks (or runs) with a noticeably improved pattern.

Lateral Locomotion

Figure 7–8 Phase I: sidestepping. (**A**) Increasing the step length causes the muscles of the weight-bearing leg (especially the gluteus medius, pes anserinus, and posterior tibialis[7]) to stabilize greater forces to maintain balance. Resistance can be added with surgical tubing. The activity can also be made more difficult by having the patient sidestep on tip-toes (**B**) with or without support. This decreases the base of support (requiring greater balance) while increasing the strength of the plantar flexors. Depending on patient ability, this activity can progress to side jumps (increased velocity) similar to the lateral motion needed to play defense in basketball.

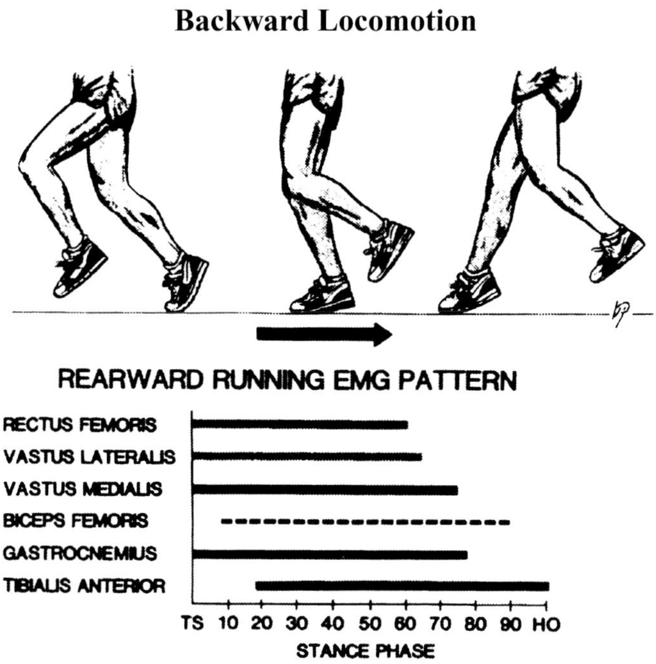

Backward Locomotion

REARWARD RUNNING EMG PATTERN

RECTUS FEMORIS
VASTUS LATERALIS
VASTUS MEDIALIS
BICEPS FEMORIS
GASTROCNEMIUS
TIBIALIS ANTERIOR

TS 10 20 30 40 50 60 70 80 90 HO
STANCE PHASE

Figure 7–9 Phase I: backward walking or retrowalking or running. Backward walking produces joint positions of the knee and hip similar to those of forward walking.[3] However, weight acceptance begins at the forefoot (instead of the heel), with footflat being controlled by the plantar flexors and peroneals.[4] When advancing to retrorunning there is an obvious pattern change (from forward running), with less hip motion being required and with the hip being maintained in flexion during the stance phase.[5] In addition, a shorter stance time[4] and a shorter step length occur during retrorunning.[2,5] The ankle plantar flexors provide the primary shock absorption, and the knee extensors are the primary source of propulsion.[2] Surgical tubing can be added to increase the resistance of either walking or running. During all backward locomotion, the altered visual input causes the body to rely more heavily on proprioceptive input to maintain balance. *Source:* Reprinted from *Journal of Orthopaedic and Sports Physical Therapy,* Vol. 17, No. 2, p. 111, with permission of the Orthopaedic and Sports Physical Therapy Sections of the American Physical Therapy Association, © 1993.

---

if the patient has protected weight-bearing orders and requires an ambulatory device, such as crutches or a cane for gait:

- negotiating around an obstacle course
- pushing open doors, pushing grocery carts, or moving furniture
- pulling open doors, pulling a golf cart, or pulling a laundry bag

If the patient is full weight bearing as tolerated or does not use an assistive device, the therapist can also use these higher-level activities to promote automatic use of the lower extremities:

- carrying a weighted milk crate, grocery bag, or laundry basket

- dribbling a basketball in all directions
- sidestepping while practicing a tennis swing

Many patients have difficulty negotiating uneven surfaces after injury to the lower extremity or due to prior balance problems. The rehabilitation specialist can simulate outdoor surface conditions by having the patient walk on and around floor exercise mats and cuff weights (Figure 7–16). This activity promotes proprioception and balance as well as the patient's ability to scan the environment.

In addition to the actual gait drills mentioned above, many patients enjoy the high-level exercise provided by the glide boards, the cross-country ski machines, and the Fitter (Figures 7–17 through 7–19). These closed-chain exercises

Carioca Stepping

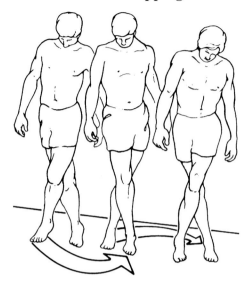

Figure 7–10 Phase I: crossover or Carioca stepping. Crossing one leg in front of or behind the other commonly occurs when one is maneuvering around an object, during many sports, and in dancing (Greek or Western line dances, Israeli hora, etc.). As the person twists to the same side as the pivot leg, tibial internal rotation of the pivot leg occurs and it is controlled by the anterior cruciate ligament.[6] The pelvis, hip, and foot also must control rotational stresses. The activity can be made more difficult by increasing the step length or speed of the activity or through providing resistance with surgical tubing. This exercise increases proprioceptive input into all weight-bearing joints, improves dynamic balance, and retrains coordination (motor control). *Source:* Reprinted from *Journal of Orthopaedic and Sports Physical Therapy* Vol. 11, No. 1, p. 16, with permission of the Orthopaedic and Sports Physical Therapy Sections of the American Physical Therapy Association, © 1989.

Circular and Figure-of-Eight Drills

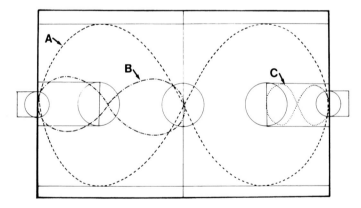

Figure 7–11 Phase I: circular and figure-of-eight drills. These walking or running agility drills require all the lower extremity joints to control rotational stresses. These are essential precursors to cutting maneuvers for sport activities but are also necessary for negotiating around everyday objects. The larger the circle or figure-of-eight pathway, the less rotational stress at the joints. The patient first walks or runs in large circles (both clockwise and counterclockwise), then in smaller circles, then in large figure-of-eights, and then in smaller figure-of-eights (shown on a basketball court). The therapist can alter velocity, step length, base of support, and resistance. *Source:* Reprinted from *Journal of Orthopaedic and Sports Physical Therapy* Vol. 11, No. 1, p. 16, with permission of the Orthopaedic and Sports Physical Therapy Sections of the American Physical Therapy Association, © 1989.

Shuttle Drills

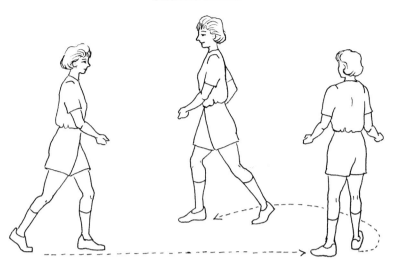

Figure 7–12 Phase I: shuttle walking or running. The shuttle drill consists of walking or running in a straight path for a short distance, planting the outside foot down, pivoting 180°, returning to the opposite direction, planting the outside foot, and repeating the back-and-forth motion. This acceleration and deceleration of the lower extremities is required in normal walking as well as in all sports and work activities. The inability to pivot and maneuver around objects and people prevents many patients who can otherwise walk from being able to walk in a dynamic environment. The maneuver consists of the sidestep cutting mechanism, in which the pivot leg initially decelerates the body through tibial external rotation, the pelvis then rotates away from the pivot leg through hip external rotation and tibial internal rotation, and the pivot leg then rotates toward the new direction before toe-off through hip internal rotation and tibial external rotation.[6,7] The lower leg musculature and ligaments must also control all foot and ankle motions. The therapist can change the intensity of the activity by altering the floor or ground surface type and the velocity.

---

promote aerobic capacity while improving strength and proprioception in a fun manner.

Phase III: Solving Functional Problems

The last phase of the gait program involves returning to everyday walking activities beyond the safe and protected therapy environment. Only by practicing gait throughout the day, even for short distances, will the activity become automatic. Practice once again refers to using similar movement patterns while attempting to solve the functional problems of everyday life and locomoting from point A to point B to point C. By experimenting with different strategies and making and correcting mistakes or inefficient motions, the patient develops the ability to walk in an efficient, pain-free manner. The patient must decide whether the benefits of improved locomotion and perhaps independent walking or running outweigh the potential risks

of falling and any injuries that may result from falling.

The nursing home patient must begin walking first with supervision and then independently along the hallways and in his or her room. The aim is no longer to walk for exercise or with a better gait pattern but to accomplish functional goals, such as getting to the dining room or the bathroom. The patient must figure out how to negotiate around beds, night tables, and moving ambulators and wheelchairs safely and in an efficient, pain-free manner.

Both the homebound patient and outpatient need to be able to move around their houses or apartments without groping for furniture and walls or tripping on chair legs or changes in carpet height. They should practice light housekeeping, including dishes, dusting, and vacuuming, as well as personal hygiene and toileting. These activities require the lower extremities to provide a stable but mobile base of support.

Low-Level Plyometrics: Basic Jumps

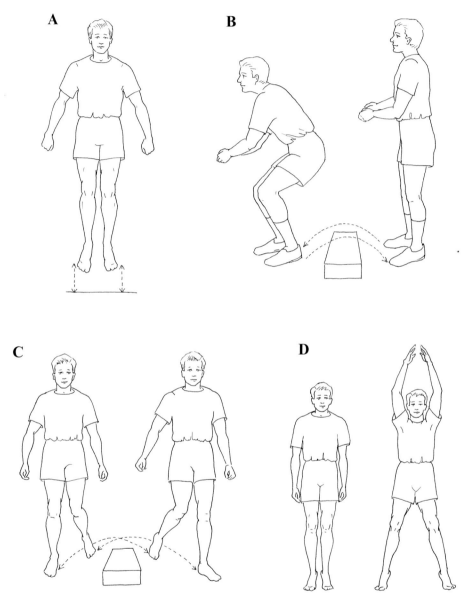

Figure 7–13 Phase I: low-level plyometrics—basic jumps. These total body exercises, which utilize the myotatic stretch response, require strength and balance and develop quickness and agility (see Chapter 6). Although athletic progressions can be quite intense, a low-level plyometric program can and should be performed by the average patient. These would consist of vertical jumps or jump roping (**A**), forward/backward jumps (**B**), lateral jumps (**C**, also called Heidens), and jumping jacks (**D**). By altering the base of support (bilateral versus unilateral jumps), the height of the jump, the distance traversed by the jump, the velocity, or the resistance (by surgical tubing or cuff weights), this basic jump advances in difficulty. For patients with balance problems, vertical jumps can be performed if a supportive surface (eg, chairs or a door frame) or clinician's manual assistance is provided. The patient with balance difficulties, however, should not progress further with these activities unless balance ability improves.

Low-Level Plyometrics: Hops and Skips

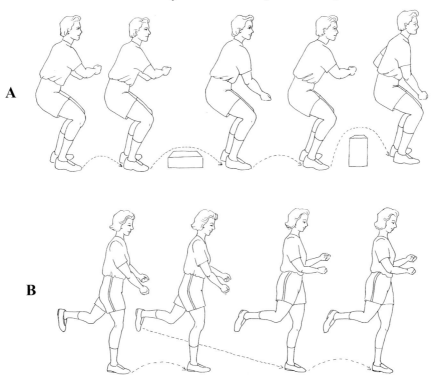

Figure 7–14 low-level plyometrics—hops and skips. (**A**) Hopping multiple times in different directions or over small obstacles or playing hop-scotch and (**B**) skipping (low to the ground, one-legged forward hops) are highly coordinated low-level jumping activities. They improve balance, coordination, and quickness. The activity becomes more difficult with increasing speed, step length, and resistance. All plyometric activities can be performed in the buoyant environment of the pool (see Chapter 6) to offset compressive joint forces.

Balance must be maintained during all locomotor and stationary aspects of the activity. Initially, the patient may choose to use a safer gait pattern (increased double support, smaller step length, wider step width, etc.) to accomplish these functional tasks. The therapist should observe the patient's solution to the functional gait problems encountered and determine whether other movement choices are available. After practicing several alternative movement solutions, the patient can decide which is best. The clinician or patient might also opt to alter the home environment.

For the patient to become a safe community ambulator, the clinician must consider the size and type of town in which the patient lives. In a study by Robinett and Vondran[9] (Table 7–2), a patient living in a rural community (population less than 10,000) needs to be able to walk a distance of about 230 m (754 ft) to walk and perform most IADLs from a handicapped parking spot (Table 7–2). These IADLs include going to the post office, bank, or doctor's office and shopping in supermarkets, department stores, or drugstores. The distances a patient needs to traverse increase to 332 m (1,089 ft) in a small town (population less than 40,000) and to 342 m (1,122 ft) in a city (population greater than 95,000).

In addition, Robinett and Vondran[9] report the average safe ambulation velocities required to cross a street in each of the communities. In the rural town, the patient needs to walk approximately 44.5 m/min (146 ft/min), in the small

Treadmill Activities

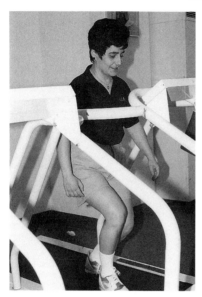

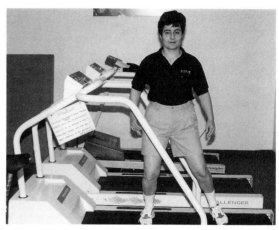

A

B

Figure 7–15 Phase I: treadmill activities. The treadmill provides a constant, preset speed with supportive handrails if needed for the patient to perform forward, backward, lateral, and crossover walking. Intensive closed-chain strengthening occurs by (**A**) Groucho walking (bent-knee walking) and (**B**) lateral stepping. For retraining quickness, small, fast steps can be substituted for large, powerful steps. Many treadmills can also simulate hill walking by increasing the gradient. In addition, the treadmill provides a protected but dynamic environment in that the patient must adjust the gait pattern temporally to the moving surface. Treadmill training has proved to be effective in improving normal gait patterns and speeds for many patients, including those with hip fractures.[8] The treadmill can also be used for a more aerobic workout.

Table 7–2 Medians and Ranges of Measurements for Specific Locations in Communities

	Population Size								
	<10,000			10,000–40,000			>95,000		
Variable	Median	Range	n	Median	Range	n	Median	Range	n
Curb height (cm)	17.0	(11.5–20.0)	14	18.0	(14.0–20.0)	9	18.5	(14.0–21.5)	11
Crosswalk									
Commercial distance (m)	15.0	(13.0–17.0)	6	19.5	(13.0–24.0)	5	16.5	(8.5–27.5)	9
Residential distance (m)	11.5	(9.0–12.0)	7	12.5	(9.0–13.0)	8	10.0	(9.0–12.0)	11
Velocity required for safe									
crossing (m/min)	44.5	(30.0–69.0)	7	58.5	(31.0–69.0)	5	63.5	(42.5–82.5)	11
Location									
Post office (m)	39.0	(13.0–65.5)	2	47.0	(44.5–49.0)	2	60.5	(36.0–84.0)	9
Bank (m)	64.0	(57.0–68.0)	3	51.0	(38.0–85.0)	5	63.0	(30.0–217.0)	10
Physician's office or medical									
building (m)	45.5	(41.5–61.0)	3	47.0	(19.5–90.0)	3	47.5	(26.5–122.0)	8
Supermarket (m)	230.0	(122.0–289.0)	4	332.0	(145.0–474.0)	5	342.0	(201.0–480.0)	9
Department store (m)	132.0	(62.0–202.0)	2	175.5	(111.0–292.0)	6	327.0	(169.0–505.0)	8
Drugstore (m)	100.0	(32.5–247.0)	4	148.0	(48.0–210.0)	6	139.5	(103.0–213.0)	7

Note: n = number of (eg, number of curbs)
Source: Reprinted from *Physical Therapy* Vol. 68, No. 9, p. 1373, with permission of the American Physical Therapy Association, © 1988.

Gait on Simulated Outdoor (Uneven) Surface

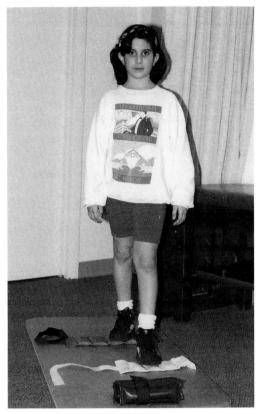

Figure 7–16 Phase II: gait activities on simulated outdoor surfaces. The therapist creates an ambulation course by using floor exercise mats of various heights and beanbag type cuff weights. The patient scans the environment and proceeds to walk on top of the different surfaces. This promotes judgment, proprioception, and balance. This activity is perfect for the patient who has difficulty with outdoor ambulation or who is homebound or institution bound. The high-level patient probably does not require this intermediary step before interacting with the outside world.

town 58.6 m/min (190 ft/min), and in the city 63.5 m/min (208 ft/min). Although these velocities are well below the normal ambulation velocity of 89 m/min (292 ft/min) for men and 74 m/min (243 ft/min) for women,[10] many patients are not trained at these velocities before returning independent to the community. In addition, high-level patients should be able to jog a small distance of about 40 ft to catch a bus or get out of the way of an oncoming car.

Aside from distance and velocity, the therapist must observe how the patient reacts to the dynamic environment of the outside world. The patient must attempt to walk on sidewalks with and against the flow of traffic, cross streets, and carry bundles outdoors first under supervision and then independently. The patient then must slowly resume everyday activities. For example, grocery shopping can be attempted first at a small farm stand or convenience store and then progressed to a supermarket. The patient reports to the clinician any problems encountered, and possible movement solutions are then discussed and simulated. As the patient builds confidence in his or her ability to walk in the real world and to independently solve everyday functional problems, ambulation returns to its original function of simply providing the body a smooth ride to its destination.

The athletic or industrial patient must be able to return to prior locomotor abilities as required by the individual sport or job. Athletes should first perform the athletic running skills needed, such as forward, backward, and lateral running, as well as cutting maneuvers when alone so that the competitive spirit does not undermine weeks of rehabilitative work. This can involve dribbling and shooting in basketball, running bases or fielding in baseball, running around obstacles in football, or playing against a backboard for tennis. After checking out the injured body part and making sure that the component tasks of the sport feel as they did before, the athlete can begin light competitive play and then progress to full intensity. A similar scenario is followed for the industrial patient trying to return to work. The walking tasks need to be assessed in full as they relate to the patient's job description. For example, some jobs, such as an airline baggage handler, require that a patient be able to carry a specified weight for a specified distance. Other occupations, such as a nurse, require the ability to walk up and down corridors pushing medication carts and assisting patients while they walk. Each job, like each sport, has its own set of locomotor skill requirements. For more information about restoring the athlete and the worker to full ability, the reader is referred to the many texts on athletic retraining and work hardening.

Glide Boards

A   B

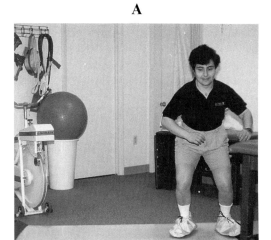   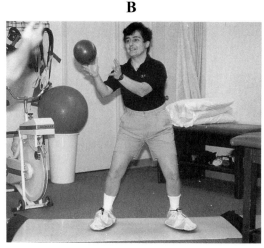

Figure 7–17 Phase II: glide board exercises. The glide board simulates the movement pattern of speed skating. (**A**) With special friction-reducing booties placed over sneakers, the patient pushes off the board's bumper laterally and rebounds off the other side. This requires balance and strength of the entire lower quarter to decelerate and stabilize the ankle, knee, and hip quickly and then immediately accelerate the body toward the other side. The farther apart the bumpers, the larger the step length and the harder the activity. The eyes should look to the horizon (not at the feet), and the knees should remain flexed with the patellae centrally tracked. The aerobic effort is great even for highly trained athletes and the patient may need frequent rests. (**B**) The activity increases in difficulty when the patient throws and catches a ball while gliding back and forth.

The rehabilitation specialist must remember that there are only small differences in restoring the locomotor skills of the elderly, debilitated patient and the young, athletic patient. They are both trying to accomplish the goal of transporting the body efficiently from one point to another in order to do something else, such as prepare a meal or score a touchdown. Although they may be at different ends of the same spectrum, it is still the same spectrum. Both patients must practice the functional activity, explore movement options, and arrive at solutions to the functional problems encountered. Walking, running, or skipping from here to there should still be an automatic, efficient movement pattern requiring minimal cerebral thought or conscious control.

Chair-to-Stand Transfers

In this age of sitting, we sit to do many activities such as toileting, watching television, riding bicycles, playing Nintendo or cards, driving a car, and, in many instances, working. The ability to get out of and into chairs safely and easily is imperative for everyday function. Lewis[11] reports that the inability to transfer independently is one of the main reasons for institutional admissions for the elderly. This act of rising and lowering a body from a chair requires greater flexibility (Table 7–3) in the joints of the lower extremity than walking or even stair climbing.[12,13] The lower the chair height, the greater the patient's need for larger hip, knee, and ankle range of motion (ROM), and the greater the need to withstand large compressive forces. In a study by Hodge et al,[14] the maximum contact pressure measured at the hip occurred during the act of rising from a chair. Twice as much force was measured during this activity than in jumping or jogging. Although the body is initially flexed at the hip, knee, and ankle, the act of rising consists mainly of an extension movement of the lower body[15] ending with the patient balancing on both legs in standing.

Although many patients can get up from a chair (some quite easily), the activity often

Cross-Country Ski Machines

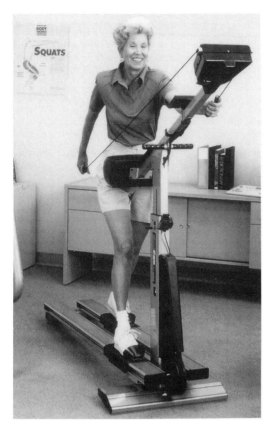

Figure 7–18 Phase II: cross-country skiing. This aerobic exercise allows a gliding, nonimpact movement pattern to emerge. The patient can adjust the step length and resistance. Many machines also work the upper extremities as well. Some patients with rotated hips have difficulty and pain (at the knees) with this machine as a result of the toe clips locking the feet straight ahead. *Source:* Photo courtesy of NordicTrak, Chaska, Minnesota.

Table 7–3 Mean ROM Needed for Chair-to-Stand Transfer from an 18-in Chair Height

Joint	Mean Motions Needed To Rise from a Chair
Hip*	112° flexion, 20° abduction, 17° external rotation
Knee†	0°–93° extension to flexion
Ankle‡	0°–12° dorsiflexion

Source: Data from *Clinical Orthopaedics and Related Research, Vol. 72, p. 208, J.B. Lippincott Co., © 1970; †Physical Therapy, Vol. 52, No. 1, p. 39, American Physical Therapy Association, © 1972. ‡Physical Therapy, Vol. 66, No. 11, p. 1709, American Physical Therapy Association, © 1986.

The Fitter

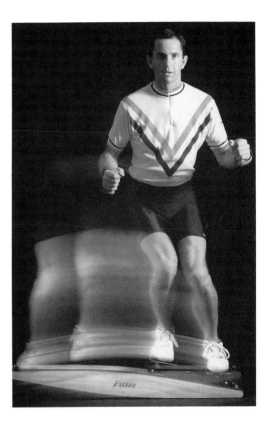

Figure 7–19 Phase II: downhill skiing on the Fitter. The Fitter somewhat simulates the motions required for downhill skiing when used as shown. Ski poles can even be used for balance. The Fitter promotes proprioception, balance, and strength and is challenging and fun for the high-level patient. *Source:* Photo courtesy of Fitter International, Inc., Calgary, Alberta, Canada.

---

causes pain in the groin or hip region. This happens often in the patient with osteoarthritis or muscle imbalance around the hip. The therapist may need to ask the patient to perform a gluteal set before rising from the chair. If the pain then disappears while getting out of the chair, the patient must work on restoring the gluteus maximus as the prime mover at the hip for this activity. Other muscles (abdominals, TFL/ITB, etc.) may be at fault instead, and the clinician should observe both initial postural alignment and any excessive movements at the back, hips, or knees that may occur during the task.

In many ways, rising from a chair is merely the continuation of a squat, and the functional program reflects that view. Instead of instructing the patient to bend forward, position the feet apart, and push to stand, the therapist merely asks the patient to slide to the edge of the chair and get up. Initially, the clinician may need to modify the environment to allow efficient, pain-free motion to emerge (Figure 7–20).

Modified Sit-to-Stand Exercise

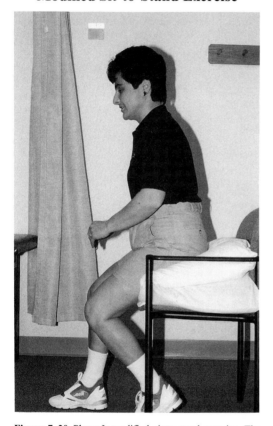

Figure 7–20 Phase I: modified sit-to-stand exercise. The therapist adds as many pillows to a chair as necessary for the patient to successfully complete the task of rising from the chair in a fluid, controlled motion without assistance and without using the upper extremities. The patient practices the task several times, exploring different movement strategies. One by one, the therapist removes the pillows until the task is too difficult to complete without loss of control. Eventually, the patient progresses to being able to rise from the unmodified seat height. Verbal cues should be kept to a minimum, but the patient can be cued to slide to the edge of the chair. As always, inefficient or dangerous postural alignments should be corrected.

Phase I: Beginning Locomotor Activity

For the patient to build sufficient lower extremity strength and gain needed flexibility, the clinician has the patient perform minisquats (Figure 7–3) and lunges (Figure 7–21). In addition, the therapist usually needs to alter the environment to allow the patient to successfully complete the task with an efficient movement pattern. This is accomplished by placing pillows in a supportive chair with arm rests, in effect raising the seat height to a level where the patient can independently explore the motion of getting in and out of the chair in a controlled fashion (Figure 7–20). As the patient progresses, the therapist removes the pillows until the patient can perform the task from the seat itself.

For the special problem of getting out of a car seat, the therapist has the patient practice simultaneous hip flexion, abduction, and external rotation from a seated position (Figure 7–22). This exercise is a needed precursor to the task of lifting one's foot up and over the car sill to place it on the street. Some patients have problems pushing off the second leg to get out of the car. The shuttle activity (Figure 7–12) of planting and reversing direction may be helpful in restoring this ability.

Phase II: Beginning Integration Program

Getting out of (or into) a chair is only a means of transporting oneself to a place or position to do something else. As such, the patient must begin the process of integrating this act into its small but important place in the scheme of things. The patient must learn how to control the activity without losing balance while environmental demands change. The demands can be spatial, in that the seat height differs (Physioball, park bench, soft sofa, toilet seat, etc.), or they can be temporal, in that the person needs to get up or down at a certain speed to accommodate a time constraint. Therefore, the therapist begins the integration program by having the patient get in and out of different height chairs, including toilet seats. At this stage, the therapist can also have the patient exercise while sitting on a large therapy ball (Figure 7–23). Although the ball's surface is supportive,

Lunges

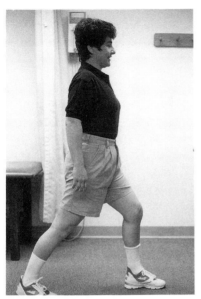
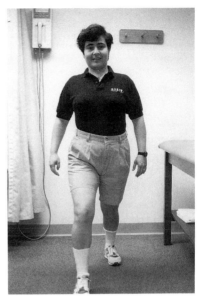

Figure 7–21 Phase I: lunges. This activity stretches the gastrocnemius component of the Achilles tendon (promoting needed dorsiflexion) and the hip flexors while simultaneously strengthening the quadriceps. The hips must remain in neutral rotation to keep the patellae centrally tracked. The deeper the lunge, the greater the stretch on the back leg and the greater the intensity of the quadriceps exercise on the front leg. Lunges should be performed in conjunction with minisquats (Figure 7–3), which further promote dorsiflexion by stretching the soleus component of the Achilles tendon.

Beginning Car Transfers:
Hip Flexion, Abduction, and External Rotation

A
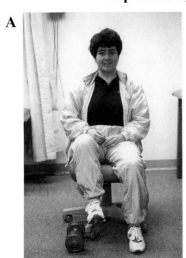

B
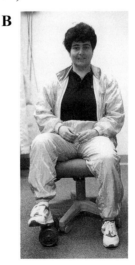
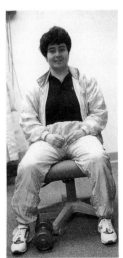

Figure 7–22 Phase I: beginning car transfers—hip flexion and abduction with external rotation. Many patients have difficulty getting the first leg in or out of the car with lower extremity dysfunction. This sitting exercise simulates lifting the leg up and over the car sill and onto the street. (**A**) First, the patient simply flexes the leg (marching) up and down. Next, the patient works on the abduction and external rotation components by sliding the leg out to the side (not shown). (**B**) Finally, the patient progresses to lifting the foot up and over a barrier, simulating the car door sill. This activity should be done in chairs without arm rests.

Sitting Exercises on the Therapy Ball

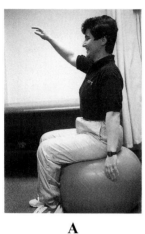
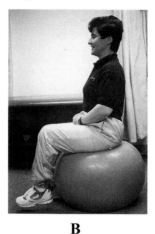
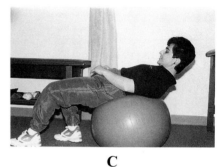

A   **B**   **C**

Figure 7–23 Phase II: sitting exercises on the therapy ball. The patient first works on simply balancing with the feet flat. (**A**) Keeping the back erect, the patient next moves the upper extremities or trunk while the legs stabilize the body, maintaining balance. (**B**) The patient then begins unilateral lower extremity open-chain exercising (hip flexion, knee extension, etc.), forcing the stabilizing leg to work harder to maintain balance. (**C**) The patient can also walk slowly (under control) away from the ball, allowing the ball to roll along the back into the bridge position and then back to sitting. This is a high-level activity requiring good strength, balance, and control.

the base of support is significantly reduced, requiring greater balance, motor control, and muscle strength.

The next step of the phase II program is to have the patient attempt the task as quickly as possible but under control and without loss of balance. Nuzik et al[15] measured the average time needed to complete the sit-to-stand transfer and found that it took 1.8 seconds. In a different study by Nevitt et al,[16] the inability to rise from a chair within 2 seconds without using the arms was one of four risk factors associated with a greater incidence of falling in the older population. This provides the clinician with a more objective guideline (and goal) for determining whether the patient is taking too long to complete the task. Of equal importance, the therapist needs to observe whether the patient can safely get up from a chair in sufficient time to answer the phone or door.

It is important to remember that, whenever possible, some aspect of the phase II program should be performed in the same treatment session as the phase I program (and not a week later). It is the integration of the basic exercises

and component task abilities into the real functional activity that causes true learning to occur.

Phase III: Solving Functional Problems

The last phase of the functional program involves the patient learning to solve independently everyday problems that arise. This requires that the sit-to-stand transfer return to being an automatic activity regardless of environmental demands in order for the person to achieve behavioral goals. The patient must therefore practice the sit-to-stand transfer independently throughout the day. If balance remains an issue, the therapist can design a supportive environment to compensate. This might entail having the patient practice standing from a sturdy chair with the dining room table placed strategically in front of the patient in case of balance loss.

The patient must also be able to do things with the upper extremities or trunk while getting out of a chair at the same time. For example, a woman standing up from a lawn chair realizes that she is being bitten by a mosquito. She stops in midactivity to swat it and then contin- ues standing up. Another example involves a man standing up from a kitchen chair while si- multaneously picking up his dishes to bring to the sink. To get up, he pushes his chair back- ward with the backs of his thighs and proceeds to the sink. To train these multiple-task actions, the therapist asks the patient to begin to stand (or sit) and then says, "Stop!" while the patient is in midactivity. The patient learns to balance under control in all positions of the task in this way. The therapist can then have the patient either return to sitting or complete the transfer to balanced standing. The task gets more difficult as the squat deepens (ie, as the patient nears the chair). The patient should also practice standing up while holding a glass or other object in the hand (Figure 7–24). As the patient progresses, the object can be made larger or heavier, or the glass can simply be filled with water.

For the special sit-to-stand activity of getting out of a car or truck, the therapist should ob- serve the patient interacting with the actual car in question. The therapist allows the patient to solve the problem alone and then may discuss different strategies to protect an area or make the activity easier. Unless compensatory methods are needed, the therapist should encourage the patient to get in and out of the car in one smooth movement (as the patient did before the injury) rather than break the activity up into its compo- nents (Figure 7–25).

Floor-to-Stand Transfer

The ability to get on and off the floor or ground voluntarily and under control is impor- tant for many high-level skills in sports and at work. It is also an imperative, even life-saving

Sit-to-Stand while Carrying an Object

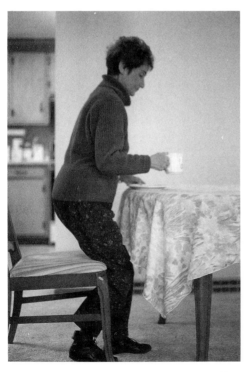
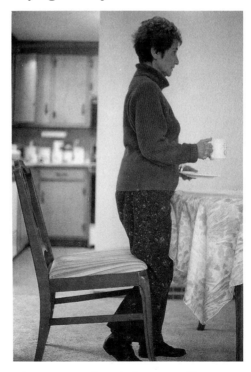

Figure 7–24 Phase III: sit-to-stand while carrying objects. The patient must now rely on the lower extremities to automati- cally come to stand while concentrating on carrying the objects (an empty mug and plate from the table). By increasing the size or weight of the plate or by filling the mug with liquid, the need to concentrate on the task becomes greater.

Car Transfers

A

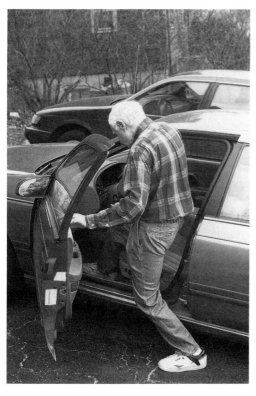

B

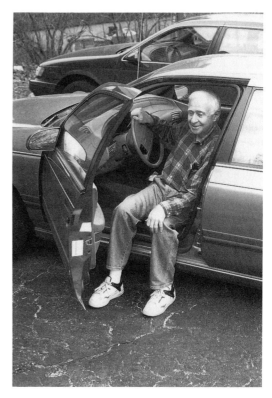

Figure 7–25 Phase III: car transfers. (**A**) The patient attempts to get into (and out of) the car in one fluid movement as he did prior to injury. (**B**) Only if pain occurs or the risk of injury is too great should the patient be forced to use the alternative strategy of breaking the activity up into its component tasks: backing up to the seat, sitting down while holding the steering wheel or seat back, slowly bringing one foot and then the other into the car, and so forth.

ability for the elderly person who falls. In the author's clinical experience, any patient who learns to get on and off the floor safely regardless of age shows an immediately improved gait pattern and stair-climbing ability. The floor-to-stand transfer requires great strength and balance. In essence, it is the last few stages of the developmental sequence taught in all therapy schools. Many orthopaedic patients never learn this important skill, however, because developmental sequence has been thought of as more of a neurologic approach. By altering which foot is placed in front or behind, the therapist can protect an injured joint. For example, when the patient is working into high kneeling, the front hip is flexed to 90° while the rear hip remains in

neutral. The front knee bears the patellofemoral load of the kneel, but the rear knee is compressed into the floor. The front ankle and foot can stay in neutral position, but the rear ankle and great toe dorsiflex.

The floor-to-stand transfer is a continuation of the lunge exercise. The therapist must carefully assess hip rotational alignment and patella tracking while the patient attempts the activity. The back should remain erect. The most common error in this activity is the failure of the patient to activate the strong rear ankle and toe plantar flexors to control eccentrically the lowering body and concentrically power the rising body. In conjunction with the front leg quadriceps action, the activity becomes easier and smoother.

Phase I: Beginning Locomotor Activity

The patient continues to work on progressively deeper bilateral and unilateral squats (Figure 7–3) and lunges (Figure 7–21). Resistive tubing can be used to increase the intensity of the exercises (Figure 7–26.)

The floor-to-stand transfer is then worked at from both ends of the activity in the following manner. On an exercise mat or plinth, the patient gets into a bilateral or low-kneeling position and works on hip extension strength while simultaneously stretching out the quadriceps by trying to sit back onto the heels and rise up (Figure 7–27). The patient only goes down toward the heels as far as can be controlled safely. The back remains erect during the activity. After about 10 repetitions or at the patient's tolerance, the activity is stopped. Next, the patient begins in standing position and, with the support of furniture, attempts to get onto the floor in a high-kneeling position. The therapist gauges the distance from the floor at which the patient loses control of the activity and stops the transfer before injury occurs. With the patient resting (from the ordeal), the clinician finds a suitable way to raise the floor height for the patient. This may entail the use of a low seat, a floor stool, aerobic steps, or (best of all) Styrofoam exercise mats (Figure 7–28). The clinician builds up the floor to a height sufficient for the patient to kneel onto the surface independently without using the hands for support (the rehabilitation specialist should measure the height or number of mats for documentation purposes). The patient then practices the activity independently, exploring different strategies of getting up and down. The therapist makes sure that optimal postural alignment is maintained and that the patient is in fact pushing off the rear foot to help

Squats and Lunges with Resistive Tubing

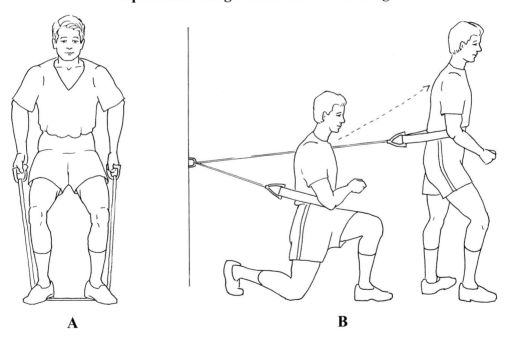

A   **B**

Figure 7–26 Phase I: squats and lunges with resistive tubing. (**A**) The patient can perform one- or two-legged squats while variable resistance is provided by surgical tubing. (**B**) Lunges progressing into kneel-downs can be resisted in various directions by surgical tubing attached to a pelvic belt. The deeper the squat, the more difficult the activity. Great care should be taken to ensure good postural alignment of the back, hips, and knees because the patient may sacrifice alignment when trying to overcome the resistance.

Sitting on Heels Exercise

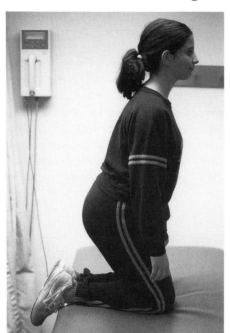 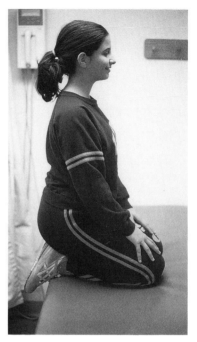

Figure 7–27 Phase I: sitting on heels exercise. From a bilateral or low-kneeling position, the patient attempts to sit back onto her heels. She stops the activity at any loss of control or from quadriceps strain. Within available range, the patient works on hip extension strengthening and quadriceps lengthening. The back should remain erect. If the patient has tight plantar flexors, the activity can begin with the feet resting in neutral position over the edge of a plinth and progress to greater range with the activity performed on the floor. This exercise also helps the chair-to-stand transfer, but it cannot be done for any length of time because of the compressive forces on the knees.

out the quadriceps. As confidence and ability build, the therapist can slowly lower the floor. Eventually (and it can take weeks), the patient regains the ability to get on and off the floor.

Phase II: Beginning Integration Program

Many activities are performed from the high-kneeling or low-squatting position, including, of course, the act of lifting. Because of the difficulty of the floor-to-stand transfer, it is better to start the phase II program after the patient can complete an independent transfer successfully and with ease. (This is the exception to the rule that the phase II program should be implemented in conjunction with the phase I program.)

The patient advances the stand-to-floor transfer by picking a light object off the floor. This progresses to larger and heavier objects (Figure 7–29). The patient also needs to do the reverse, that is, getting onto the floor while holding a weight, such as a tool chest or even just a dust rag. In addition, the patient can then carry the activity one step further by dusting a low shelf while kneeling and then rising back to standing.

(*Author's personal note:* I would not choose to dust *anything* while regaining my own functional capacity. Nevertheless, it is amazing to me how many of my patients view cleaning obscure places of their home as being of vital importance.)

Phase III: Solving Functional Problems

The final phase of the floor-to-stand program involves performing the transfer while achieving other more important functional goals. Many functional activities utilize this transfer:

- washing the floor
- changing a tire
- playing with children

Modified Floor Height for Floor-to-Stand Transfer

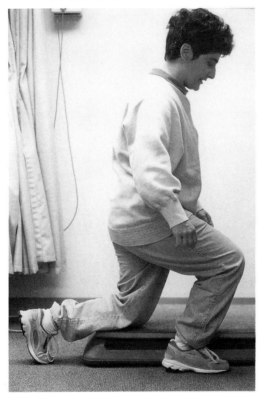

Figure 7–28 Phase I: modified floor height for floor-to-stand transfer. By having the patient kneel onto a raised floor, the activity becomes easier and doable. The modified floor can be as high as a chair, as low as a pillow on the floor, or any height in between by using sturdy building blocks, such as aerobic steps or Styrofoam exercise mats. Initially the patient can use the support of furniture, but this must be discontinued quickly so that the proper movement pattern emerges. The hips must be kept in neutral rotation so that the patellae will centrally track and the rear foot plantar flexors must activate to help eccentrically lower the patient and concentrically power the patient back up. The back should remain erect. The floor height is lowered until the patient can perform the activity from the ground. This often takes weeks to accomplish and should not be rushed.

- gardening
- getting things out of a low cupboard
- looking for contact lenses
- painting the walls

The patient needs to return to these types of activities to return to normal function at home. If needed, they can be simulated initially in the clinic under supervision. However, the patient has to begin solving the functional problems independently and that involves just getting up and down whenever the situation calls for it (instead of avoiding the activity).

For the institutionalized patient, the actual activity of getting on and off the floor is only needed in the event of a fall (which can be a good reason to learn it). In many cases, the institution itself frowns on the patient taking the risk to participate in such a transfer. Therefore, if the patient desires to learn this task, the clinician should continue the training under supervision.

Many patients, especially the frail elderly, wish never to get onto the floor for the rest of their lives. If the patient never desires to wash the floors, simply kneeling on and off the floor once a day is usually enough to maintain the ability if it is ever needed (as when the patient may fall down). If the therapist determines that the patient is unsafe to perform this activity independently, a family member or personal attendant may wish to assist with the exercise. If no one is available to help, a compensatory solution (eg, Lifeline communications) may be needed in the event of an emergency.

Stair Climbing

Although ramps are now more readily available, the ability to climb or descend stairs and curbs is still a prerequisite for normal function. Often no railings are present, especially on small sets of steps. The standard stair pitch is approximately 7 in and can easily reach as high as 11.5 in while still conforming to building codes.[17] The average curb height is also about 7 in and ranges from 4.5 to 8.4 in (11.5 to 21.5 cm), depending on the community setting.[9]

Lifting from the Floor

A   B

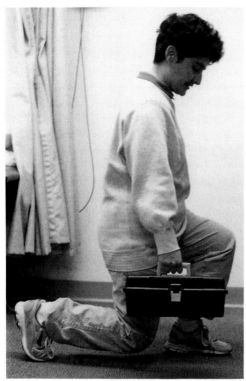
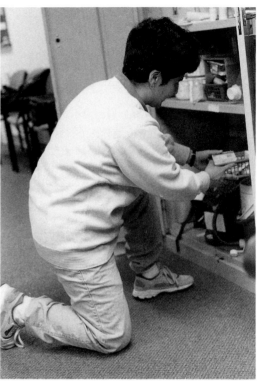

Figure 7–29 Phase II: lifting from the floor. The activity of lifting an object off the floor or of placing one on the floor is an important advancement of the floor-to-stand transfer. Without the use of the hands, the patient must balance and slowly lower herself to the floor. (**A**) The patient can practice the activity using a pocketbook, a toolbox, or a milk crate. (**B**) The patient can also spend a small amount of time in the kneeling position performing another task, such as cleaning out a bottom shelf. The time spent stationary in the kneeling posture makes the act of getting up more difficult.

Negotiating the average 7-in stair (step over step) requires moderate amounts of flexion and full extension of both the knee and the hip. The joint motion needed can be reduced by having the patient climb and descend one step at a time (Table 7–4). The joint reaction forces are greatest at the hip (3 to 6 × body weight [BW]) and at the patellofemoral joint (3.5 × BW) during stair-climbing activities. Without sufficient power of the gastrocnemius, quadriceps, and gluteus maximus, the patient accomplishes the task of stair climbing by inefficient compensatory actions. These alternative strategies include pulling the body up the stairs with the upper extremities anchored to a railing and using excessive pelvic and back oscillations.

The functional program therefore emphasizes strengthening of the lower extremities and improving the ability to balance dynamically. Modification of the environment in the form of reducing the stair pitch greatly helps reduce the joint motions and forces needed to perform the activity.[17] Altering the step height allows the patient to immediately utilize efficient movement patterns while strength and balance levels return.

Phase I: Beginning Locomotor Activities

To achieve sufficient strength of the entire lower limb, the patient begins bilateral and unilateral heel-offs (Figure 7–2) and squats (Figure

Table 7–4 Mean ROM Needed To Negotiate 7-in Stairs One Step at a Time

One Step at a Time	Mean Hip Motions*	Mean Knee Motions[†]
Up		
First leg	67° flexion, 7° extension, 8° abduction, 10° external rotation	0°–73°
Second leg		0°–62°
Down		
First leg	36° flexion, 7° abduction, 5° external rotation	0°–43°
Second leg		0°–76°

Note: To ascend and descend stairs step over step requires slightly more flexion: approximately 80° of both hip and knee flexion.
Source: Data from *Clinical Orthopedics and Related Research*, Vol. 72, p. 209, J.B. Lippincott Co., ©1970; [†]*Physical Therapy,*
Vol. 52, No. 1, p. 38, American Physical Therapy Association, © 1972.

7–3). Resistance can be added with rubber tubing (Figure 7–26). In addition, the patient should begin basic plyometric jumps on level surfaces (Figure 7–13).

During this phase, the patient also begins step-ups. Initially, the therapist chooses a low-pitched sturdy step, such as a 4-in-high aerobic step. The patient steps up and down in all directions: forward, backward, and laterally (Figure 7–30). Postural alignment must be maintained. The patient should not bend the trunk forward excessively or allow the hips to rotate. The patellae must remain centrally tracked or patello-femoral dysfunction will occur (or worsen). Lateral step-ups have been shown to increase quadriceps activity significantly[18] and should be especially used to increase knee extensor strength. During forward step-ups, the therapist must make sure that the patient is activating the gastrocnemius muscle at the ankle. Oftentimes, the patient is so afraid of falling while on the stairs that the entire foot, instead of just the ball of the foot, is placed in contact with the step. When the ball of the foot is placed properly and the patient uses the powerful ankle plantar flexors to assist with the task, stair climbing and descending can become easier. Because the base of support is reduced, however, this method requires a greater ability to balance.

If available, stair-climbing machines can be used for additional strengthening of the quadriceps and gastrocnemius (Figure 7–31). In a study by Cook et al,[18] stepping machines were found to cause high gastrocnemius activity compared with lateral step-ups. In any event, the therapist needs to examine the many models

of stair-climbing machines used by patients. Some machines allow the step heights to be customized, some allow both concentric and eccentric work, and some have railings for balance support. If the perfect machine cannot be found, the patient can simply use an available flight of stairs and functionally exercise the old-fashioned way.

Phase II: Beginning Integration Program

Once again, the patient should work on phase II program skills during the same session as the phase I program to promote carryover into the actual activity of negotiating stairs and curbs. The patient progresses from climbing (or descending) one step at a time to the step-over-step technique. The therapist can make the activity more difficult by increasing the pitch of the stair. Excessive trunk lean indicates insufficient strength of the lower extremities. Ambulation devices and railings can be used as needed. The patient should be able to stop at any time while on the stairs without loss of balance or control. Although safety is the paramount issue on the stairs, the need to get from one level to another in a reasonable amount of time cannot be overestimated. Patients often complain of the horrible feeling of holding up faster-paced individuals on the stairs and the pressure to go faster lest they be pushed over by impatient ambulators. Therefore, under the protective supervision of the rehabilitation specialist, the patient should practice climbing and descending the stairs at different paces. To have the power and balance to increase speed safely on the stairs,

Step-Ups and Step-Downs

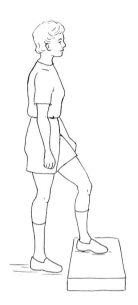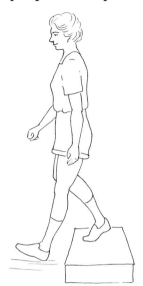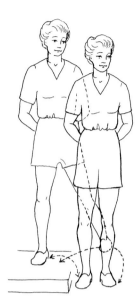

Figure 7–30 Phase I: step-ups and step-downs. Beginning initially on a 4-in aerobic step, the patient performs forward, backward, and lateral step-ups and step-downs. The therapist must make sure that proper alignment is occurring and that the hips remain in neutral with the patellae tracking centrally. The patient must activate the ankle plantar flexors if she can balance on the ball of her foot (ie, a reduced base of support).

Stair-Climbing Machines

A

B

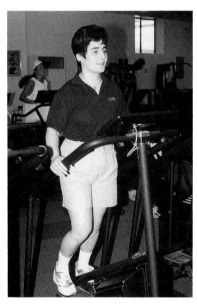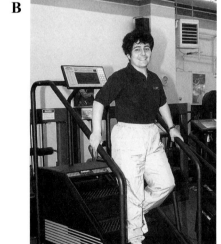

Figure 7–31 Phase I: stair-climbing machines. **(A)** Exercising on a stair climbing machine simulates, but does not duplicate, the functional activity of ascending and descending stairs. Utilizing a stair climber increases activity of the quadriceps but especially increases activity of the gastrocnemius.[18] **(B)** Depending on the machine, eccentric work of the quadriceps and gastrocnemius can be elicited by turning around and walking down the rising stairs.

the patient can progress the low-level plyometrics program by advancing the jumps off a 4-in-high surface (Figure 7–32). Although athletes will progress to higher box jumps, the average patient with orthopaedic problems can accomplish the highly skilled goal of lightly running the stairs by performing the plyometric exercise of jumping off a low platform, such as an aerobic step.

Phase III: Solving Functional Problems

The last portion of the stair-climbing program involves problem solving by the patient: how to get up the stairs holding a laundry basket or bag of groceries, how to get safely onto the sidewalk after crossing the street, how to climb a ladder to paint the wall while holding a wet paint brush, and the like. The patient can surely practice some of these activities in the clinic or at home. Once the basics are cognitively learned or relearned, however, the patient must figure out life's stair problems by simply doing them as each occasion arises.

Patients in nursing homes or long-term care settings should be able to negotiate the fire stairs before being discharged from therapy. Because of the need to move large numbers of people quickly, fire stairs usually have larger pitches than general purpose stairs, making them harder to use.[17] The patient should be trained on these exact stairs while being taught how to exit the building during an emergency.

Athletes and other high-level patients should be able to run up and down stairs under control. Railings can be used initially for safety pur-

Low-Level Plyometrics: Advanced Jumps

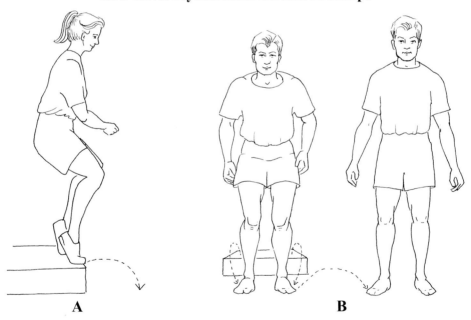

A   **B**

Figure 7–32 Phase II: low-level plyometrics: advanced jumps. (**A**) The jumping program progresses to jumping off and on various heights in all directions and is also called box jumping. The patient must first demonstrate the ability to control stepping off and on the height before initiating this exercise. The average patient (as opposed to the athlete) only needs to use a small increase of 4 in in vertical height (such as provided by an aerobic step) to achieve an enormous change in the intensity of the program. (**B**) Adding a lateral cutting maneuver at the end of a forward jump increases the difficulty of the exercise. Aside from increasing the height of the platform, the therapist can increase the difficulty of the program by changing the base of support (bilateral versus unilateral jumps), the velocity, and the resistance. These high-level activities help restore the ability to run up or down a flight of stairs.

poses. Although running the stairs is a high-skill activity, most able-bodied people get up and down stairs in this fashion without even realizing that they are running. Since it is a normal functional skill, the therapist should not balk at teaching the patient how to go quickly on the stairs if the patient has the ability and desire to do so.

Each patient will identify areas other than standing, walking, transfers, and stair climbing that he or she deems necessary to regain normal function. With the clinician's help, a more individualized functional program can be developed to augment the basic program presented here.

ADAPTATIONS FOR SPECIFIC MUSCULOSKELETAL DISORDERS

Although the general functional program helps restore the patient's ability to interact with the environment regardless of the actual diagnosis or physical impairment, the rehabilitation specialist should be aware that individual modifications are necessary to protect injured sites and to optimize the benefits of the program for each patient. A sampling of some common lower extremity impairments and the associated adaptations to the functional program is presented. The list is by no means exhaustive or all inclusive and should be used only as a guide for individualizing the functional treatment program.

Hip Disorders

The hip is an inherently stable ball-and-socket joint with a strong joint capsule and ligamentous support system. The muscles surrounding the hip are massive and provide additional stability when the primary movers maintain dominance over the secondary movers. The hip normally withstands joint reaction forces many times the body weight during everyday activities as well as during work and sports activities.

When dysfunction occurs at the joint itself, the ability to absorb and transmit forces dimin-

ishes and can become painful. These dysfunctions include:

- osteoarthritis
- rheumatoid arthritis
- total hip arthroplasty
- aseptic necrosis of the femoral head
- postural dysfunction
- hip fracture

Exercises and activities that place excessive compressive forces or torque should be minimized (done bilaterally or in a water environment) but do not have to be avoided. Patients with total hip arthroplasties need to be more cautious because an artificial joint with different characteristics has replaced their own joint (Table 7–5). For each individual patient with hip joint problems, the known disadvantage of increasing the hip joint reaction force needs to be weighed against the potential benefits realized by walking briskly, getting out of a chair without arm rests, going hiking, lifting weights, playing sports, etc.

Often, initial painful episodes at the hip joint set off a cascade of muscular changes including altered length, strength, and firing patterns. The reverse of course is true in postural dysfunction, with poor postural alignment altering the length of the surrounding musculature, thereby causing joint problems. The therapist must therefore restore the muscular support system while protecting the hip joint as well as the low back and knee. Whenever possible, the patient should attempt to achieve:

- hip extension to neutral or hyperextension to 10° controlled by the gluteus maximus
- hip abduction controlled by the gluteus medius
- hip in neutral rotation controlled by balance of internal and external rotators
- hip flexion controlled by the iliopsoas

While implementing the full body program, including the functional component, the clinician must step back and see how the patient is interacting with the environment. Only when the patient begins to solve problems independently to achieve behavioral goals does the person emerge from the therapeutic process ready to get on with life again.

Knee Disorders

The knee consists of two separate joints: the patellofemoral joint and the tibiofemoral joint. The same functional activities and exercises affect them differently. Modifications to the program to protect injured sites also differ depending on which joint is impaired.

Patellofemoral Problems

The patellofemoral joint consists of the patella riding along the trochlear groove of the femur. Although the patella is covered with the thickest cartilage in the body,[19] it can be eroded by poor tracking and lack of nutrition. Many impairments fall under the collective heading of patellofemoral disorders:

- chondromalacia patellae
- patella alta or baja
- patellar osteoarthritis
- patella tracking problems
- anterior knee pain
- patella fracture
- patellofemoral malalignment
- plica syndrome
- quadriceps tendinitis

Postural considerations can affect the patellofemoral joint. Femoral rotation influences the ability of the patella to remain within the groove. In addition, foot position (as in excessive pronation) can alter patella tracking. The soft tissue structures that influence patella tracking include the following:

- quadriceps femoris
- TFL and ITB
- hamstrings
- gastrocnemius
- patella retinaculum
- plica (embryological seam of the knee synovium)

Proper muscle length and postural alignment help restore this joint to optimal functioning. Specific treatments to correct patella tracking

Table 7–5 Functional Exercises and Total Hip Precautions

Functional Exercise	Total Hip Precautions
Crossover or Carioca stepping	Avoid; no simultaneous flexion, adduction, internal rotation
Circular and figure-of-eight drills	Large circles only; begin after postoperative (PO) week 3
Shuttle walking	Plant and pivot on unaffected side only
Fitter and glide board	High level; avoid up to PO month 4; check with physician
Sit-to-stand transfers	Chair/toilet height must be sufficient to prevent dislocations
Car transfers	Avoid initially; keep modified to prevent dislocation
Therapeutic ball exercises	Need sufficient height; may substitute stool on wheels
Sitting on heels	Avoid; dislocation danger too great
Floor-to-stand transfers	Keep affected hip in neutral (back leg on high kneel)
Lifting	Avoid heavy lifting; maintain hip in neutral

Note: For a lateral or posterolateral approach, the patient should avoid simultaneous hip flexion, adduction, and internal rotation. In addition, many physicians routinely order no flexion beyond 90° or no adduction and internal rotation beyond neutral. Most functional exercises can be done with only slight modifications to the program to ensure that proper positioning is maintained. The greatest danger of dislocation is within the first 3 weeks following surgery. After 4 months the capsule is considered healed, and some physicians remove the precautions whereas others leave standing orders forever. In any event, the patient should always avoid maintaining any torqued position during functional exercises and activities. Questions should be referred to the surgeon, who knows the condition of the bone stock, the amount of motion safely achieved in surgery, and any complications that may have occurred.

include the use of ultrasound, biofeedback, stretching, myofascial release, taping or bracing, and exercises to balance the musculature. More detailed information about exact treatments for these disorders can be found in the literature.[20]

Adaptations of the functional exercise program are needed to protect this joint from excessive forces caused by antigravity activities, such as sit-to-stand transfers, squats, stair climbing, and others. The patellofemoral joint bears excessive compressive forces when the knee flexes beyond 20°.[21] If improper tracking is occurring, the compressive forces are concentrated on small portions of the patellar cartilage, causing accelerated destruction. During the acute stage of injury, beginning functional activities and exercises should avoid that motion.

When the pain and swelling subside, the patient can initiate other parts of the functional program as long as proper patella alignment is maintained through postural correction or taping (Table 7–6). In fact, pain-free exercising throughout range will actually help correct the problem, since proper tracking allows the com-

pressive forces to be spread over a larger surface, promoting cartilage nutrition. During this subacute stage, the patient should initiate backward running before forward running because it has been shown to increase quadriceps strength and power while decreasing eccentric loading.[22] With increased pain as a simple indicator of improper technique, the patient with patellofemoral problems can participate fully in the general functional rehabilitation program. It is imperative that the patient control hip rotational alignment as well as foot alignment when performing the functional program.

Tibiofemoral Problems

The tibiofemoral joint is the joint of weight bearing. Damage to this joint generally causes pain during walking and standing activities. Tibiofemoral joint problems encompass a wide variety of musculoskeletal disorders:

- meniscal tear
- tibial spine or plateau fracture
- osteoarthritis

Table 7–6 Adaptations of the Functional Program for Patellofemoral Dysfunction

Functional Exercises	Acute Stage	Subacute Stage
One-legged standing balance	Keep hip in neutral, pelvis level, patella central	Keep hip in neutral, pelvis level, patella central
Bilateral minisquats	1/4 squat, small ball between knees to recruit adductors	1/2 squat, can add resistance with rubber tubing
Unilateral minisquats	Avoid initially	1/4 to 1/2 squat
Treadmill	All directions walking	Begin retrorunning, progress to forward running
Lunges	Small; keep patella positioned over second toe	Larger; keep patella positioned over second toe, add resistance
Sit-to-stand transfer	Modify for pain-free function (use pillows to increase seat height)	All chairs, including toilets
Floor-to-stand transfer	Progress to deeper lunge pain-free	Progress lunge to high-kneel position
Lifting	From waist height	From floor height
Step-ups and step-downs	4-in step only	7-in step, progress to full flight of stairs

Note: The patient must concentrate on optimal hip, knee, and foot alignment to ensure central tracking of the patella. In the acute stage, knee flexion beyond 20° is discouraged. As the patient improves, the same exercises are performed in increased flexion or with resistance. Vastus medialis oblique (VMO) strengthening is emphasized because the VMO functions to pull the patella medially. The functional program can be performed with patella taping or bracing and biofeedback if desired.

- rheumatoid arthritis
- osteochondral lesions or fractures
- osteochondritis dissecans
- ligament sprains or tears (cruciates and/or collaterals)

In the acute stage, the tibiofemoral joint forces can be mitigated during the functional program to protect the injured structures and allow them to heal. This can be accomplished by limited weight bearing (by using crutches or a pool environment) or by limited exercising (slow, submaximal effort without resistance).[23] For the patient with anterior cruciate ligament (ACL) deficiency, the closed-chain component of the functional program is particularly helpful in restoring prior abilities without causing undue anterior tibial displacement.[24]

The functional program augments the special protocols established for different disorders, such as ACL reconstruction. In many instances, portions of the functional program are found within these rigid protocols (Table 7–7). For all tibiofemoral dysfunctions, the therapist needs to progress the functional program carefully to prevent further degeneration of the joint. In general, planting and pivoting of the injured leg as well as plyometric activities can further damage already weakened tibiofemoral joint structures and are contraindicated in the acute stage.[25–27] As healing occurs, the patient progresses to these more stressful types of activities. Many patients, however, especially those with arthritis, should continue to limit impact loading and pivoting maneuvers in daily life, work, and sports.

Table 7–7 Accelerated ACL Reconstruction Rehabilitation Protocol (Activities in Boldface Indicate Correlations of the Exercise Program with the Functional Program)

Time after Reconstruction	*Rehabilitation Program*
Day 1	Continuous passive motion (CPM), rigid knee immobilizer in full extension for walking, weight bearing as tolerated without crutches
2–3 days	CPM, passive ROM 0° to 90° (emphasis on full extension), weight bearing as tolerated without crutches
2–4 days	Discharge from hospital; CPM at home. *Note:* Prerequisites to discharge are satisfactory pain management, full extension symmetric to nonoperated knee, able to do SLR for leg control, full weight bearing with or without crutches
7–10 days	ROM terminal extension, prone hands (2 lb) if patient has not achieved full extension, towel extensions, wall slides, heel slides, active-assisted flexion, strengthening—**knee bends, step-ups, calf raises;** weight bearing partial to full; gradual elimination of required use of knee immobilizer
2–3 weeks	ROM (0° to 110°), **unilateral knee bends, step-ups, calf raises, StairMaster 4000, weight room activities: leg press, quarter squats and calf raises in the squat rack,** stationary bicycling, swimming, custom-made functional knee brace with no preset limits (to be used at all times out of the home for the next 4 weeks)
5–6 weeks	ROM (0° to 130°), isokinetic evaluation with 20° block at 180°/sec and 240°/sec. When strength is 70% or greater than the opposite unoperated knee, the patient can begin **lateral shuffles, Cariocas, light jogging, jumping rope, agility drills, weight room activities,** stationary bicycling, and swimming. *Note:* Functional brace discontinued (except for sports activities) when muscle tone and strength are sufficient.
10 weeks	Full ROM; isokinetic evaluation at 60°/sec, 180°/sec, and 240°/sec, KT-1000, increased agility workouts, sport-specific activities
16 weeks	Isokinetic evaluation, KT-1000, increased agility workouts
4–6 months	Return to full sports participation (*if* patient has met criteria of full ROM, no effusion, good knee stability, and has completed the running program)

Note: SLR = straight leg raise
Source: Reprinted from *The American Journal of Sports Medicine*, Vol. 18, No. 3, p. 294, with permission of the American Orthopaedica Society for Sports Medicine, © 1990.

Combined Patellofemoral and Tibiofemoral Problems

Due to the proximity of the two joints to each other, many problems commonly affect both joints of the knee. Most open surgeries damage the extensor mechanism, requiring rehabilitation of the patellofemoral joint in addition to whatever injury was surgically repaired. Even arthroscopic surgery can affect patellofemoral function. The therapist needs to be aware that loss of ROM or painful movement at the knee can easily be attributed to dysfunction at the patellofemoral joint, even if the diagnosis or impairment is clearly located at the tibiofemoral joint.

The ACL-deficient knee requires special rehabilitation to protect the ligament while ensuring patellofemoral integrity. The tension on the posterolateral and intermediate bundles of the ACL increases as the knee moves into extension.[28] Many ACL protocols limit terminal knee extension in the acute stage to prevent excessive forces from acting on the reconstruction. However, terminal knee extension is the preferred ROM to begin rehabilitation of patellofemoral dysfunction. Therefore, the best treatment compromise for the patient with ACL reconstruction is to perform the ACL exercises without sacrificing central tracking of the patella. Rehabilitation of this problem is not complete until the strength, stability, and motor control of the extensor mechanism are restored.

Patients with total knee arthroplasties (TKAs) also have to rehabilitate both the patellofemoral and tibiofemoral joints. Therapists tend to concentrate treatment efforts on the tibiofemoral joint, but the patellofemoral joint is often the cause of stiffness, pain, and loss of function. The degree of constraint built into the arthroplasty (totally constrained, semiconstrained, or unconstrained) as well as the fixation method (cemented or uncemented) determine the patient's ability to participate in the functional program (Table 7–8). In general, the lesser the constraint, the greater the available ROM and the greater the ability to perform high-level ambulation skills, including stair climbing. Patients with fully constrained TKAs should only perform minimal functional programs to restore basic ADL skills. Patients with cemented TKAs have immediately stable knees that can withstand most stresses from the functional program without prosthetic loosening.

Ankle and Hindfoot Problems

The calcaneus is the first skeletal part to contact the ground during normal ambulation activities. The invertors and evertors control the forces transmitted to the subtalar joint, and the dorsiflexors and plantar flexors control the ankle (talocrural) joint. In addition, the deltoid ligament and three lateral ligaments (calcaneofibular and anterior and posterior talofibulars) help maintain stability. Although large joint reaction forces occur during gait (3 to 6 × BW), the large surface area of the ankle mitigates the force per unit area.[29] Lateral displacement of the talus on the tibiofibular mortise by as little as 1 mm, however, reduces the weight-bearing area by 42%,[30] thereby doubling the loading on the remaining cartilage.[31] Many patients with ankle and hindfoot injuries avoid both heel strike (weight acceptance) and toe-off (push) during the stance phase of the gait cycle, as these two activities cause high joint reaction forces. Injuries to this region of the body include:

- ligament sprain or tear
- ankle fracture
- plantar fasciitis
- osteoarthritis
- rheumatoid arthritis
- total ankle arthroplasty
- Achilles tendon strain or rupture
- calcaneal bursitis
- painful calcaneal heel pad

In the acute stages of ankle and hindfoot injury, the patient must protect the injured structures from excessive weight-bearing forces. The functional program can be performed bilaterally or in a pool environment; the basic exercise program is done in the sitting or supine position. Some conditions, such as severe ankle sprain,

Table 7–8 Functional Exercises and TKA: Guidelines To Modify Functional Program for Different Types of TKAs

Functional Exercise	Cemented TKA: Semiconstrained and Unconstrained	Uncemented TKA: Semiconstrained and Unconstrained
Standing program: balance, toe-offs, heel-offs, squats, etc.	Safe; progress to unilateral as tolerated	Safe bilaterally; maintain weight-bearing (WB) precautions, avoid torque
Walking: all directions	Safe; velocity as tolerated	Maintain WB precautions
Agility: Carioca, figure-of-eights, shuttle walking	Safe, but slow velocity, gentle pivots	Pivots on unaffected side only, maintain WB precautions
Plyometrics: basic jumps	Light vertical leaps, emphasis on ankle muscles	Contraindicated except in water environment
Treadmill: walking	All directions, velocity as tolerated	All directions, use railings to maintain WB status
Glide board/Fitter	Avoid; excessive lateral forces	Contraindicated
Lunges	Helps achieve flexion, maintain patella tracking	Maintain WB precautions and patella tracking
Sit-to-stand	Important; builds strength, maintains patella tracking	Important; builds strength; use arm rests to maintain WB
Car transfers	Modify; back up into seat	Modify; back up into seat
Therapeutic ball exercises	Strengthens knee muscles, increases ROM	Strengthens knee muscles, increases ROM, protects WB
Sitting on heels	Contraindicated	Contraindicated
Floor-to-stand	Progress lunge to high-kneel with affected knee forward	Progress lunge slowly, maintain WB precautions
Lifting	Light weights only, <20 lb	After full WB, light weights
Step-ups/downs and stairs	Begin 4 in, progress to regular stair height (7 in)	Begin 4 in to 7 in, use railings to maintain WB

Note: As more constraint or stability is built into the TKA, available motion is reduced. For fully constrained TKAs (eg, as Waldius hinge, spherocentric, etc.), the patient should perform the most minimal functional program possible to restore ADLs. Excessive motion and activity loosen the fully constrained TKA. Although good functional results occur equally after semiconstrained and unconstrained TKAs, patients with totally unconstrained TKAs (eg, Cloutier) consistently perform better during stair-climbing activities.

ankle fracture, or Achilles tendon rupture, may be casted initially to prevent excessive motion and to allow the structures to heal. Compressive wrapping and modalities such as ultrasound or electrical stimulation may be used as needed to reduce swelling and promote healing.

As the injury improves, the functional and exercise programs become more intensive. The patient trains to maintain postural alignment of the entire lower chain, stretches out shortened structures, and strengthens weakened ones. The therapist fully examines and recommends the need for alternative footwear, orthotics, and protective padding or doughnuts to relieve excessive forces. In many instances of fracture or severe strain, full weight bearing is not resumed until 6 to 8 weeks after injury.[31] Table 7–9 sum-

marizes the general progression of the functional program in relationship to the healing stages of injuries to the ankle and hindfoot. As always, specific adaptations need to be made to these guidelines to customize treatment for the individual.

Forefoot and Toe Problems

The forefoot and toes work with the rest of the foot to absorb ground reaction forces (during pronation) and to provide a rigid framework for propulsion (during supination). The beam action of the metarsophalangeal joint (MTP) takes up 25% of the static weight-bearing stress on the foot, while the plantar aponeurosis (fas-

Table 7–9 Functional Exercises in Relation to Healing Stages of Ankle and Hindfoot Injuries

Functional Exercise	Acute Condition: Protected Weight Bearing	Mostly Healed: Full Weight Bearing
Standing program: balance, wobble board, toe-offs, heel-offs, squats, etc.	In sitting or protected standing or in pool environment	Begin bilaterally, progress to unilaterally
Walking: straight in all directions	Protected weight bearing, slow velocity	Walk on toes, on heels, normally, progress velocity
Running	Contraindicated	Begin retrorunning first, progress to all directions
Agility: Carioca, figure-of-eights, shuttle walking	In pool only, large gentle circles, slow velocity	Progress to smaller circles, faster velocity
Plyometrics	Contraindicated	Basic to advanced jumps
Glide board/Fitter/StairMaster	Contraindicated	Progress intensity as needed
Sit-to-stand	Injured foot in front, most weight on unaffected foot	Feet even, or injured foot in rear to accept more weight
Sitting on heels	Avoid if painful	Excellent plantar flexion stretch
Floor-to-stand	Only if protected weight bearing	Progress lunge into high kneel
Step-ups/downs and stairs	Maintain weight bearing with crutches or railing	Progress from foot-flat to ball of foot (using plantar flexors)

Note: Partial weight bearing must be maintained in the acute and subacute stages. When full weight-bearing orders are received, the patient can progress the intensity of exercise and functional programs as tolerated.

cia) takes up approximately 60%.[32] Dynamically, these structures take up more force through the windlass effect caused by toe extension.[32] This ability to extend at the MTP joint maintains the integrity of the foot into supination, providing the needed leverage for push-off. The forefoot also is active in negotiating stairs, curbs, and uneven terrain. The ability or inability of the foot to provide shock absorption as well as power affects the amount of joint motion and strength needed in the knee and hip joints during functional activities. Common injuries to the forefoot and toes include:

- metatarsalgia
- march fracture
- splay foot
- rheumatoid arthritis
- fat pad pain
- plantar neuroma
- Morton's toe (short first toe)
- hallux valgus (bunion)
- hallux rigidis
- hammer toe

Postural alignment, especially the maintenance of the longitudinal and transverse arches of the foot, is the key to most treatment of forefoot disorders. The clinician must correctly place pads or design orthotics so that proper foot motion can occur. Initially, protective weight bearing can allow the injured structures the necessary time to heal. In addition, the patient must strengthen the dynamic stabilizers of the foot: the intrinsic foot muscles as well as the posterior tibialis, flexor hallucis longus, and peroneal muscles. Ankle dorsiflexion, foot inversion, and MTP dorsiflexion must also be restored for more efficient and pain-free foot motion to occur.[33]

As the patient improves and returns to full weight bearing, he or she can begin to place more pressure onto the MTP region. The ability to move on the balls of the feet greatly increases agility and function. The clinician should progress the functional program slowly because many of the functional activities place high stress on the midfoot and forefoot regions. Plyometrics and backward running[4] transmit enormous forces to this region and are not recommended until the last stage of rehabilitation. Table 7–10 summarizes the general progression of the functional program in relation to the healing of forefoot and toe dysfunctions.

FUNCTIONAL EXERCISE PROGRESSION AND MUSCULOSKELETAL DYSFUNCTION

The modifications presented above to protect injured structures apply to the exercise portions (phases I and II) of the functional program. As the patient improves, the key to independent function involves having the patient perform actual ADLs or activities of work or sport (phase III). If dysfunction still exists, the patient's options for solving functional problems are restricted by the need to allow the injury to heal. In this common case, the clinician needs to teach the patient how to progress the functional and exercise programs independently.

The therapist must be able to predict the rate of improvement and convey this to the patient on paper. If the therapist continues to treat the patient until healing is mostly complete (even at the frequency of once every 2 weeks), the patient can report any successes or failures while attempting new or old functional tasks. The transference from performing functional exercises to truly interacting with the environment is the key to successful restoration of functional independence.

REFERENCES

1. Perry J. The mechanics of walking: a clinical interpretation. In: Perry J, Hislop H, eds. *Principles of Lower-Extremity Bracing.* Washington, DC: American Physical Therapy Association; 1967: 9–32.

2. Devita P, Stribling J. Lower extremity joint kinetics and energetics during backward running. *Med Sci Sports Exerc.* 1991;23(5):602–610.

3. Winter DA, Pluck N, Yang JF. Backward walking: a simple reversal of forward walking? *J Mot Behav.* 1989; 21:291–305.

Table 7–10 Functional Exercises in Relation to Healing Stage of Forefoot and Toe Injuries

Functional Exercise	Acute and Subacute: Protected Weight Bearing	Fully Healed: Full Weight Bearing
Standing program: balance, wobble board, toe-offs, squats, etc.	In protected standing or sitting, heel-offs (plantar flexion), open-chain only	Begin bilaterally, progress to unilaterally
Walking: straight in all directions	Protected weight bearing, avoid toe-off (push)	Normal gait, heel walking, light toe-walking
Running	Contraindicated	Jogging forward first, running, avoid retrorunning
Agility: Carioca, figure-of-eights, shuttle walking	Protected weight bearing, pivot on unaffected side	Progress to smaller circles, faster velocity
Plyometrics	Contraindicated	Small, basic jumps only
Glide board/Fitter	Contraindicated	Progress velocity
Stair or ski machines	Contraindicated	Foot flat initially, progress to MTP dorsiflexion
Sit-to-stand	Injured foot in front, most weight on unaffected foot	Feet even, progress to injured foot in rear with MTP dorsiflexion
Floor-to-stand	Protected weight bearing, injured foot in front	If injured foot in rear, MTP dorsiflexion necessary
Step-ups/downs and stairs	Foot flat, protected weight bearing	Use balls of feet (MTP joint), activate foot supinators and ankle plantar flexors

Note: Partial weight bearing must be maintained in the acute and subacute stages. When full weight bearing is allowed, the patient slowly increases the stresses to the region as tolerated.

4. Threlkeld AJ, Horn TS, Wojtowicz GM. Kinematics, ground reaction force, and muscle balance produced by backward running. *J Orthop Sports Phys Ther.* 1989;11(2);56–63.

5. Gray GW. Chain reaction (course notes). Adrian, Mich: Wynn Marketing, Inc.; 1990.

6. Cross MJ, Gibbs NJ, Bryant GJ. An analysis of the side-step cutting maneuver. *Am J Sports Med.* 1989;17(3): 363–366.

7. Andrews JR, McLeod WD, Ward T, et al. The cutting mechanism. *Am J Sports Med.* 1977;5:111–121.

8. Baker PA, Evans DM, Lee C. Treadmill gait retraining following fracture of the femur. *Arch Phys Med Rehab.* 1991;72:649–652.

9. Robinett CS, Vondran MA. Functional ambulation velocity and distance requirements in rural and urban communities. *Phys Ther.* 1988;68(9):1371–1373.

10. Blessey RL, Hislop HJ, Water RL, et al. Metabolic energy cost of unrestrained walking. *Phys Ther.* 1976;56: 1019–1024.

11. Lewis CB. Documentation and functional assessment (course notes). Sarasota, Fla: Advanced Educational Seminars; 1992.

12. Laubenthal KN, Smidt GL, Kettelkamp DB. A quantitative analysis of knee motion during activities of daily living. *Phys Ther.* 1972;52(1):34–42.

13. Johnston RC, Smidt GL. Hip motion measurements for selected activities of daily living. *Clin Orthop.* 1970;72: 205–216.

14. Hodge WA, Carlson KL, Fijan RS, et al. Contact pressures from an instrumented hip endoprosthesis. *J Bone Joint Surg Am.* 1989;73-A (9):1378–1386.

15. Nuzik S, Lamb R, VanSant A. Sit-to-stand movement pattern: a kinematic study. *Phys Ther.* 1986;66(11): 1708–1713.

16. Nevitt MC, Cummings SR, Kidd S, et al. Risk factors for recurrent nonsyncopal falls: a prospective study. *JAMA.* 1989;261:2663–2668.

17. Kling VG. Architectural barriers. In: Erligh G, ed. *Rehabilitation Management of Rheumatic Conditions.* 2nd ed. Baltimore, Md: Williams & Wilkins; 1986:314–329.

18. Cook TM, Zimmermann CL, Lux KM, et al. EMG comparison of lateral step-up and stepping machine exercise. *J Orthop Sports Phys Ther.* 1992;16(3):108–113.

19. Evans P. *The Knee Joint.* Edinburgh, Scotland: Churchill Livingstone; 1986.

20. Shelton GL, Thigpen LK. Rehabilitation of patello-femoral dysfunction: A review of literature. *J Orthop Sports Phys Ther.* 1991;14:243–249.

21. Frankel VH, Nordin M. *Basic Biomechanics of the Skeletal System.* Philadelphia, Pa: Lea & Febiger; 1980.

22. Flynn TW, Soutas-Little RW. Mechanical power and muscle action during forward and backward running. *J Orthop Sports Phys Ther.* 1993;17(2):108–112.

23. Goldstein T. *Geriatric Orthopaedics: Rehabilitative Management of Common Problems.* Gaithersburg, Md: Aspen; 1991.

24. Yack HJ, Collins CE, Whieldon TJ. Comparison of closed and open kinetic chain exercise in the anterior cruciate ligament–deficient knee. *Am J Sports Med.* 1993;21(1):49–53.

25. Anderson MA. Rehabilitation of the athletic knee following articular cartilage injury. *Sports Med Update.* 1993;8(3):8–28.

26. Terrell J. Management of a tibial plateau fracture. *Sports Med Update.* 1993;8(3):12–16.

27. Engle RP, and Giesen DP. Anerior cruciate ligament reconstruction rehabilitation. In: Engle RP, ed. *Knee Ligament Rehabilitation.* New York, NY: Churchill Livingstone; 1991:117-134.

28. Seto JL, Brewster CE, Lombardo SJ, Tibone JE. Rehabilitation of the knee after anterior cruciate ligament reconstruction. *J Orthop Sports Phys Ther.* 1989;11(1):8–18.

29. Soderberg GL. *Kinesiology Application to Pathological Motion.* Baltimore, Md: Williams & Wilkins;1986.

30. Ramsey PL, Hamilton W. Changes in tibio-talar area of contact by lateral talar shifts. *J Bone Joint Surg Am.* 1976;58A(3):356–357.

31. Morris M, Chandler RW. Fractures of the ankle. *Tech Orthop.* 1987;2(3):10–19.

32. Donatelli R. Normal biomechanics of the foot and ankle. *J Orthop Sports Med.* 1985;7:91–95.

33. Cailliet R. *Foot and Ankle Pain.* 2nd ed. Philadelphia, Pa: Davis;1983.

ADDITIONAL READING

Albert M. *Eccentric Muscle Training in Sports and Orthopaedics.* New York, NY: Churchill Livingstone; 1991.

Andrews JR, Harrelson GL. *Physical Rehabilitation of the Injured Athlete.* Philadelphia, Pa: Saunders; 1991.

Engle RP. *Knee Ligament Rehabilitation.* New York, NY: Churchill Livingstone; 1991.

Smythe R. *Acceleration: An Illustrated Guide.* Portland, Ore: Speed City; 1988.

Smythe R. *Plyometrics: An Illustrated Guide.* Portland, Ore: Speed City; 1987.

8

Functional Exercises for the Upper Extremities

The upper extremities function to manipulate the environment. The hands interact intricately with the world by grasping, gesturing, holding, touching, etc. The shoulder, elbow, and wrist act primarily to place the hand in the desired position. The upper body collectively must be stable and strong enough to lift and carry heavy weights, mobile enough to reach desired objects, and coordinated enough to perform fine work.

GENERAL FUNCTIONAL PROGRAM

When designing the functional program, the therapist addresses the barriers to function mentioned in Chapter 6 through correctional exercises (phase I) and goal-oriented exercise (phases II and III). First, the therapist considers the interrelationships of the upper extremities to themselves as well as to the other body segments. Proper alignment of body segments must be accomplished before functional activities are initiated. The lower body segments need to provide a stable base for proper upper body motion. Oftentimes, a dysfunction in the thorax or pelvic segments is the initial cause of a cascade of motor events that results in upper extremity injury and pain.[1] In addition, many glenohumeral

instabilities and painful conditions arise from loss of scapular positioning on the thorax.

Janda[1] reports muscle imbalance patterns that occur commonly in the proximal part of the upper body and are observed as part of the classic forward-head posture. Muscles that tend to develop tightness are:

- pectoralis major
- pectoralis minor
- upper trapezius
- levator scapulae
- sternocleidomastoid

Muscles that tend to develop weakness include:

- serratus anterior
- rhomboids
- middle trapezius
- lower trapezius
- deep neck flexors
- suprahyoid
- mylohyoid

By the stretching of tight muscles and the strengthening of weak ones, a stable proximal base will develop from which to launch the functional program without inhibitory shoulder

109

pain. The therapist must observe the quality of the movement patterns to ensure that the intricate ballet of efficient scapulohumeral motion occurs with all upper extremity motion and function. The altered movement pattern of reverse scapulohumeral rhythm so commonly seen in shoulder dysfunctions, such as frozen shoulder syndrome, must be corrected during the phase I program. Oftentimes, the patient can correct the pattern simply by using a mirror for additional biofeedback and by controlling the excessive scapular motion. The therapist can also assist by manually stabilizing the scapula while the patient practices elevation activities (Figure 8–1). Klein-Vogelbach[2] calls this a buttressing mobilization.

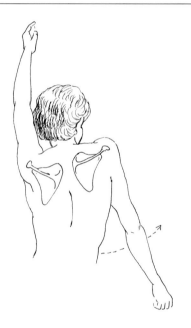

Figure 8–1 Reverse scapulohumeral rhythm. The clinician can easily recognize the altered movement pattern (right arm) commonly seen in frozen shoulder syndrome through the abnormally elevated right scapula and trunk side bend to the left (which allows the patient some arm movement, although the glenohumeral joint remains relatively motionless). This movement pattern must be corrected before pain-free shoulder function can return. To begin retraining scapulohumeral rhythm, the patient can attempt to keep the clavicles horizontal (using a mirror as biofeedback), while moving the humerus through small excursions of range in both flexion and extension. The therapist may help by manually stabilizing the scapular as the patient attempts arm movement.

Sahrmann[3] describes other faulty muscle patterns of the elbow and wrist that can lead to painful disorders. One example is the extensor carpi radialis longus acting as the prime mover in elbow flexion instead of the biceps brachii and the brachialis muscles. This pattern can lead to the development of a lateral epicondylitis (tennis elbow).

The patient begins phase I of the upper extremity functional program by first working on exercises to correct postural alignment, to strengthen and stabilize the weakened musculature, and to establish more efficient motor patterns. These exercises must then immediately blend into a total body program (phase II), which begins to integrate the upper body segments back into the rest of the person. Examples of phase II integration types of activities are:

• reaching
• lifting
• carrying
• pushing
• sport tasks

The patient must consistently practice the exercises and activities of phases I and II at home or in the hospital room. The home program should be of short duration (5 to 15 minutes) but done throughout the day. The patient then incorporates these efficient movement patterns into true functional activities (phase III). A true functional activity is an action taken by a person to achieve a goal. The phase II activity of reaching overhead becomes a phase III true functional activity when the patient reaches overhead to get a book off a shelf to read it. Through trials and practice, the patient independently figures out how to overcome functional problems in a safe and efficient way. Phase III functional activities include basic activities of daily living (ADLs), instrumental ADLs, work activities, and sports/recreational activities. Solving problems in the real world involves an element of risk that the patient must choose to undertake. These interactions are the only road to true functional independence.

Phase I Exercises

The patient begins the upper extremity correctional program by attempting the following scapular stabilization activities at the proper ability level (basic through advanced):

- humeral elevation in the scapular plane, or scaption (Figure 8–2)[4]
- chair press-ups (Figure 8–3)
- push-ups with a plus (Figure 8–4)
- scapular adduction or rowing (Figure 8–5)

Mosley et al[5] determined that the above four exercises were the most efficient in returning

Scaption

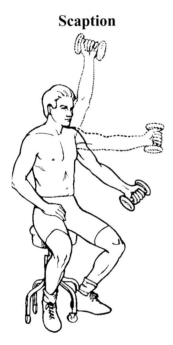

Figure 8–2 Phase I: Scaption, or humeral elevation in the scapular plane. This exercise promotes strength in the scapular stabilizers and supraspinatus as well as in the deltoid, pectoralis major, and latissimus dorsi while protecting the glenohumeral joint from excessive impingement.[4] The exercise can be performed best in sidelying, sitting, or standing position. Supine lying is not recommended as the scapula becomes pinned to the mat by the body weight. Resistance with dumbbells, cuff weights, surgical tubing, or isokinetic machines can be added. *Source:* Reprinted with permission from *Clinical Management* (1991;11[6]:44), Copyright ©1991, American Physical Therapy Association.

Chair Press-Ups

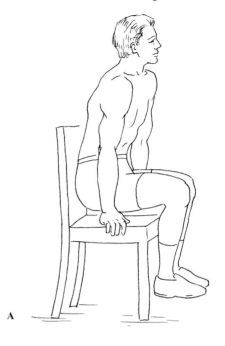

A

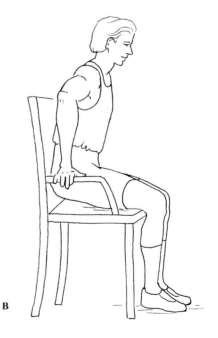

B

Figure 8–3 Phase I: Chair press-ups. **(A)** This exercise strengthens the scapular stabilizers as well as the deltoid, pectoralis major, and the latissimus dorsi.[4] **(B)** For weaker patients, the exercise can be performed from an armchair with the feet on the floor for stability. The exercise becomes more like a *dip* with the triceps contracting as well.

Push-Ups With a Plus

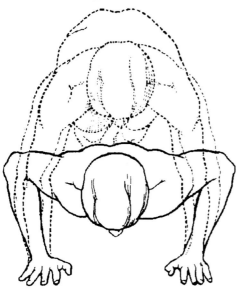

Figure 8–4   Phase I: Push-ups with a plus. This exercise strengthens the scapular stabilizers, including the serratus anterior, pectoralis minor, levator scapulae, and upper trapezius. Mosely et al[5] have shown electromyographically that the plus action, or scapular protraction, is the most beneficial arc of the exercise. The push-ups are started against a wall and progressed to the floor. Modified push-ups from the quadruped position accomplish the same goal. In addition, this exercise is extremely similar to the bench press or Nautilus upper body press machine, which can be substituted for the push-up. *Source:* Reprinted with permission from *Clinical Management* (1991;11[6]:45), Copyright ©1991, American Physical Therapy Association.

Rowing (Scapular Adduction)

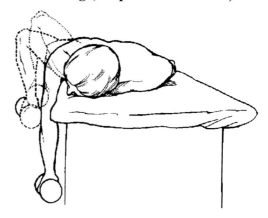

Figure 8–5   Phase I: Rowing, or scapular adduction. This exercise strengthens the trapezius, levator scapulae, and rhomboids.[4] The exercise can be performed prone (shown), in sitting with resistive tubing, or on the Nautilus rowing machine. *Source:* Reprinted with permission from *Clinical Management* (1991;11[6]:44), Copyright ©1991, American Physical Therapy Association.

needed strength to the scapular stabilizers. As mentioned previously, the therapist makes sure that the joints are properly aligned and that the lower scapular depressors are working efficiently. If they are not, additional exercises for the lower trapezius (Figures 8–6 and 8–7) should be added to the program.

As the scapula begins to resume a more optimal position on the thorax, dysfunctions of the glenohumeral joint may disappear spontaneously. Additional strengthening and stabilizing exercises for the rotator cuff should be included in the program as needed (Figures 8–8 to 8–10). In general, the rotator cuff muscles require only light resistance for strengthening. Heavy resistance will cause the body to recruit the larger sur-

rounding musculature and will diminish the rotator cuff program. Special attention should be paid to improving the strength and endurance of the small external rotators (infraspinatus and teres minor), which often fatigue during prolonged activity. During many sport activities, such as throwing a ball or serving in tennis, the loss of eccentric control of internal rotation results in glenohumeral instability.

The phase I program easily adjusts to dysfunctions of the elbow, forearm, wrist, and hand through simple modifications. Initial protection of these joints involves relieving them of pressure. For example, knuckle push-ups (Figure 8–11) maintain a neutral wrist position, and cuff weights can be used instead of dumbbells. If additional work is required at the distal joints, the program can be altered to intensify their input. For example, push-ups on a wobble board or medicine ball (Figure 8–12) or fingertip push-ups can replace standard push-ups, forcing the fingers, hands, wrists, and elbows to stabilize an unsteady surface to accomplish task. In addition, specific exercises for the distal upper extremity can be initiated while the shoulder complex is protected. Strengthening and stability

Facelying/Arm Lifts

Facelying/Arm Lifts

Purpose: strengthen muscles of the middle and lower back
and prevent use of the muscles of the upper shoulder.

Starting position: Lie face down with a towel roll under
your forehead.

Support your shoulder with a towel roll placed under the
shoulder.

____ Place a pillow under your abdomen.

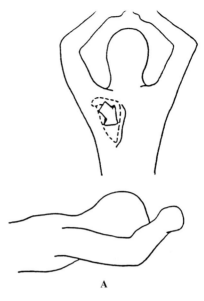

(A) Assume starting position.

Place your arms overhead with your elbows bent slightly.

Bring your shoulder blade *back* and *down* toward your
spine.

Do not let your shoulder shrug.

Hold this position for 3 seconds, then relax.

   Repeat ____ times   R.   L.

A

(B) Assume starting position.

Place your arms overhead with your elbows bent slightly.

Bring your shoulder blade *back* and *down* toward your
spine, then gently lift your arms from the table.

Keep hand at same level as elbow.

Do not let your shoulder shrug.

Hold this position for 3 seconds, then relax.

   Repeat ____ times   R.   L.

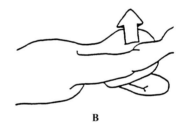

B

(C) Assume starting position.

Place your arms overhead, elbow *straight* and thumb pointing to the ceiling.

Bring your shoulder blade *back* and *down* toward your
spine, then gently lift your arm from the table (1–2 in).

Do not let your shoulder shrug.

Hold for 3 seconds, then relax.

   Repeat ____ times   R.   L.

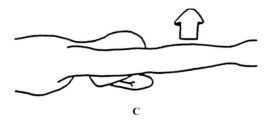

C

Figure 8–6   Phase I: Facelying/arm lifts. This exercise, developed by Sahrmann,[3] is designed to improve the performance of the lower trapezius, primarily when there are faults in strength and muscle length. The exercise is performed with the muscle at its shortest length and initially with a small load (**A**, with elbow flexed). The difficulty of the exercise is increased by progressing from scapular adduction and depression without humeral motion (**A**) to scapular adduction and depression with shoulder flexion and the elbow extended (**C**). The exercise is intended to deemphasize upper trapezius and rhomboid activity. *Source:* Reprinted with permission from *Exercises for Correction of Muscle Imbalances* by S. Sahrmann, St. Louis, Missouri.

Standing Lower Trapezius Exercise (Facing Wall)

Purpose: To strengthen and shorten the lower trapezius, the muscle that turns the shoulder blade upward.

Position: Standing facing a wall with the arms overhead and slightly out to the side. The thumbs should point away from the wall.

Method: With the arms overhead, pull the shoulder blades back or together.

    Hold for count of _____.

    Repeat _____ times.

    Option: _____ Bring the arms down and relax before repeating the exercise.

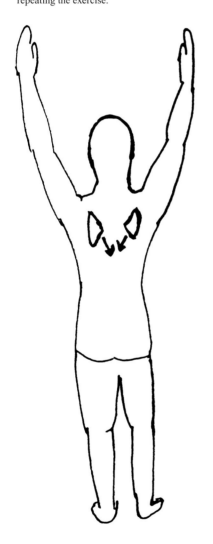

Figure 8–7   Phase I: Standing lower trapezius exercise facing the wall. *Source:* Reprinted with permission from *Exercises for Correction of Muscle Imbalances* by S. Sahrmann, St. Louis, Missouri.

Supraspinatus Exercise

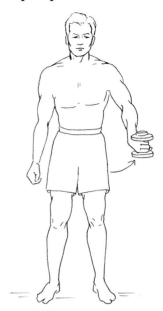

Figure 8–8   Phase I: Supraspinatus, or empty can, exercise. This exercise has been found to emphasize, but not necessarily isolate, supraspinatus activity.[a] With the thumb pointing downward, the humerus is elevated in the plane of the scapula to 60°. *Caution:* Because of the position of humeral internal rotation, impingement can occur even at low elevations, especially if the patient presents with a round-shouldered posture. For patients with impingement problems, scaption (with humeral external rotation) can be substituted (Figure 8–2). Resistance can be added with dumbbells, cuff weights, and surgical tubing. For low-level patients, resistance should not exceed 3 lb. For high-level patients, resistance should be initiated at 1 to 3 lb but should not exceed 10 lb.

[a]Jobe FW and Moynes DR. Delineation of diagnostic criteria and a rehabilitation program for rotator cuff injuries. *Amer J Sports Med.* 1982;10:336–339.

exercises for the fingers and hand with the PowerWeb, Eggserciser, DigiFlex, Theraputty, and the like (Figure 8–13) can easily be performed with the shoulder held in neutral position (see Chapter 14 for more information about functional exercise equipment).

Other alterations in the environment change the intensity of the program, allowing minute adjustments to be made for individual needs. Debilitated patients may only be able to perform wall push-ups instead of floor push-ups and chair press-ups with both feet on the ground in-

Infraspinatus and Teres Minor Exercise (Lying Ls)

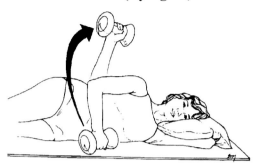

Figure 8–9   Phase I: Lying Ls for external rotator strengthening. The patient lies on the unaffected side with the elbow flexed 90° and placed adjacent to ribs and then externally rotates the arm against gravity. The eccentric lowering back into internal rotation is the most important component of the exercise because the infraspinatus and teres minor act to maintain glenohumeral joint stability during high-intensity internal rotation activities such as throwing. If necessary, the teres minor can be further isolated by prone-lying shoulder extension exercises performed in external rotation. *Source:* Reprinted with permission from *Clinical Management* (1991;11[6]:43), Copyright ©1991, American Physical Therapy Association.

Subscapularis Exercise

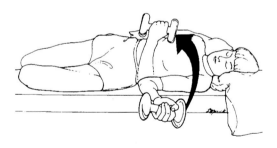

Figure 8–10   Phase I: Subscapularis or internal rotator strengthening. With the elbow bent by the side, the patient brings the forearm across the chest into internal rotation while sidelying on the affected side. In general, the subscapularis (assisted by the pectoralis major and latissimus dorsi) is rarely weakened. This muscle's strength should be assessed properly before the patient initiates this exercise so that a greater imbalance in muscle strength does not occur between the shoulder internal and external rotators. *Source:* Reprinted with permission from *Clinical Management* (1991;11[6]:43), Copyright ©1991, American Physical Therapy Association.

Knuckle Push-Ups

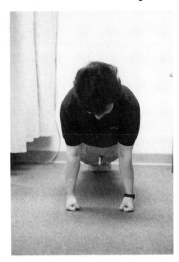

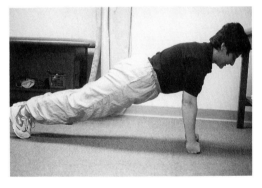

Figure 8–11   Phase I: Knuckle push-ups. This modification of the push-up should be performed if the patient has insufficient wrist dorsiflexion to perform the push-up in the standard fashion (palms on the floor). This exercise requires greater wrist stabilization in neutral position than the standard push-up.

stead of off the ground. The programs are still working on the same goals of restoring muscular strength, joint stability, and postural alignment.

Phase II Functional Integration Program

The phase I exercise program lays the foundation for the phase II functional integration program. Individual muscles and joints are no longer isolated to be stretched or strengthened.

Push-Ups on Unstable Surface

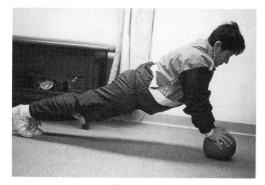

Figure 8–12   Phase I: Push-ups on an unstable surface. This exercise retrains proprioception and stability of the entire kinetic chain. By altering the base of support, the intensity of the exercise increases dramatically. This exercise is also helpful in retraining more distal joints in the upper extremity as the hand, wrist, and elbow must maintain their relative positions.

Hand-Strengthening Exercises

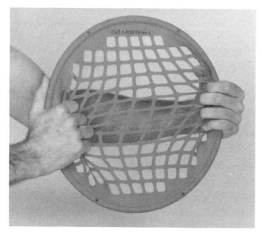

Figure 8–13   Phase I: Hand-strengthening exercises. Many simple exercise devices, such as the PowerWeb (shown), Eggserciser, or Theraputty exist on the market specifically to strengthen and stabilize the fingers and hands. These exercises may be needed precursors to the power and precision grip functional work of the phase II program. *Source:* PowerWeb photo courtesy of Fitter International, Inc., Calgary, Alberta, Canada.

In this part of the functional program, the activities encourage total body participation. The rest of the body must now properly balance and stabilize all loose segments to accomplish functional tasks in a protected environment. During the phase II program, the patient can explore alternative movement strategies under professional supervision. Depending on the physical impairments present, the patient can attempt any or all of the following 10 functional activities:

1. beginning program (protected function)
2. lifting
3. carrying
4. reaching
5. pushing
6. pulling
7. forearm rotations
8. power grip
9. precision grip
10. throwing

By adjusting the environment and the patient's motion, the therapist can safely progress the phase II program as the patient heals. This list of phase II activities is not inclusive of all upper extremity activities but instead represents a general sampling of functional tasks. Specific tasks may be added as the patient's situation requires.

Beginning Program (Protected Function)

The first group of functional activities includes light shoulder depression work with the glenohumeral joint kept in neutral position. This is a safe position for even acute shoulder conditions because it entails light weight bearing through the upper extremity joints. The patient tries to accomplish any of the following closed-chain tasks:

• light dusting (waist high)
• rinsing of sink basins with a cloth
• light sanding of wood
• cleaning off counter tops and tables
• dribbling a basketball
• writing on a pad of paper

The key to the successful return to these activities is allowing only a small arc of glenohumeral motion to occur while simultaneously maintaining a light compressive force into the upper extremity joints to help stabilize the kinetic chain. The patient progresses the activities by experimenting with a greater range of motion (eg, rinsing the faucets and taps) or applying a greater compressive force (scrubbing or sanding harder). As the patient gains confidence, he or she can spend increasing amounts of time on these activities. The patient reports to the therapist any problems or increase in symptoms encountered while attempting these low-level functional tasks. Most patients should be able to perform some or all of the beginning program activities from the onset of the rehabilitation program.

Lifting

An important everyday functional task is the ability to lift objects to manipulate or transport them. This is a full-body activity requiring coordinated effort of the lower body segments, pelvis, and thorax to balance and stabilize the body so that it can position itself to lift. In addition, the upper body segments must possess the stability and coordinated movement to perform the lift without injuring the healing joints. The patient progresses the activity by lifting heavier weights or transporting the lifted object over a greater area (which requires both a greater joint range of motion and a greater degree of stability). An example of a functional progression for lifting is as follows:

1. Lift a 1-lb weight off the floor to waist or table height (empty milk crate, cuff weight, etc.).
2. Lift a 1-lb weight off the floor and hang it on a coat hook (shoulder height).
3. Lift a 1-lb weight off the floor and put it on an overhead shelf.
4. Progress to a 5-lb weight (heavy book, half-full tea kettle, hammer, pocketbook, half-gallon of milk, coat, weighted milk crate, plyoball, etc.).
5. Progress to light plyoball activities:
   • underhand throw and catch (Figure 8–14)

Plyoball: Underhand Throw and Catch

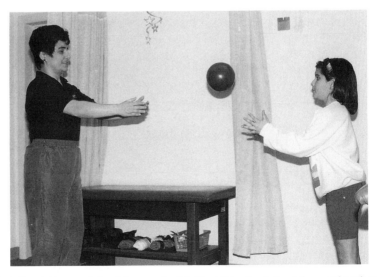

Figure 8–14   Phase II: Light plyoball activities—underhand throw and catch. The bilateral underhand throw and catch requires only minimal glenohumeral excursion, but the patient must adjust the whole body to participate in the game. The patient needs to absorb the forces imposed on the system by the incoming weighted ball without incurring any injury. In addition, the patient needs to act quickly enough to accommodate the changing temporal environment. Although this activity sounds difficult, most patients enjoy playing catch and automatically engage in the game without realizing the level of skill needed to participate.

- juggle (Figure 8–15)
- shot-put position (Figure 8–16)
- military press

6. Progress to a 10-lb weight (grocery bag, gallon of milk, briefcase, infant, etc.).
7. Progress to a 25-lb weight (suitcase, heavy grocery bag, small toddler, etc.).

As the patient progresses to lifting heavier weights, the therapist must make sure that the patient is using proper body mechanics. The milk crate is an inexpensive but excellent training device for practicing weight lifting because it can be held by any angle or by its handles. This provides the patient with alternative hand holds to practice different ways of lifting the crate.

The plyoball activities begin the advanced portion of the program as they add a temporal constraint on the system. The entire body has to

Plyoball: Shot-Put Position into Military Press

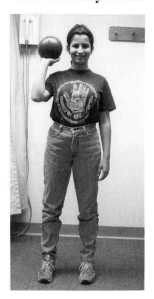

A

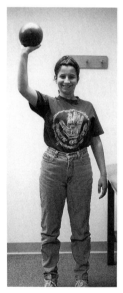

B

Figure 8–16   Phase II: Light plyoball activity—shot-put position into military press. (**A**) Initially the patient holds the plyoball in the shot-put position (balanced in the palm on the shoulder) as shown. For many patients, especially the elderly, simply stabilizing the shoulder complex in this position is stressful, even though the glenohumeral joint is in a relatively neutral and therefore safe position. (**B**) If the patient wishes to progress the activity, the plyoball can be lifted slowly into an overhead or military press. Increasing the weight of the plyoball increases the intensity of this exercise.

Plyoball: Juggle

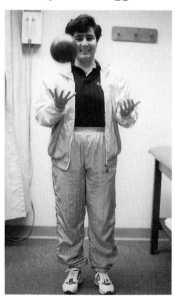

Figure 8–15   Phase II: Light plyoball activity—juggle. The patient stands or sits comfortably and lightly tosses the plyoball from one hand to the other. The patient begins juggling the ball with a small arc of flight and increases the difficulty of the activity by throwing the ball higher. To increase the intensity of the task further, the patient can progress to heavier plyoballs or can throw the ball faster.

react in time to catch a weighted ball, requiring the absorption of forces up along the entire kinetic chain without the body losing balance. Similar constraints occur in lifting a baby or toddler who squirms and wriggles (Figure 8–17). The upper extremities and entire body must counter and stabilize each unexpected movement of the child.

Carrying

Oftentimes the ability to lift an object is not as important as the ability to transport it or carry it somewhere else. This total body functional task first requires the ability to lift but then requires the endurance to carry the object about. Many true functional activities require the ability to carry in the following contexts:

- grocery shopping
- traveling (carrying suitcases)
- cooking (carrying pots, food, measuring cups, etc.)

Lifting a Squirming Child

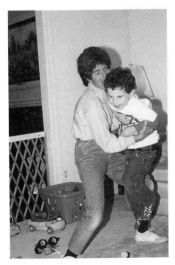

Figure 8–17   Phase II: Lifting a squirming child. A toddler not only weighs a considerable amount (25 to 50 lb) but adds to the difficulty of the lift by moving about. This moving environment requires high-level abilities on the part of the patient to stabilize and maintain balance with both the upper extremities and the whole body.

- cleaning
- parenting (carrying a child, toys, playpen, etc.)
- laundry
- working (carrying lumber, tools, briefcases, etc.)

The list is endless. People are forever carrying objects to and fro. One sport even requires a person dressed in a modern suit of armor to carry a brown oval ball 100 yards while being chased and attacked by other players.

After demonstrating the safe ability to lift an object, the patient then carries it a specified distance, which the therapist measures. The clinician initially documents progress by recording the patient's ability to carry a certain weight over a certain distance. Objects of different shapes (eg, bulky, long, fragile, etc.) and different weights should be used. The patient should experiment with different methods of carrying an object based on its contour and weight and his or her level of physical impairment. Some patients may prefer to carry a bag in one hand, whereas others will grasp both hands together and pull it against the torso (Figure 8–18). Often it is easier to sling a heavy object onto the top of one's shoulder, the way a waitress or waiter carries a serving tray. In fact, there are many right, or efficient and pain-free, ways to carry things. The patient must determine through trial and error the optimal movement pattern based on his or her physical body build, the actual thing being carried, and the environment.

To increase the difficulty of the task, the therapist can change the surroundings. Instead of the patient carrying the object in the safe, protected setting of the clinic, the therapist can make the environment more dynamic by having the patient carry the item onto an escalator or by having the patient maneuver around an obstacle course or through a crowded corridor. This advanced step is a necessary precursor to true return to function because many patients can become frightened of a complicated environment and refuse to interact with it, even though they have the so-called ability to perform independently in a static or safer setting.

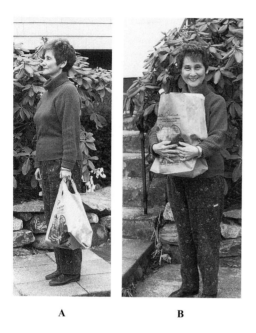

A   B

Figure 8–18   Phase II: Two different but correct ways to carry a bag. **(A)** This woman carries the shopping bag by its handles in one hand or **(B)** grasps the bag to her body for additional support while interlocking her hands together. There are many correct and safe ways to carry objects, depending on their contour and weight, the availability of hand holds, the patient's current abilities, and the environment.

Reaching

The ability to reach for items in whatever inconvenient place they may be located is another function of the upper extremity. Although functional reach is often measured as how far someone can reach in front of the body, the fact is that people reach in all different directions to perform the most basic tasks of daily living. People reach in front to get clothes out of the closet, under chairs to pick up a fallen pencil, in the back seat of a car for a briefcase, to the side to answer the telephone, to the back and front of the body to get dressed and perform personal grooming and toileting, overhead to change a ceiling light bulb, and so on.

The shoulder girdle and elbow/forearm are the joints most responsible for placing the hand within reach of any desired object. Patients tend to be extremely creative when attempting

to get to an item with a dysfunctional upper extremity and use whatever movement is possible to get the job done. These unorthodox movement patterns (eg, reverse scapulohumeral rhythm or trunk bending) generally will cause future dysfunctions and should be discouraged by the therapist, even though the patient may in fact accomplish the task. Reaching activities should follow immediately after the phase I work of correcting motor sequencing problems. The patient may need to practice reaching activities and humeral elevation with a mirror for visual feedback to maintain proper clavicle (and therefore scapular) positioning. The therapist must ensure that proper scapular stabilization and rotation are occurring along with glenohumeral elevation during the reaching activities in all directions. The patient should only reach as far as the body can move in a pain-free, efficient manner.

In addition, the rehabilitation specialist must place special emphasis on the ability to reach behind the body (shoulder extension and internal rotation combined with scapular adduction and trunk rotation). This motion is necessary for the most personal ADLs: wiping oneself after a bowel movement as well as pulling up one's pants and putting on one's bra. Because of embarrassment, many patients fail to mention a lack of ability in this area unless asked directly.

If the patient can reach safely to a certain level, the next step is to be able to lift the object from that place and either move it somewhere else or manipulate it. When the humerus is elevated and the elbow is extended, there is a great levering force at the glenohumeral joint, which requires stabilization. By adding further mass to the most distal end of the lever (the hand), the shoulder girdle may struggle to lift a seemingly inconsequential weight, such as a 1-lb can of beans. Only by performing the reaching activities in combination with the stabilization exercises in phase I will the patient regain the functional ability of reaching and manipulating objects.

Lastly, the most difficult object to reach for is the one that is moving. In the dynamic environment, the patient must now visually track the trajectory of the elusive item, have the physical ability to reach into the particular coordinates of space that the object will occupy, and time the action to reach the object when it arrives. Then the patient must have the ability to decelerate the object with the upper extremity musculature without causing further injury to any joints. This scenario is of course what occurs when one plays catch with a ball or Frisbee. In a more mundane but equally functional setting, this occurs when a grocery bag splits open and the person gropes wildly for the contents that are spilling about in random vectors. To train for such an event, which happens with much more frequency than one might first think, the patient and therapist can simply play ball. The object of this game is to purposely throw the ball away from the patient so that the patient in fact must spontaneously reach for the errant throw. The difficulty of the activity increases with the use of a smaller ball or a plyoball.

Pushing

Pushing is another indispensable function of the upper extremity. People are forever pushing papers, carriages, vacuums, doors, brooms, lawn mowers, shopping carts, and of course other people around. (In general, we are very pushy people.) After working on the phase I activities of push-ups or bench presses, the patient is ready to integrate the rest of the body into the activity. Now the lower body segments, pelvis, and torso must provide a stable base from which the upper extremities can push. If the load being pushed is heavy or if the person is attempting to push uphill (against the additional force of gravity), the rest of the body leans in and provides the bulk of the power to move the object.

Some examples of phase II activities to promote pushing ability include:

- plyoball chest passes (Figure 8–19)
- milk crate pushes on a table top (Figure 8–20)
- isometric pushes into a wall (Figure 8–21)
- drop push-ups (Figure 8–22)
- baby stroller pushes
- carpet sweeper or broom pushes

Plyoball Chest Pass

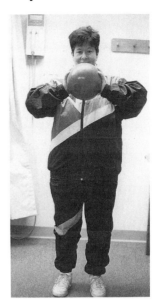

Figure 8–19   Phase II: Plyoball chest pass. The patient holds the ball in both hands close to the chest and forcefully pushes the ball to a partner or ball rebounder. During the catching portion of the game, the patient attempts to reverse the motion and eccentrically control the object by making a chest catch. The patient can warm up initially with a basketball and progress to weighted plyoballs. The patient strives to have the ball achieve a horizontal flight path.

Although initially most pushes are in the forward direction, patients should also learn to push to the side and overhead. The overhead push is the same as the overhead reaching activity or military press (see Figure 8–16).

Pulling

Another functional activity of daily life is pulling. Often it is performed immediately after a pushing activity, such as sawing wood or vacuuming a carpet. People also pull doors open, pull golf carts behind them, and pull window shades down. The action should involve both shoulder extension and scapular adduction. Failure to involve the scapular muscles can cause increased pressure into the anterior capsule of the glenohumeral joint, leading to a painful anterior instability. Some phase II activities that involve pulling include:

Milk Crate Push on Table Top

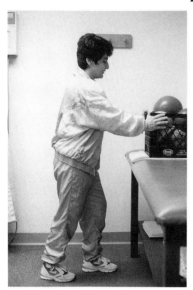

Figure 8–20   Phase II: Milk crate push across a table top. With a towel placed under the milk crate both to reduce friction and to protect the furniture, the patient stands next to the table and pushes the milk crate forward or to either side. The crate can be weighted with household items or any other type of weight to alter the movement pattern needed to accomplish the task. Learning to predict the amount of push needed for moving an object is important for regaining true function. This exercise is also good for the low-level patient who has difficulty with the phase I push-ups or the other phase II pushing activities.

- rowing with free weights or on machines
- vacuuming
- pulling a bag or suitcase
- rowing with surgical tubing (Figure 8–23)
- pulling a rope in a tug-of-war

The last two activities of pulling against a variable opposing force are higher-level exercises because they involve a more dynamic environment. Similar occurrences happen in real life when a dog pulls away quickly on a leash or a toddler suddenly decides to go off in another direction.

Forearm Rotations

The forearm longitudinal rotations of pronation and supination are helpful in placing the

Isometric Wall Push

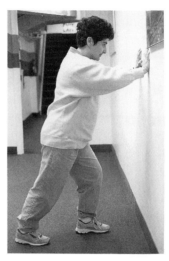

Figure 8–21   Phase II: Isometric wall push. Unlike the wall push-up, which focuses on moving the body away from the wall, the isometric wall push is a powerful closed-chain exercise that mimics trying to move the wall. Using the strength of the entire body (not just the upper extremities), the patient attempts to push through the wall. The isometric exercise is held for 5 seconds and is followed by a rest period. This exercise will help build strength and stability of the entire upper extremity. Care must be taken not to overpower any weakened body structures.

---

wrist and hand in necessary positions for manipulating objects. Even with proper shoulder stabilization, a person would be unable to lift, carry, or reach many items without the ability to position both the elbow and the forearm. The more commonly thought of functions for supination involve the functional tasks of turning a doorknob and using a screwdriver. During these activities, the triceps also contracts to counter the flexion moment produced by the biceps brachii.[6] The rotations can be trained in isolation with the elbow locked by the side and a dumbbell placed in the hand, but the phase II program involves total body work. Aside from using a Baltimore Therapeutic Equipment (BTE) (Figure 8–24) if available, phase II types of activities are the functional tasks of:

- turning doorknobs
- brushing one's hair
- making Tai Chi arm movements

Drop Push-Ups

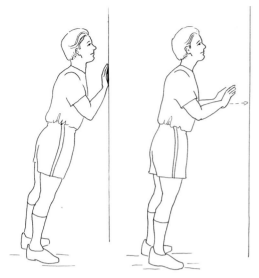

Figure 8–22 Phase II: Drop push-ups. This exercise is a plyometric activity that activates the myotatic stretch reflex. The patient falls from a standing position into a nearby wall. The hands contact the wall as the upper extremity muscles eccentrically control the body weight to prevent the person from smashing into the wall. The person then pushes off the wall quickly, performing a push-up. This exercise helps re-train the ability to absorb the forces that occur when one loses one's balance and falls. To advance this activity, the therapist can stand behind the patient and push him or her into the wall. This eliminates the patient's ability to antici-pate the activity. Another advancement for the high-level pa-tient is to perform clap push-ups on the floor. Boxers often use this type of plyometric push-up in their training.

- using a screwdriver
- using a racquet (Figure 8–25)
- batting

The last two activities can involve a temporal component by making the patient actually hit a moving ball with either the racquet or the bat. During all these activities, the therapist needs to make sure that the patient is not substituting shoulder rotations.

(Author's note: Although elbow flexion and extension are not specifically mentioned in the phase II program, these motions are obviously important to upper extremity function. Many of the phase II activities call for closed-chain and open-chain elbow work, such as push-ups, chest

Plyometrics: Pulling Against Surgical Tubing

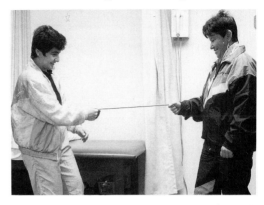

Figure 8–23 Phase II: Plyometrics—pulling against surgi-cal tubing. The variable resistance offered by the elasticity of the rubber tubing forces the body to make constant minute adjustments in the activity. This prepares the patient for pulling against moving objects (eg, a dog on a leash), which occurs in the real world.

BTE Work Simulator

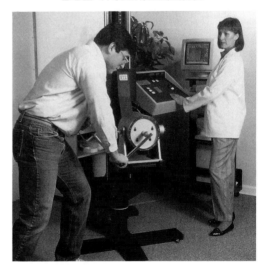

Figure 8–24 BTE work simulator. The BTE works many upper extremity motions, including pronation and supina-tion. This unit is readily available in most work-hardening centers and hand clinics. *Source:* Photo courtesy of Balti-more Therapeutic Equipment Company, Hanover, MD.

passes, lifts, and the like.) The clinician must assess whether to design specific activities for flexion and extension in addition to the ones al-ready mentioned.)

Racquet Work

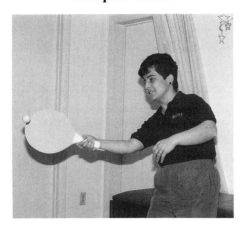

Figure 8–25 Phase II: Racquet work. By using either a racquetball racquet or a beach paddle, the patient can work on improving pronation and supination (tennis and squash racquets can be used, but they are larger and may cause damage in a small clinic). The racquet can be weighted or attached to surgical tubing for additional resistance. The therapist can make the environment dynamic and fun by throwing a foam or light rubber ball toward the patient and having the patient hit it back. This same activity works well if a baseball (or Wiffleball) bat is substituted. If batting is the preferred activity, the therapist must make sure that the patient bats both right-handed and left-handed.

Power Grip

The ability to grasp objects is one of the major functions of the hand and the entire upper extremity. Grasping or prehension is divided into two major functional categories: power grip and precision grip. The power grip is the one used in holding onto the racquet in Figure 8–25. The cylindrical racquet handle is clamped by flexed fingers into the palm while counterpressure is applied by the adducted thumb. A sustained isometric contraction is required to hold the object while the wrist or forearm provide the movement.[7] Examples of this are the forearm pronation and supination described previously and the act of hammering. As a result of the length-tension relationships of the area muscles, the wrist is considered the key joint in the physiological unit of the hand/wrist/forearm.[7] The wrist must be held in neutral position or dorsiflexed for the finger flexors to possess the strength to hold the object with a power grip.

Some aikido self-defense movements use this knowledge of flexing the wrist (and thereby extending the fingers) to free a weapon from an assailant's hand.

Phase II activities for improving the power grip are:

- racquet work (Figure 8–25)
- grasping a ball
- hammering
- opening jars
- golfing
- batting
- holding a hairdryer

The list is endless. The patient needs to begin by holding unbreakable objects and build from there.

Precision Grip

During precision grip, the object is manipulated between the thumb and fingers but is not compressed against the palm. Pound for pound, the precision grip or pinch causes five times the pressure in the tendons of the carpel tunnel as the power grip.[8] Three basic classifications of precision grip are commonly used:

1. tip grip: tip-to-tip opposition of digits (Figure 8–26)
2. palmar grip: pad-to-pad opposition of digits
3. lateral grip: thumb tip or pad opposition of the radial side of the index finger[6] (Figure 8–26)

The phase II program involves having the patient manipulate common objects, as follows using the various precision grips:

- picking up a pencil
- placing a key in a keyhole
- tying shoelaces
- turning bolts
- using eating utensils
- writing
- threading a needle

In all but the most simple hand injuries (eg, sprain or strain), the proper care of any hand-

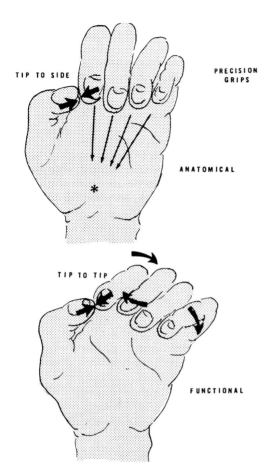

Figure 8–26 Motion of the fingers in functional movements. Precision grip requires tip-to-tip finger approximation. If pure finger flexion is used, the fingers flex toward the palm causing the thumb to first finger approximation to be tip-to-side (lateral grip). To cause tip-to-tip approximation, the fingers must rotate and deviate in an ulnar direction. *Source:* Reprinted from HAND Pain and Impairment, ed. 2 (p. 37) by R Cailliet with permission of F.A. Davis Company, © 1975.

injured patient should be undertaken by a certified hand therapist, who has specialized knowledge and equipment to manage this complex physiological unit appropriately. If a patient displays any difficulties with either the power or precision grip activities mentioned above, a referral should be made to a hand specialist.

Throwing

Throwing is a much studied activity in the field of sports medicine. It is used as part of the phase II program because it involves high-level coordination, is common to many sports, requires shoulder stability in an elevated range, and is fun and because most people already know how to do it. The larger surrounding shoulder musculature (deltoid, pectoralis major, latissimus dorsi, etc.) must accelerate the humerus[9] while the scapular stabilizers and rotator cuff maintain joint integrity. Throwing also involves the distal upper extremity: The hand must be able to grasp the ball while the wrist and elbow provide additional accelerating movement. During the phase II throws, the therapist must make sure that the patient does not put in the snap component and only lobs or tosses the ball. The phase II activities involving different types of throwing include:

- bilateral to unilateral underhand throw (see Figure 8–14)
- chest pass (see Figure 8–19)
- modified wrist toss with the glenohumeral joint in neutral
- light throw (glenohumeral joint cocked into abduction and external rotation)
- bilateral overhead throw (Figure 8–27)
- Frisbee throw (Figure 8–28)

The size of the ball (baseball, play ball, football, etc.) and its weight (Nerf ball, rubber ball, plyoball, etc.) will affect the type of hand grasp and movement pattern of the entire upper extremity. Therefore, the patient should throw (and catch) different types of balls as well as Frisbees so that many types of movement patterns can emerge spontaneously.

Phase III Functional Problem-Solving Program

The phase III portion of the program involves the patient performing functional tasks to achieve behavioral goals. As mentioned previously, this involves the patient experimenting with alternative movement patterns to find or create a movement that is fluid, effortless, and pain free and gets the job done. During this

Bilateral Overhead Throw

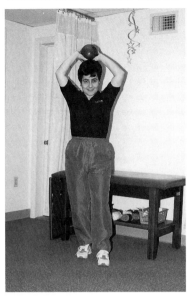

Figure 8–27 Phase II: Bilateral overhead throw. This throw requires full range of motion of the entire upper extremity with the ability to stabilize the shoulder girdle in a highly elevated (and therefore potentially unstable) position. The intensity of the activity can be increased by altering the size or weight of the ball.

Frisbee Throw

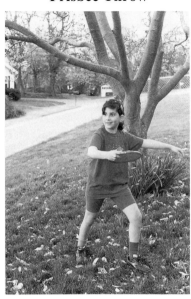

Figure 8–28 Phase II: Frisbee throw. The mechanics involved in throwing a Frisbee or discus place much less stress on the glenohumeral joint but more stress on the acromioclavicular joint and wrist. It is generally a fun way to begin throwing activities without damaging the glenohumeral joint. Other ways of throwing the Frisbee (with less horizontal adduction) are equally acceptable and encouraged.

phase, the patient practices activities, makes mistakes, and, by eliminating unprofitable patterns, eventually learns how to function independently. The therapist, nurse, or family member may have difficulty *letting go* of the patient and may try to help, but only by doing things independently will the patient regain true independence.

Inpatient Setting: Optimizing Functional Independence

Nursing home residents and inpatients in acute and rehabilitation hospitals should be encouraged to take care of themselves and their personal belongings. All basic activities of daily life require the use of the first nine phase II activities (throwing is not necessary). Whether from the stable position of a chair or from a standing position, residents should be able to perform all personal hygiene, grooming, toileting, and dressing activities within their present

physical limitations. Dressing alone involves some of the following upper extremity activities:

- opening and closing drawers (power gripping, reaching, forearm rotations, pushing, and pulling)
- getting out the clothes (power gripping, reaching, forearm rotations, lifting, and carrying)
- doffing the pajamas (power gripping, lifting, forearm rotations, and pulling)
- donning the new clothes (power gripping, lifting, carrying, pulling, forearm rotations, and precision grip)

The therapist observes the patient a few times to make sure that no safety issues exist and then allows the patient to explore the movements alone. The therapist can later ask the patient whether any problems or increase in symptoms occurred when he or she was trying the task. The nursing home or hospital staff should be discouraged from placing a temporal constraint on the patient (as in "hurry up already") except when absolutely necessary. In addition, the staff should also refrain from doing the activity for the patient simply because it is easier and takes less time. (This is difficult when personnel are short-staffed, but in the long run a patient independent in ADLs helps out an overworked nursing staff.)

Outpatient Setting: Restoring ADL

Outpatients should begin to perform all ADLs, household chores, and instrumental ADLs with their new found and changing capabilities. Laundry (lifting, carrying, reaching, pulling, forearm rotation, and power gripping) should be started with small manageable loads; groceries can be bagged light, shopping can begin at a fruit stand or butcher shop as the patient figures out how best to perform the activities. Although initially the patient should be slow and cautious while exploring a new movement, it is important for the patient to resume the activities at a quicker pace. Any problems are brought to the attention of the rehabilitation specialist who may recommend alternative movement strategies. The therapist should warn the patient that the activities must be performed hundreds of times before they will become automatic and that the functional program must be done for months to reestablish normal movement.

Outpatient Setting: Restoring Work Capacity

Patients returning to work need to evaluate their workstations for possible causes of cumulative trauma. These may range from chairs that offer no lumbar support and therefore result in poor neck and shoulder posture to repetitive upper extremity activities such as[10]:

- holding a flexed elbow and/or supinated forearm
- excessive or maintained wrist flexion and/or ulnar deviation

- sustained power or precision grip
- excessive thumb work
- cold, vibration, and/or direct compression to the wrist

If questioning of the patient produces no insight into any potential problems at the job, a worksite inspection may be necessary. The reader is referred to the many texts on industrial rehabilitation for further information about this subject and for treatment strategies for specific work-related disorders.

Outpatient Setting: Restoring Athletic Capacity

For the athlete, a high-level rehabilitation program may be needed. The plyometric work performed with surgical tubing and the plyoball can be done twice a week, slowly building up to 100 or more throws each session.[11] In addition, other high-level exercise such as upper extremity work on the Fitter (see Chapter 14), one-arm push-ups, and the like can be initiated. When the athlete is returning to throwing, an interval training program may be helpful in reducing injury (Table 8–1). The object of each phase is for the athlete to throw the ball the specified distance without pain.[11] Interval training has also been helpful in restoring the upper extremity for other sports, such as golf and tennis. For golf, the patient begins chipping and putting (with rest intervals) the first week, progresses to the short and long irons the second week, adds the woods on the third week, plays 9 holes the fourth week, and plays 18 holes by the fifth week.[12] The patient should also take a motorized golf cart (or a caddy) for the first month because many injuries are exacerbated by carrying or pulling the clubs, not by the actual sport itself.

ADAPTATIONS FOR SPECIFIC MUSCULOSKELETAL DISORDERS

Although the general functional program helps restore the patient's ability to interact with

Table 8–1 Interval Throwing Program

Distance	Step 1	Step 2
45-ft phase	A. Warm-up throwing B. 45 ft (25 throws) C. Rest 15 minutes D. Warm-up throwing E. 45 ft (25 throws)	A. Warm-up throwing B. 45 ft (25 throws) C. Rest 10 minutes D. Warm-up throwing E. 45 ft (25 throws) F. Rest 10 minutes G. Warm-up throwing H. 45 ft (25 throws)
60-ft phase	A. Warm-up throwing B. 60 ft (25 throws) C. Rest 15 minutes D. Warm-up throwing E. 60 ft (25 throws)	A. Warm-up throwing B. 60 ft (25 throws) C. Rest 10 minutes D. Warm-up throwing E. 60 ft (25 throws) F. Rest 10 minutes G. Warm-up throwing H. 60 ft (25 throws)
90-ft phase	A. Warm-up throwing B. 90 ft (25 throws) C. Rest 15 minutes D. Warm-up throwing E. 90 ft (25 throws)	A. Warm-up throwing B. 90 ft (25 throws) C. Rest 10 minutes D. Warm-up throwing E. 90 ft (25 throws) F. Rest 10 minutes G. Warm-up throwing H. 90 ft (25 throws)
120-ft phase	A. Warm-up throwing B. 120 ft (25 throws) C. Rest 15 minutes D. Warm-up throwing E. 120 ft (25 throws)	A. Warm-up throwing B. 120 ft (25 throws) C. Rest 10 minutes D. Warm-up throwing E. 120 ft (25 throws) F. Rest 10 minutes G. Warm-up throwing H. 120 ft (25 throws)
150-ft phase	A. Warm-up throwing B. 150 ft (25 throws) C. Rest 15 minutes D. Warm-up throwing E. 150 ft (25 throws)	A. Warm-up throwing B. 150 ft (25 throws) C. Rest 10 minutes D. Warm-up throwing E. 150 ft (25 throws) F. Rest 10 minutes G. Warm-up throwing H. 150 ft (25 throws)
180-ft phase	A. Warm-up throwing B. 180 ft (25 throws) C. Rest 15 minutes D. Warm-up throwing E. 180 ft (25 throws)	A. Warm-up throwing B. 180 ft (25 throws) C. Rest 10 minutes D. Warm-up throwing E. 180 ft (25 throws) F. Rest 10 minutes G. Warm-up throwing H. 180 ft (25 throws) I. Return to position

Source: Adapted from *Preventive & Rehabilitative Exercises for the Shoulder & Elbow,* ed. 4, (p. 20) by KE Wilke with permission of the American Sports Medicine Institute, ©1993.

the environment regardless of the actual diagnosis or physical impairment, the rehabilitation specialist should be aware that individual modifications are necessary to protect injured sites and to optimize the benefits of the program for each patient. A sampling of some common upper extremity impairments and the associated adaptations to the functional program is presented. The list is by no means exhaustive or all inclusive, but it should help the clinician individualize the functional treatment program for each patient

Shoulder Complex Disorders

The shoulder complex is an extremely mobile physiological unit with sparse connections to the thorax at the sternoclavicular joint. Although the shoulder is not usually considered a weight-bearing joint, humeral elevation can cause glenohumeral joint reaction forces of up to 89% of body weight.[12] Although pain is commonly experienced at the deltoid insertion on the humerus or at the anterior glenohumeral joint, dysfunction can be occurring at any of the four joints that make up the shoulder complex:

- glenohumeral joint
- acromioclavicular joint
- sternoclavicular joint
- scapulothoracic joint (not a true joint)

Some of the common disorders which affect the shoulder complex include:

- osteoarthritis
- rheumatoid arthritis
- total shoulder replacement (TSR)
- postural dysfunction and muscle imbalance
- instability
- impingement syndrome
- frozen shoulder
- hemi-shoulder
- humeral fracture

Postural dysfunction and muscle imbalance contribute to many other shoulder problems,

such as osteoarthritis, instability, and impingement syndrome. Even a lot of the pain associated with rheumatoid arthritis and hemi-shoulder derives from postural faults or faulty timing patterns causing rotator cuff tendinitis or tears (impingement syndrome). The entire functional program can be performed safely if proper posture is maintained with scapulohumeral rhythm. The accessory motions at the sternoclavicular and acromioclavicular joints should be checked to make sure that free scapular rotation can occur. Biofeedback over the scapular muscles or over the infraspinatus belly (Figure 8–29) can be used to retrain the musculature further to ensure proper firing patterns and glenohumeral stability. If the pain is coming from the glenohumeral joint, the distal functional program of forearm rotations and gripping should be performed first, allowing the glenohumeral joint to remain in a relatively neutral and therefore pain-free position. As elevations are added (lifting, reaching, pushing, pulling, etc.), they should be done first in the scapular plane, which causes less impingement.

Rehabilitation after shoulder surgery for TSR, instability, humeral fracture, acromioplasty, etc., requires thorough knowledge of

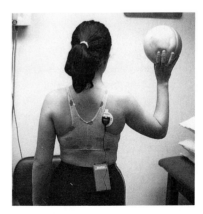

Figure 8–29 Biofeedback on the infraspinatus. For additional work of the external rotators to help with glenohumeral stabilization, biofeedback can be placed over the infraspinatus. After the patient has mastered the ability to contract the muscle with the shoulder held in neutral, the patient proceeds with elevation activities, maintaining tension in the infraspinatus. Biofeedback unit is a Myotrac™ by Thought Technology Ltd., West Chazy, New York.

which muscles were compromised or split. Although initial protection of these structures is necessary, the therapist must strive to rebalance the muscles after sufficient healing has occurred. Unskilled passive stretching (including self-stretching with a pulley) of the shoulder to regain range of motion needs to be discouraged if the scapula is not moving in concert with the humerus. In addition, heavy lifting (more than 25 lb) may cause injury to a TSR and should be discouraged for at least 1 year postoperatively. For patients with an uncemented TSR, even light lifting may cause micromotion at the implant-bone interface and should be performed with caution.

Elbow/Forearm Disorders

The elbow is made up of three synovial joints: the ulnohumeral, the radiohumeral, and the radioulnar. Collateral ligaments provide medial and lateral stability and the annular ligament keeps the proximal radius in articulation with the ulna. The skeletal structure also provides good joint stability in both flexion and extension.

Morrey et al[13] report that most ADLs can be performed with 30° to 130° of elbow flexion and 50° of both forearm pronation and supination. Opening a door or getting in and out of a chair requires less than 90° of flexion, and eating or holding a telephone requires around 130° of flexion. Most eating activities require both supination and pronation, except for cutting with a knife, which requires around 40° of pronation. Getting in and out of a chair also requires only pronation.

Motions of the elbow influence both the shoulder and the forearm as a result of muscular and skeletal attachments. Injury to the elbow will therefore affect wrist and hand function distally and may interfere with normal shoulder function. Common injuries to this area include:

• fracture
• medial or lateral epicondylitis
• dislocation
• ligamentous sprain

The elbow plays a prominent role in the ability to perform functional tasks. Exercises along with the phase II program help restore this joint with minimal risk of reinjury. Patients with elbow fracture, sprain, or dislocation travel quickly through the functional program. Care needs to be taken in the amount of resistance applied during activities (even isometrics) because the joint reaction forces can exceed two times the body weight (in this so-called non–weight-bearing joint).[6] During throwing, snap should be avoided until all structures are completely healed. For patients with epicondylitis, the clinician should pay careful attention to postural alignment at the elbow and changes in motor fiber recruiting sequence as possible causes of this overuse injury. Sahrmann[3] has found that overuse of digits 4 and 5 when grasping a tennis racquet can lead to a medial epicondylitis.

Part of the functional program involves looking for problems in the environment that are preventing independent, pain-free function from occurring. Simple changes, such as using a tennis elbow band to alter the biomechanical stresses on the muscles or using an electric screwdriver to decrease the torque at the elbow,[14] may be needed.

Wrist and Hand Disorders

It is perhaps important here to reiterate that injuries to the wrist and hand should be referred to a certified hand specialist. To treat the hand properly, the clinician requires a thorough knowledge of the complex anatomy and biomechanics of these areas as well as of the process of scar maturation, even for simple injuries. Because the hand is used as the major tactile and manipulating center for the body, it often comes in contact with a dangerous environment. Hammers smash thumbs, finger pads get burned, fists run into windows or faces, and so forth. In addition to human error, the workplace has been unkind to the hand, with major impairments occurring (degloving incidents, amputations, crush injuries, severed tendons and nerves, etc.). Some common musculoskeletal disorders which affect the wrist and hand include:

- osteoarthritis

- rheumatoid arthritis

- scaphoid fracture

- Colles' fracture

- sprains and strains

- dorsal ganglion

- carpal tunnel syndrome

- Dupuytren's contracture

- tendon rupture

The hand and wrist may require protective splinting to maintain both proper muscle length and functional position while injured structures heal. The so-called position of function has the wrist dorsiflexed, the fingers flexed, the thumb abducted, and the index and middle fingers opposed to the thumb.[15] Many conditions need surgical correction to reestablish the intricate mechanical relationships in the wrist and hand. Swelling and scarring must be kept to a minimum. The majority of the functional program can be performed, with special care, for all types of grasping and manipulating. Because a strong grip is associated with improved functional performance, gripping should not be avoided but progressed cautiously. Many types of hand exercise equipment exist that can slowly increase the strength and stability of the hand (see Chapters 14 and 15). To perform common ADLs, a grip of 20 lb and pinch of 6 lb are required; normal grip and pinch strength are three to four times greater than the functional strength required for ADLs.[16]

For overuse (versus traumatic) injuries, the clinician must assess the activity or environment causing the problem. If the technique cannot be changed, perhaps the surroundings can be made less harmful. Many pieces of equipment exist now to modify the stresses of our world: padded grippers, shoulder straps, electric appliances and tools, vibration-absorbing gloves, and so forth. The occupational therapist or hand specialist is most qualified to address these issues.

REFERENCES

1. Janda V. Cervicogenic pain syndromes. In: Grant R., ed. *Physical Therapy of the Cervical and Thoracic Spine.* New York, NY: Churchill Livingstone; 1988: 153–166.

2. Klein-Vogelbach S. *Functional Kinetics.* Berlin, Germany: Springer-Verlag; 1990.

3. Sahrmann S. *Diagnosis and treatment of muscle imbalances associated with regional pain syndromes* (Course notes). Presented at Massachusetts Chapter of the American Physical Therapy Association Annual Conference, Danvers, Mass, 1990.

4. Pink M, Jobe F. Shoulder injuries in athletes. *Clin Manage.* 1991;11:39–47.

5. Mosley JB, Jobe F, Pink M, et al. EMG analysis of the scapular muscles during a shoulder rehabilitation program. *Am J Sports Med.* 1992;20:128–134.

6. Soderberg GI. *Kinesiology: Application to Pathological Motion.* Baltimore, Md: Williams & Wilkins; 1986.

7. Hertling D, Kessler RM. *Management of Common Musculoskeletal Disorders.* Philadelphia, Pa: Lippincott; 1990.

8. Hebert LA. *The Neck Arm Hand Book.* Bangor, Me: IMPACC; 1989.

9. Bartlett LR, Storey MD, Simons BD. Measurement of upper extremity torque production and its relationship to throwing speed in the competitive athlete. *Am J Sports Med.* 1989;17:89–91.

10. Albert M. *Eccentric Muscle Training in Sports and Orthopaedics.* New York, NY: Churchill Livingstone; 1991.

11. Middleton K, ed. *Preventive and Rehabilitative Exercises for the Shoulder & Elbow.* Birmingham, Ala: American Sports Medicine Institute; 1989.

12. Poppen NK, Walker PS. Forces at the glenohumeral joint in abduction. *Clin Orthop.* 1978;135:165–170.

13. Morrey BF, Askew LJ, An KN, et al. A biomechanical study of normal functional elbow motion. *Am J Bone Joint Surg.* 1981;63:872–877.

14. LaCroix E. *Treatment of problems of elbow, forearm, and wrist joints.* In: Goldstein T, ed. *Geriatric Orthopaedics.* Gaithersburg, Md: Aspen; 1991: 203–213.

15. Cailliet R. *Hand Pain and Impairment.* Philadelphia, Pa: Davis; 1975.

16. Phillips C. Management of the patient with rheumatoid arthritis: the role of the hand therapist. *Hand Clin.* 1989; 5:291–309.

9

Lumbar Functional Stabilization Program

Beverly Biondi

Low back pain and its conservative care historically have been challenging and vexing problems for clinicians. Many physicians would agree that finding an accurate diagnosis for a low back patient often is a difficult task. It is not uncommon for a patient to complete extensive and expensive diagnostic testing with all tests negative only to have the same disabling back pain.

The rehabilitation of low back patients is also often frustrating for the clinician. Passive therapy protocols such as heating pads, ultrasound, and massage all have their place in effectively treating pain and dysfunction. None of these treatment methods, however, addresses the cause of pain or dysfunction; thus it is common that patients who are treated with solely passive therapy experience repeat episodes of pain. These patients return to the clinic seeking more pain relief, their episodic pain often growing more severe with each incident.

Recently, active and functional approaches to back rehabilitation are becoming the standard of care. Back pain, although often initiated with acute onset, is most often due to cumulative and detrimental stresses imposed on the spine.[1] Back pain can be considered a movement disorder that has resulted in symptoms and dysfunction.[2] It would seem appropriate, then, that a movement disorder be treated with movement

therapy and not exclusively with passive care. Otherwise the patient will probably resume faulty movement patterns and postures, and symptoms will perpetuate themselves. Studies have shown that back injury can be prevented or incidences reduced by patients learning proper body mechanics.[3] Additional studies have shown that there is a great decrease in the need for back surgery when stabilization methods are used.[4] Stabilization training is simply a method of retraining patients' faulty movement patterns from stressful ones to safe and efficient ones, so that the patient can return to functional daily activities. In physical learning situations, the body responds to repetition and to auditory, tactile, and visual feedback. As mentioned in Chapter 4, stabilization training incorporates this type of learning and may be the most successful way of changing movement patterns to promote patient safety. Learning proper and specific body mechanics, reestablishing functional movement patterns, and facilitating the most efficient movements should form the basis for recovery stages and prevention of further recurrences.[5] A careful patient evaluation, then, should include assessment of daily movement patterns, habitual postures, and whether activities of daily living (ADLs) are potentially traumatic to the patient's spine and therefore are contributing to the back condition (see Chapter 13). Patients must understand how their daily postures and movements contribute to their pain. As early in the rehabilitation process as possible, the patient must not become dependent on the therapist as the fixer; instead, the patient should view the therapist as the facilitator in the rehabilitation process.[6] So that patients take more responsibility for managing their conditions, it is important that patients develop a practical understanding of the anatomical and biomechanical aspects that relate to their condition. Increasing patients' knowledge about their back problems will result in less fear or hesitance in carrying out a desired treatment program.

REVIEW OF ANATOMY

Vertebrae, Facet Joints, and Discs

The spinal column consists of three distinct regions: cervical, thoracic, and lumbar spine. The evolutionary process of coming from a quadruped to a two-legged stance has given these three regions curves: a cervical lordosis, a thoracic kyphosis, and a lumbar lordosis. With these healthy curves, the spine is 10 times stronger than if it were straight.[7] The lumbar spine, with its connections to the pelvic ring, is the main support and load-bearing region of the body during upright postures. The lumbar spine consists of five large vertebrae, and it is this collection of bones that is responsible for most of the physical strength of the spine. Where each bone overlaps is the facet or apophyseal joint. Where the bones articulate with each other, there is a smooth cartilage lining that secretes lubricating fluid. This lubrication prevents friction as the joint glides in movement. The function of the facet joint is to guide and limit the motion of the vertebrae. As the lumbar segments are stacked on top of each other, a hole or opening, called the intervertebral foramen (IVF), is created. It is here that the spinal nerves are allowed to exit the spinal cord to give nerve supply to muscles and viscera. Lumbar extension, or an increase in lumbar lordosis, will tend to narrow the IVF, and the lumbar flexion, or

forward bending of the spine, will slightly enlarge the IVF. In between each vertebra is an intervertebral disc. This structure acts as a shock absorber between both bones. The disc is made up of many thin, oblique layers of fibrous tissue called the annulus fibrosus. The annular layers encase a gelatinous nucleus pulposus. Spinal movements and body postures influence the pressure within the disc. Because of nuclear migration, forward bending or lumbar flexion is thought to increase pressure on the posterior wall of the disc, and backward bending or lumbar extension may increase pressure on the anterior wall of the disc.

Muscles

Trunk posture and position are influenced by the muscles which attach to the lumbar spine and pelvis. The abdominal muscles consist of three groups: the rectus abdominis, the transversus abdominis, and the internal and external obliques. One of the key functions of the abdominal muscles is to provide strong support for the spine. Contraction of these muscles can reduce the lumbar lordosis to various degrees, depending on the amount of muscle contraction. The obliques, which run around the sides of the trunk, are the trunk's primary rotators. The gluteus maximus is a large and powerful muscle and is the strongest extensor muscle controlling lifting activities. The therapist must make sure that the hamstrings do not substitute for the gluteus maximus during hip extension activities.

The low back extensors are divided into those that attach to the lumbar vertebrae and act directly on the spine and those that do not attach to the vertebrae, but still exert an action on the spine. Extensive studies have been done to determine the exact function of each of these muscles, and several theories exist. It seems that a common role of the extensors is to balance the intersegmental shear stress, or translational stress, as the body moves in space via other larger muscular contractions. The extensors may be considered fine tuners in movement control. It appears that the multifidus, once thought to be a pure trunk rotator, actually lies too close to the midline to contribute to pure rotation. Instead, the multifidus may act to oppose the flexion moment when the oblique abdominals contract to produce rotation.[9] The thoracolumbar fascia, the midline ligaments of the spine, and the transversus abdominis all have attachments that are thought to act as corsets when contracted.[10]

There are many other muscles with attachments on the pelvis that play a significant role in lumbopelvic posturing. The iliopsoas, hamstrings, quadriceps, and iliotibial band all have muscle attachments and can be likened to guy wires that attach to the pelvis. The pelvis is the platform that supports the spinal column. Decreased mobility in any of these muscles can change the angle of the platform and, therefore, the position of the spine.[11] It becomes important, then, to have adequate length of the lower-quarter muscles that attach to the lumbopelvic region.

PATHOLOGICAL CONSIDERATIONS

With proper posture and a healthy spine, the lumbar vertebrae are aligned in such a way that the facet joints have adequate intracapsular space, disc pressure is symmetric, and the IVF has adequate space for the exit of nerve roots. Congenital factors, poor posture, or abnormal movement patterns during everyday activities may alter proper posture and promote degenerative trauma.

Liu et al[1] have suggested that, under cyclic torsional fatigue loads, synovial fluid may leak from the facet joints and that in the absence of adequate fluid the joint may exhibit more bony contact and higher friction Under these fatiguing loads to the spine, the rate of damage may exceed the rate of repair by cellular mechanisms in the body. Hardy et al[11] studied the effects of repeated axial compressive loads on the lumbar spine and found that the vertebral body, disc, annulus, and vertebral end plates were damaged as a result of this type of load. Adams and Hutton[12] studied the lumbar motion segment and applied forces that would simulate a day's

heavy labor. Twenty-four of the 41 discs studied showed distortions in the lamellae of the annulus, and a few showed complete radial fissures on the posterior annulus. Dunlop et al[13] performed detailed studies of the facet joints and concluded that decreased disc space, extension maneuvers, and extension and torsional maneuvers all narrowed the IVF and increased pressure on the facet joints.

McKenzie[8] has recognized three factors predisposing to low back pain: frequent poor sitting posture, loss of extension range, and frequency of flexion. All three factors create increased pressure on the posterior wall of the annulus and may mechanically deform pain-sensitive structures.

To avoid or halt further degenerative change to the lumbar motion segment, it seems to be of the utmost importance to assist low back patients in establishing movement patterns that do not involve repetitive flexion, torsion, extension, or cyclical axial loading.

HISTORY OF STABILIZATION TRAINING

Stabilization training has become a common treatment tool among physical therapists in the United States. It has gained the support of patients, clinicians, and physicians. One study demonstrated that by using stabilization training with an appropriate patient population the need for surgery was reduced by as much as 90%.[4] The term *stabilization* is actually misleading; it may suggest to the clinician that the patient is expected to hold the spine rigid while moving about in space. This is actually an undesirable, if not unattainable, expectation for any person. Instead, stabilization training is a movement therapy designed to help patients exercise and increase physical capacity while developing coordinated movement patterns that will not lead to or perpetuate pathology. The fundamental concept of stabilization is that each patient must develop a stable and controlled trunk as a base for movement. Peripheral movements are then superimposed on a stable base. Proprioceptive neuromuscular facilitative (PNF) techniques and neuromuscular reeducation techniques form an integral part of the stabilization program and are necessary tools to assist patients in safe motor planning skills.

GOALS OF TRAINING

Every back patient seen in the clinic deserves to receive therapy that includes back education with an active stabilization and conditioning program. Studies show that 1 day of bed rest results in a 3% loss of muscle strength.[14] Other studies indicate that 3 weeks of bed rest leads to a 27% loss of maximum oxygen uptake.[14] Back patients who are instructed to rest in bed gain no skills in self-management of their condition and will deteriorate physically. Epidural injections,[15] physical modalities such as ice, and/or nonsteroidal antiflammatory agents should be employed during the acute stage of injury. Training and active therapy should commence at the subacute stage. Training techniques are designed to improve patients' physical capacity by increasing strength, endurance, coordination, and flexibility.[2] All training techniques should help patients control and eliminate painful symptoms. Many low back patients have learned to abstain from previously pleasurable exercise because of exacerbation of symptoms with movement. When the patient finds he or she can move and exercise in ways that control or even eliminate symptoms, exercise training becomes a success, and willingness to commit to exercise increases. Once the patient is engaged in active therapy, giving patients tools to help them recognize functional and efficient movement will allow them the opportunity to establish better movement habits during all ADLs and thereby attain independence from therapy. A major goal of therapy is to have patients move efficiently throughout the day.

GENERAL PRINCIPLES OF TRAINING

Stabilization training actually begins by asking appropriate and specific questions in a subjective evaluation. Pertinent information must be gained as to what stresses the spine can withstand, how functional the patient is at present, and what the patient's tolerances are to movement. Long-term goals must be established; exercise therapy for an older, sedentary woman will differ greatly from that for a young athletic firefighter.

In addition, the therapist must evaluate each patient for functional loss characteristics.[16] In other words, is the patient sensitive to position, weight bearing, pressure, or stasis?

Treatment techniques vary greatly according to these findings. For example, a patient with a weight-bearing sensitivity would do better with exercises in recumbent or antigravity positions than in upright, loaded postures. A patient with a significant pressure sensitivity over the lumbar spinous process would have exacerbation of symptoms with exercises in supine positions but would succeed with exercise using padding, bolsters, or postures that alleviate pressure on the sensitive tissue Exercise training should be initiated in stable, supported positions with movements that are gross and simple. As the patient gains confidence, coordination, and proprioceptive skills, exercises can then be progressed to less stable or unstable postures and smaller, more complex movements.

Progression of Exercise

After having learned basic body mechanics, the patient is asked to get down onto the floor using good body mechanics. In a supine position, the patient is asked to produce lumbopelvic motion. It is imperative that the patient not only learn this motion but also understand what muscle control is required to produce these motions. Facilitation techniques such as tactile cueing, visual cueing, and associated movements may assist patients in learning these motions.

Once the patient has discovered how to move the lumbar region in space, he or she is asked to move through the range slowly and to discover the painless or least painful range of motion

(ROM). Some patients will have a narrow range and will need to develop a high level of proprioceptive skill to move safely. Other patients may discover a wide range of painless motion and will progress with stabilization training with greater ease. This functional range or neutral spine posture varies from patient to patient, may vary from posture to posture, and varies depending on the stage of pathology.[2] Therefore, evaluating and discovering this neutral range should become automatic for every patient as posture, positions, and pathology change.

Once the patient becomes familiar with finding and discovering the functional range, he or she is asked to move about in space while maintaining a neutral spine. It makes sense to begin with easy functional movements such as getting in and out of bed or a chair, bending over the sink, etc. Once the patient has mastered these skills and has felt success, more complex movements can be added. As coordination improves, the patient can be challenged and prepared for dynamic activities by the introduction of exercises on unstable surfaces, such as physioballs, foam rollers, or balance boards. The use of unstable surfaces will provide afferent stimulation in an effort to improve automatic postural reactions.[17] The patient is asked to superimpose isolated motion on a stable trunk to test coordination training further. As the patient improves, strength and endurance training continues with increased use of weights, repetition, pulleys, and aerobic equipment. Making exercise and movements as functional as possible will make the recovery phase more meaningful for the patient.

Stretching

A major goal in stabilization training is for the patient to develop safe and stress-free postures and movements. The physical therapist must evaluate patient posture and body mechanics during all functional tasks. If faulty positions are noted, the therapist must then ascertain the cause of dysfunctional movement and eliminate these barriers to function (see Chapter 6). Oftentimes, restrictions in soft tissue mobility will cause poor postures. For example, to complete a safe and functional squat to the floor, one must have full ROM of the hip, knee, and ankle joints and adequate flexibility in the hip extensors, lumbar fascia, adductors, hip rotators, and soleus muscles. Muscle stretching must become an integral part of the recovery phase, and both therapist and patient are responsible for increasing patient flexibility.

Stretching techniques vary widely, and superiority of a specific technique has not been demonstrated. Static stretching, held for 15 to 90 seconds, seems to be the safest method of stretching.[18] Holding for longer than this has not proved to be of any more benefit.[19] Stretching poses must be so specific that selective muscles will be well stretched without jeopardizing the safety of surrounding body parts. In the clinic, careful positioning and use of belting greatly enhance manual stretching (Figure 9–1).

After manual stretching, a careful and specific home stretching program must be employed by the patient to maintain new muscle length. Studies have shown that PNF techniques such as hold-relax and contraction of antagonists will further increase flexibility.[20] In addition, stretching after activities appears to be important in attaining and maintaining flexibility.[21]

Assessing potential joint restriction is also an important aspect of flexibility evaluation. Joint restriction in the hips, knees, or ankles could

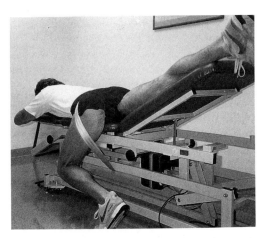

Figure 9–1   Careful positioning and use of belting greatly enhance manual stretching.

place excessive stress on the back and would require mobilization techniques. Restrictions in the rib cage, thoracic spine, or thoracolumbar junction are not uncommon and would also need manual therapy and a home mobilization program. Once restrictions have been alleviated and flexibility is adequate, the patient must become responsible for maintaining this range as a preventive measure.

SETTING UP A FUNCTIONAL STABILIZATION PROGRAM

Who Should Teach Stabilization Training in the Clinic?

Because training a back patient in the clinic requires a detailed and thorough assessment, a wide range of clinical skills is necessary to facilitate the training phase most thoroughly. The licensed physical therapist, with a background in evaluation and treatment of spinal pathologies and exercise physiology, is the most qualified to teach the stabilization program. In addition, the therapist must have detailed, hands-on instruction in stabilization training since it is impossible to have training expertise via commercial videotapes or by reading a book about stabilization training. The therapist should also possess advanced expertise in the areas of PNF and neurodevelopmental training (NDT) as they are frequently used in the training process. Constant observation, continual reassessment, careful cueing and reinforcement, and constant change of exercise routine are needed and require the skill of an experienced therapist. The whole rehabilitation process will surely fail if stabilization training is performed via exercise handouts and videotapes. Also, because of the detailed, hands-on therapy required in training a back patient, the student:instructor ratio should be no more than 4:1. The therapist must be familiar with each patient's abilities, special problems, and limitations and must develop the skill and creativity to adapt exercise training to meet these needs.[2]

Equipment Needed

Stabilization training utilizes some basic, inexpensive pieces of equipment, but most gym equipment can be utilized as long as stabilization principles are adhered to and care is taken to adapt equipment and exercise to patients' needs. The most important ingredient in stabilization training is providing adequate space for movement therapy to occur. A padded but firm floor surface is ideal, although patients with pressure sensitivities may require bolsters, pillows, or other props to accommodate their needs. A fully mirrored wall will enable a patient to obtain valuable visual feedback when learning new and perhaps foreign movement patterns. Other common pieces of equipment include straps for stretching, dumbbell and cuff weights for strengthening, physioballs, foam rollers, and balance boards for creating unstable, dynamic, and challenging surfaces (see Chapter 14).

Adjustable pulleys are the most adaptable piece of gym equipment, and they can be used to simulate numerous activities and functional tasks. They are also well suited to accommodate each person's functional loss characteristics. For example, an advanced patient may be challenged by simulating a tennis serve with pulleys adjusted overhead (Figure 9–2). Another patient with a sacral pressure sensitivity and a weight-bearing intolerance may be challenged by lifting pulleys and at the same time accommodated by being exercised in an antigravity posture with no pressure on the posterior sensitivity (Figure 9–3). Exercise training with isokinetic machinery is not commonly used for the back patient because such machinery most often offers sitting and loaded postures and do little to create strength training in functional postures.

Setting up Stabilization Training in the Clinic

Several methods have been attempted for setting up a stabilization training program in the clinic, and there is certainly no one right or wrong way to do so. Each clinic has a certain amount of available floor space, a certain number of therapists available to teach, and certain

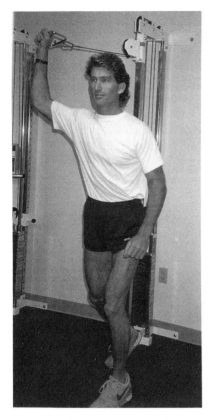

Figure 9–2 Use of adjustable pulleys to simulate a tennis serve for an advanced patient.

requirements of staff. One method of teaching that has proved to be successful in the clinic is providing group classes, with groups formed according to patients' abilities. Group situations have been valuable in the clinical setting. Patients have the chance to see others who are in the same situation and may find that a supportive atmosphere motivates them to exercise. Placing patients according to expertise will help keep the class running smoothly.

If forming a group class is not possible in the clinic because of space limitations, reimbursement problems, or staffing limitations, physical therapy patients will need individual stabilization training. It is wise to begin training very early in the rehabilitative phase, even when manual therapy or modalities form part of the treatment session. In this manner, the patient will start to gain control of the spine early on, and the dependency of pure hands-on treatment will be diminished.

Level 1 Class

A level 1 class is geared for patients with relatively sedentary goals (eg, sitting or non–labor-intensive jobs) and patients with no desire or need to return to sporting life. Activities in level

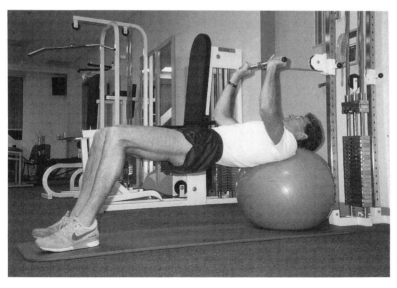

Figure 9–3 A patient with both posterior-pressure sensitivity and weight-bearing intolerance can exercise in an unloaded posture without direct pressure on sensitive tissues.

1 involve postures that are stable: supine, prone, quadruped, sitting, kneeling, and standing. Exercises are prescribed first in the cardinal planes. Exercises are performed relatively slowly with minimal or no weights. The basics of stabilization are taught: finding neutral, maintaining neutral while performing mass body movements, and performing simple, gross, isolated movement patterns.

Early on in the rehabilitation process, it is important that each patient understand the functional importance of every posture and exercise. For example, an exercise such as lifting an arm in quadruped position with good form will be similar to an activity such as scrubbing the floor. An exercise as simple as lifting the arms overhead will simulate overhead task work or sport-specific movement patterns. When a patient understands that a specific exercise performed in class will be meaningful and useful outside class, compliance in class will be enhanced.

When a level 1 patient can perform all exercises with good form and of adequate duration, he or she is ready to be progressed out of class. The goals of training will need to be reevaluated. Does the patient have adequate coordination, strength, flexibility, and endurance to carry out everyday needs? If so, the patient is ready to be discharged with a thorough home program and is expected to continue exercising on a regular basis. If the patient has higher-level needs for either job or recreation, it becomes important to place the patient into a level 2 class.

Level 2 Class

The level 2 exercise class differs in that strong emphasis is placed on endurance training, more detailed coordination training, and instruction on protecting the spine while moving around combined axes. Specific exercises are employed using longer lever arms, increased speed, weight, and repetition. Exercises are performed in more upright postures and in less stable, or even unstable, postures. For example, in level 1 a simple exercise for hip and back extensors may be performed in a bridging posture (Figure 9–4A). In level 2, that same exercise can

be made more challenging by using a less stable base, such as on one foot instead of two or with an exercise physioball under the foot (Figure 9–4B and C).

In level 2 exercises, creativity is used to make exercising specific to the patients' needs. For example, instead of a sea kayaker's oblique abdominal muscles being trained in a nonfunctional supine position, the patient can be trained on an unstable foam roller to simulate ocean activity while pulling on surgical tubing pulleys to simulate paddling (Figure 9–5). Training the

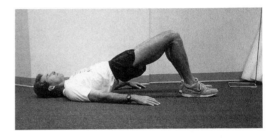

A

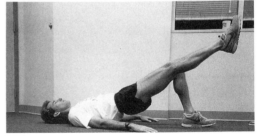

B

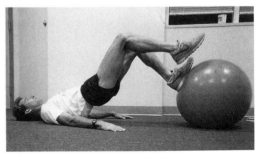

C

Figure 9–4 Exercises begin in stable postures **(A)**, and advance to less stable postures **(B** and **C)** as patient's expertise improves.

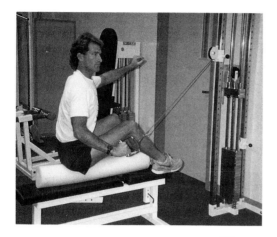

Figure 9–5 Use of unstable surfaces (Ethafoam™ roller) and adjustable pulleys can closely simulate a kayaking stroke in advanced functional training.

Level 3 Class

The next level of training, then, would be actual sports training or high-level job simulation. Level 3 stabilization training should be started when the patient has successfully completed level 2 training. In sports training, therapist and patient work together on the field or court or in the training room, and stabilization techniques are employed during sport. It is important that the therapist see the patient in action (not just talk about it in the clinic) and be there to assess and facilitate safe movement patterns. Simulating job tasks using stabilization philosophy should be carried out with the level 3 patient who is training to return to a physical labor occupation.

muscles specific for the activity is imperative, as is assessing safe postures during all high-level activities.

Finally, in level 2 patients should undergo cardiovascular training. Finding a meaningful aerobic activity is as important as prescribing any other exercise. Asking a stenotic patient to work on a cross-country ski machine may be unwise; a bicycle may be a smarter choice for this patient. A patient with significant weight-bearing sensitivity would not tolerate a treadmill or bicycle but may succeed with the use of a bike tipped on its side (Figure 9–6) or by exercising in a swimming pool.

ASSESSMENT AND DOCUMENTATION METHODS

Assessing a patient's needs for type, dose, and kind of exercise should begin with proper questioning on initial subjective evaluation and a thorough objective examination. Not only will such assessment result in success in training, but documenting these assessments will surely result in expedient insurance reimbursement. In a subjective examination, specific questioning will help the clinician know what exercises to avoid and which ones to encourage. What activ-

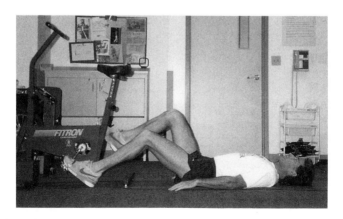

Figure 9–6 Standard exercise equipment can be used in unconventional ways to accommodate weight-bearing sensitivities.

ities aggravate the pain and need to be avoided? What postures ease symptoms and should be emphasized in exercise training? How much load tolerance will a patient withstand, and how can exercise training be modified to accommodate this limitation? Subjective examining lays the groundwork for proper exercise planning.

The initial objective examination should include some baseline data from which to document patient progress. Specifically, baseline flexibility should be noted, including muscle length and joint ROM important in safe function and posturing. Length of hip extensors, hip rotators, lumbar fascia, adductors, iliopsoas, hamstrings, gastrocnemius, soleus, and quadriceps should be noted. Documenting ROM of hips, knee, and ankle joints as well as thoracic and lumbar ROM is crucial for safe posture and safe movement patterns. A baseline strength assessment should be noted initially and monitored as the patient progresses through rehabilitation. Gross testing of the major stabilizing muscles is a good place to begin. Testing for strength in the abdominals, quadriceps, gluteals, upper extremity, and back extensors is of prime importance. In addition, testing patients for strength during functional movements is encouraged. Such activities can include (but are not limited to) squatting to floor, carrying a box, getting out of a chair, lifting an object from the floor to overhead or from shelf to shelf, placing a box on the floor, and the like. Adding functional activity to the strength test that will be meaningful for the patient's return to safe ADLs or work functioning may be prudent.

As the patient progresses in stabilization training, charting objective progress will ensure reimbursement. Such progress can include length changes in shortened soft tissues or joint ROM, strength changes in primary muscle stabilizers, or improved body mechanics or movement patterns while in good stabilization form. If insurance carriers are not familiar with the terms and techniques used in stabilization training, it becomes imperative to educate the carrier by sending relevant research articles or inviting the carriers into the clinic for some physical therapy education. There is no reason why insurance should cover weeks and weeks of hot packs and massage while denying coverage of such valuable and practical active therapy (for more information about documentation, see Chapter 13).

CONCLUSION

Functional stabilization training is an important treatment technique that should be utilized by all physical therapists in the treatment of low back disorders. It is in the patient's best interest to get to the source of his or her back problem rather than rely solely on pain-relieving treatments. Patients will feel empowered when treatment actively involves them and when they discover painless ways of moving and maintaining physical fitness. The clinician benefits because the patient learns to become independent from therapy. Finally, insurance carriers benefit because stabilization training cuts health care costs enormously by getting patients out of the clinic earlier and by giving patients methods of avoiding costly surgeries.

REFERENCES

1. Liu Y, Goel V, DeJong A, et al. Torsional fatigue of the lumbar intervertebral joints. *Spine.* 1985;10:894–900.
2. Morgan D. Concepts in functional training and postural stabilization for the low back injured. *Top Acute Care Trauma Rehabil.* 1988;2:8–17.
3. Nachemson A. Work for all. *Clin Orthop Relat Res.* 1983;179:77–85.
4. Saal J. Non-operative treatment of herniated lumbar intervertebral disc with radiculopathy. *Spine.* 1989;14:431–437.
5. Morgan D. The industrial back patient: a physical therapist's perspective. *Top Acute Care Trauma Rehabil.* 1988;2:38–46.
6. Schacht WD. The special patient–therapist relationship created by "handson" practitioners. *Phys Ther Forum.* 1990;2–5.
7. White A. *Conservative Care of Low Back Pain.* Baltimore, Md: Williams & Wilkins; 1991.
8. McKenzie R. *The Lumbar Spine: Mechanical Diagnosis and Therapy.* Waikanae, New Zealand: Spinal Publications Limited; 1981.
9. Gracovetsky S, Farfan H. The optimum spine. *Spine.* 1986; 11:543–573.

10. Saal J. Rehabilitation of football players with lumbar spine injuries. *Physician Sportsmed.* 1988; 16:117–125.

11. Hardy W, Cissner H, Webster J, et al. Repeated loading tests on the lumbar spine. *Surg Forum.* 1958;9:690–695.

12. Adams M, Hutton W. The effect of fatigue on the lumbar intervertebral disc. *J Bone Joint Surg Br.* 1983;65:199–203.

13. Dunlop R, Adams M, Hutton W. Disc space narrowing and the lumbar facet joints. *J Bone Joint Surg Br.* 1984;66:706–710.

14. Sanders V. *Inactivity: Physiological Effects.* New York, NY: Academic Press; 1986.

15. White A. Epidural injections for the diagnosis and treatment of low back pain. *Spine.* 1980;5:79–82.

16. Volowitz E. Furniture prescription for the conservative management of low back pain. *Top Acute Care Trauma Rehabil.* 1988;2:18–37.

17. Jull G, Jantz V. *Muscles and Motor Control in LBP Assessment and Management.* New York, NY: Churchill Livingstone; 1987.

18. Saal J. Rehabilitation in sports related lumbar spine injuries. *Phys Med Rehabil.* 1987;1:613.

19. Knotte F, Pauley D, Ptak R. The rationale for prolonged stretching for correction of shortening of connective tissue. *Arch Phys Med Rehabil.* 1966;47:345–352.

20. Knott M, Voss PE. *Proprioceptive Neuromuscular Facilitation.* New York, NY: Harper & Row; 1956.

21. Moller M, Oberg B, Gillquist J. Stretching exercise and soccer: effect of stretching on range of motion in lower extremities. *Arch Phys Med Rehabil.* 1985;66:171–173.

10

Geriatric Functional Rehabilitation

There is a dramatic increase in musculoskeletal symptoms with advancing age. In one study of both men and women older than age 65, musculoskeletal problems were the leading daily symptom, with arthritis being the most common chronic condition reported. In addition, there is evidence to suggest that the increase in disability associated with age correlates in part with the presence of musculoskeletal disorders. Progression of hand impairments leads to losses in basic activities of daily living (ADLs), and lower extremity impairments tend to affect negatively the performance of instrumental ADLs (IADLs).[1]

ELIMINATING THE BARRIERS TO FUNCTION

As mentioned in Chapter 6, the barriers to function that can be addressed by rehabilitation therapists consist of physical impairments and environmental constraints. Other barriers that are prevalent among the elderly include psychological issues such as fear and depression as well as other chronic diseases. Patients with these impairments should be appropriately referred to other health professionals.

Improving the Physical Impairments

There are many physiological changes associated with aging and hypokinetics or disuse syndromes (Table 10–1). In many instances, full correction of the physical impairments present may not be possible. Exercise, however, has been shown to have an effect on the body's systems even in the old elderly (>85 years).[2] The patient will be better able to participate in the phase I and II portions of the functional program if the following physical impairments are improved first:

- postural alignment and base of support
- flexibility and mobility
- strength and dynamic stability
- sensory input
- sequence of movement and coordination/ motor control

Postural Alignment and Base of Support

There is great variability in individual posture regardless of age as well as a definite progression of postural deviations from the young elderly (>65 years) to the oldest old (>85 years). The typical age-related changes occurring at the

Table 10–1 Comparison of Physiological Characteristics Associated with Aging and Disuse Syndromes

Characteristic	Aging	Disuse*	Characteristic	Aging	Disuse*
Body composition			**Musculoskeletal system**		
Lean body mass	⇓†	⇓	Muscle fiber number and size (type II > type I)	⇓	⇓
Fat mass	⇑	⇑,⇓	Muscle strength	⇓	⇓
Bone mass	⇓	⇓	Capillary density	⇓	⇓
Total body water	⇓	⇓	Muscle oxidative capacity	⇓	⇓
Bone marrow fat	⇓	⇑	Intramuscular fat and connective tissue	⇑	⇑
			Cartilage water content	⇓	–
Cardiovascular function			Connective tissue elasticity	⇓	⇓
Exercise capacity (VO₂ max)	⇓	⇓	Tensile strength of bone	⇓	⇓
Cardiac output (resting, maximal)	⇓,–	⇓			
Stroke volume, resting	–,⇓	⇓	**Nervous system**		
Stroke volume, maximal	⇓,⇑	⇓	Nerve conduction velocity	⇓	⇓
Heart rate, resting	–,⇑	–,⇑	Reaction time	⇓	⇓
Heart rate, maximal	⇓	⇑	Auditory thresholds	⇑	⇑
Blood pressure, supine	⇑,–	–	Visual acuity (near vision)	⇓	⇓
Blood pressure, after tilt	⇓	⇓			
Baroreceptor function	⇓	⇓	**Psychologic function**		
Venous pooling	⇑	⇑	Anxiety, depression	⇑,–	⇑
Capillary fragility	⇑,–	⇑	Insomnia	⇑	⇑
Peripheral vascular resistance	⇑	–	Appetite	⇓,–	⇓
A–VO₂ difference	⇓,–	⇓,–	Fatigue, apathy	⇑,–	⇑
			Metabolic/hematologic systems		
Pulmonary function			Basal metabolic rate	⇓	⇓
Total lung capacity	–	–	Exercise-induced hyperthermia	⇑	⇑
Vital capacity	⇓	–	Glucose tolerance	⇓	⇓
Residual volume	⇑	–	Insulin sensitivity	⇓	⇓
Tidal volume	–	–	Calcium balance	⇓	⇓
Forced expiratory volume	⇓	–	Red cell mass	⇓,–	⇓
Elastic recoil	⇓	–	Lymphocyte reactivity	⇓	⇓
Chest wall compliance	⇓	–	Phagocytosis	–	⇓
Expiratory muscle strength	⇓	⇓	Fibrinogen, coagulability	⇑,–	⇑
			Cholesterol levels (low-density lipoproteins)	⇑	⇑,–

*Disuse data were taken from studies of hypokinesia, immobilization, bed rest, or weightlessness.
†⇑, increased; ⇓, decreased; –, no change in a majority of studies to date.
Source: Reprinted from *Topics in Geriatric Rehabilitation* (1990;5[2]:64), Copyright © 1990, Aspen Publishers, Inc.

axial skeleton and the extremities are depicted in Table 10–2. Although the actual range of motion (ROM) measurements at each joint may be normal or minimally impaired when taken in the supine test position, the elderly patient's actual standing or sitting posture may show greater deviations.[3]

Unlike younger persons, who often improve posture simply through awareness and voluntary control, many elderly patients have significant restrictions in the soft tissues (muscle, joint capsule, fascia, etc.) in both distensibility and strength that need to be addressed. Kauffmann[3] recommends a short exercise program to work

these areas, as shown in Figure 10–1. In addition to this program, Lewis[4] has elderly patients perform lumbar extension exercises (Figure 10–2), pelvic tilts, and hip and knee extension exercises to improve static posture.

Flexibility and Mobility

Internal restrictions causing loss of flexibility and ROM include muscle shortening, insufficient muscle strength, and shortening of ligaments, joint capsules, and fascia. These soft tissue structures collectively are called periarticular connective tissue (PCT) and are pri-

These exercises are to be started gradually. Work at your own pace and level of ability. Start with 5 or 10 repetitions, and do fewer or more if you must or can. Slowly increase by adding 2 to 4, or more, repetitions every 5 to 10 days. Progress until you can do approximately 15 to 25 repetitions of each exercise. Do these exercises at least three times weekly.

1. **High step**
   Hold onto chair for balance; stand up straight. Raise one foot off the floor so that your knee is as high as your hip. Reverse legs. Try not to lean on the chair too much. As you get stronger, you may be able to raise your leg higher, hold for count of 5 (less if necessary), and decrease amount of leaning on chair.

   Purpose: To increase hip and leg strength and balance.

2. **Side step**
   Hold onto chair for balance, stand up straight. Move one leg out to your side and hold it in the air. Don't bend at the waist. Hold leg for 5 seconds, or less if necessary. Reverse legs. At first, you may be unable to hold your leg in the air. If so, simply move your foot out to the side.

   Purpose: To increase hip and leg strength and balance.

3. **Stand up–sit down**
   This is the key to being independent. Simply stand up, then sit down. To do this, you must get your feet under the front of the chair. Move your center of gravity forward and then up. If necessary use the chair's arm rest. As you get stronger, decrease the amount of push that you need from your arms.

   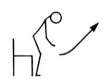

   Purpose: To improve strength, balance, coordination, and joint motion.

4. **Shoulder shrug**
   Sit up or stand up straight. Shrug your shoulders up high and release. Pull your shoulders back. You should feel your shoulder blades pull together.
   Purpose: To strengthen back, stretch chest muscles, and improve posture.

5. **Cervical range of motion**
   Sit up or stand up, head erect but not forward.
   a. Turn your chin to your left shoulder and reverse to the right.
   b. Lean your ear to your left shoulder and reverse to the right.
   c. Lightly place your finger on your chin and push your chin backward. DO NOT roll your head backward as if
      looking up at the ceiling.
   Purpose: To improve posture, balance, and ROM.

6. **Walk, walk, walk**
   Walk at whatever level of ability you have. If you can walk only 50 ft, start at that level and try to increase the distance and improve your gait speed. Avoid stops and starts. If you are walking longer distances, such as a half mile or longer in 5 to 10 minutes, do a little stretching before starting. When finishing your walk, cool down by simply walking slowly, stretching, and doing a few of these exercises or your favorite ones.
   Purpose: To enhance overall health of muscles, bones, joints, circulation, heart, lungs, digestion, bowels, and mind.

If you need help getting started or if you have any concerns about your health, show these exercises to your physician.

Figure 10–1   Postural exercises for persons 55 years and older. *Source:* Reprinted from *Topics in Geriatric Rehabilitation* (1987;2[4]:27–28), Copyright © 1987, Aspen Publishers, Inc.

1. **Prone-lying**
   Lie prone to tolerance (20 seconds to 20 minutes). If necessary, place pillow(s) under pelvis. Remove pillow(s) gradually (over days or weeks) to tolerance. If you cannot tolerate prone-lying at all, begin with back bends in standing position.

2. **Prone-on-elbows**
   Use this developmental sequence position to increase the lumbar lordosis. You may tolerate it more easily than prone-lying.

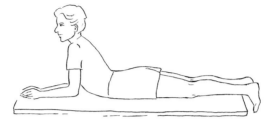

3. **Modified press-up**
   Place hands ahead of shoulders as shown. Push upper body but not pelvis off plinth using arms only. This is a *passive* back exercise! Repeat until symptoms decrease or are eliminated. Number of press-ups is limited by upper extremity strength and endurance.

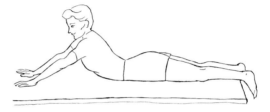

4. **Standing back bends**
   Place feet shoulder-width apart. Place hands in the small of back. Lift upper torso up and over hands while keeping neck in neutral and knees straight.

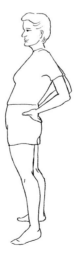

5. **Walking**
   Walk, walk, walk!
   Do not sit for more than 45 minutes at a time without getting up and walking around.
   Begin a daily walking program. Gradually build up endurance.

Figure 10–2   Modified extension postures and exercise. *Source:* Reprinted from *Geriatric Orthopaedics* (p. 156) by TS Goldstein, Aspen Publishers, Inc., © 1991.

Table 10–2 Typical Age-Related Changes in Axial and Extremity Posture

Body Segment	Typical Age-Related Changes
Axial skeleton	Forward head posture
	Increased thoracic kyphosis
	Decreased lumbar lordosis
Upper extremities	Round shoulders (scapular protraction)
	Increased elbow flexion
	Increased wrist ulnar deviation
	Increased finger flexion
Lower extremities	Increased hip flexion
	Increased knee flexion
	Decreased ankle dorsiflexion
	Increased (widened) base of support

Source: Data from Kauffmann T. Posture and age. *Topics in Geriatric Rehabilitation* 1987;2(4):15–18.

marily made up of the proteins collagen and elastin as well as extracellular ground matrix and water. The viscoelastic properties of PCT do appear to change with increasing age. Based mainly on animal studies, the increased stiffness in PCT probably results from the increased number of cross-links between adjacent tropocollagen molecules.[5]

The therapist uses both modalities and manual therapy in addition to active and passive stretching exercises to restore maximal distensibility to the soft tissues. The geriatric patient generally needs to perform a more prolonged stretch to achieve a lasting effect without causing further injury.[3] Restoring the minimal joint functional ROMs mentioned in Chapters 7 and 8 is a necessary building block for regaining independent function in the elderly patient. Of particular importance to this population is the need to restore hip extension to at least neutral and ankle dorsiflexion to at least 5°. Lack of adequate dorsiflexion is associated with an increase in falls in the elderly,[6] and stretching to regain ankle motion is an important safety as well as functional issue.

Strength and Dynamic Stability

Although it is not known how much strength is required to perform functional activities, the loss of strength associated with aging and disuse is known to affect functional performance adversely. The relationship of strength to function is magnified in the frail elderly.[7] Because rising from a chair often exceeds the strength of octogenarians, Fiatrone and Evans[2] report that the elderly should engage in strength training to maintain functional ability.

Judge[8] recommends that geriatric patients stretch properly before engaging in resistance training. He believes that this population should strengthen the lower extremity motions of hip abduction and extension, knee flexion and extension, and ankle dorsiflexion. In addition, he proposes that elderly patients should work the following upper extremity motions to maintain functional status: finger and elbow flexors, triceps, and combined shoulder/triceps/biceps.

The exact risk involved in strength training in the elderly is not known, and much research is needed. Risks in the elderly can be categorized as cardiovascular (ischemia, dysrhythmia, cardiac arrest, hypertension, etc.), musculoskeletal (muscle soreness, fracture, ligament strain, etc.), and metabolic (dehydration, hypoglycemia, heat stroke, etc.). Adequate warm-ups and cooldowns are imperative in this population. In addition, the therapist should encourage the elderly patient to drink adequate amounts of water during or after exercise periods to prevent dehydration. Because many elderly patients have diminished control of homeostasis, they should not be allowed to exercise in extremes of temperature.[2]

Although muscle strengthening is of great importance, especially in the elderly patient, the therapist should remember the importance of also building dynamic stability for these patients. Only through control of the joints does true function reemerge.

Sensory Input

There is evidence to support a disheartening list of dysfunctions in the sensorimotor system associated with aging (Table 10–3).[9] Changes occur in the brain cells, the neurotransmitters, and the special senses, resulting in distorted input and processing of the surrounding environment and the internal workings of the body. Much more research on these changes associ-

Table 10–3 Examples of Age-Related Changes in the Sensorimotor System

Sensory System	Age-Related Changes
Visual	Decline in visual acuity
	Decline in visual accommodation
	Decrease in peripheral and upper visual fields
	Decrease in retinal photoreceptors
	Decrease in neurons in the primary visual cortex
	Decrease in dark adaptation
	Decrease in color vision (shorter wavelengths)
	Decrease in depth perception
Auditory	Slow, progressive bilateral hearing loss
	Decline in function of cochlea
Vestibular	Decline in hair cells of saccule and utricle
	Decline in hair cells of semicircular canals
Somato-sensory	Change in morphology and decrease in density of peripheral receptors
	Loss of some peripheral nerves
	Loss of some vibratory sense in lower extremities
	Possible loss of some proprioceptive sense

Note: Better testing and more experiments are needed to substantiate the reported decline in the sensory systems with age. Also, because aging is an individual process, these declines cannot be generalized to the entire aging population.
Source: Information from *Geriatric Physical Therapy* (pp. 80–85), Mosby-Yearbook, © 1993.

ated with aging needs to be done before conclusive evidence appears. In any event, there is a consensus that the sensorimotor system declines with age, affecting the way the body functions. There is not a linear correlation with the presence of sensory impairments and the resultant functional loss. The varied combinations of these types of changes in different individuals may cause different motor patterns to emerge in the elderly. In other words, with aging each person attempts to solve life's problems within his or her own remaining abilities.

When these changes occur (and they do not occur for all individuals), they are mostly irreversible. When treating the older adult, the therapist should take these possible impairments into account and treat accordingly. In general a higher stimulus is necessary to activate impaired systems. Therefore, it is reasonable to suppose that by improving sensory perception the elderly patient may make gains in functional performance.

To enhance vision, the therapist should make sure that passageways and treatment areas have proper lighting and that the elderly patient leaves a light on at night either at the bed side or in the bathroom. Too much lighting is not necessarily a good thing, however, because the elderly patient may have problems with glare. In addition, colorless surfaces, such as the gray fire stairs in nursing homes, should have contrasting black treads placed upon them to clarify the edge of the step. If the patient has difficulty grasping the handles of a walker or cane (gray-on-silver contrast), the therapist can outline the handles in colored (red, orange, etc., but not blue) electrical tape.

For patients with hearing loss, the clinician should try to enunciate words more clearly and speak more loudly without yelling. If distracting background noise can be minimized, as in a quiet gym, it will be easier for the older patient to understand what is being said. In addition, the rehabilitation specialist should encourage the elderly patient with hearing loss to seek help for this disorder. Many elderly patients think that nothing can be done for this condition and that it is just a part of getting old.

Patients complaining of dizziness should immediately be referred back to the physician for reevaluation. Many vestibular complaints are treatable if properly diagnosed.

Tactile input, especially in the feet and hands, is imperative for safe function. A good athletic shoe with a flexible but supportive shank can allow an elderly person to feel the ground better and therefore balance and walk more easily. Additional tactile input can also improve the proprioceptive response of the joints. Weighting the ankles with small cuff weights or putting compressive bandages or even McConnell tape on the knees can cause increased kinesthetic awareness. Lower extremity proprioceptive retraining on wobble boards should start in a seated position (Figure 10–3) before progressing to standing in a door frame or within parallel bars for support. The clinician should not be afraid to place the elderly patient on the wobble board because it is generally a challenging experience and a welcome break from boring exercise. If the patient is too frail, the therapist can provide manual assist at the pelvis for additional support.

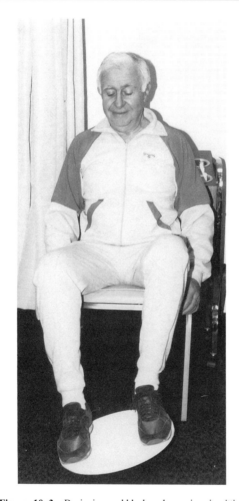

Figure 10–3 Beginning wobble board exercises in sitting. The movement of the unsteady surface stimulates the mechano-receptors in the joints of the foot and knee without placing the older patient in jeopardy by also having to maintain balance. When ready, the patient can progress to supported standing wobble board exercises. *Source:* Reprinted from *Geriatric Orthopaedics* (p. 119) by TS Goldstein, Aspen Publishers, Inc., © 1991.

Sequence of Movement and Coordination/ Motor Control

As mentioned in Chapter 4, the elderly generally use different motor patterns from those of their younger counterparts. This is easily seen in gait patterns but also in other ADL patterns, such as getting out of bed (see Figures 4–2 and 4–3). Even though occurring automatically, many of the changes in pattern are attributable to making the elderly patient safer in performing activities. (In other words, the elderly patient does not say to him- or herself, "I think that to maintain better balance I will now walk with a wider base of support and take smaller steps." The new patterns simply emerge with changes in the patient's physical abilities.) Because these motor patterns are only now being studied for different age groups, complete information is unavailable to the clinician as to what motor patterns are good or bad and which should therefore be left alone and which should be corrected. The clinician will have to rely on experience and common sense to strike a balance between a higher level of function and safety.

In general, no harm can come from having the patient perform coordination type exercises, even if there is presently no proof that the patient's everyday movements will improve. Activities such as tandem walking or performing proprioceptive neuromuscular technique (PNF) skill patterns can help increase the patient's motor control. A good exercise for motor control for the elderly (and, for that matter, all age groups) is the Chinese exercise form known as Tai Chi Chuan (Figure 10–4). When this exercise is performed properly, the patient must coordinate both upper and lower extremity movements with trunk movements and breathing while maintaining balance and good posture. The movements are slow and gentle, but the exercise requires a high degree of skill and is therefore challenging. In other words, it is an absolutely perfect exercise. If the rehabilitation specialist is unqualified, which is most often the case, the patient needs to seek out a good martial arts instructor. Although Figure 10–4 is provided for reference, the reader should under-

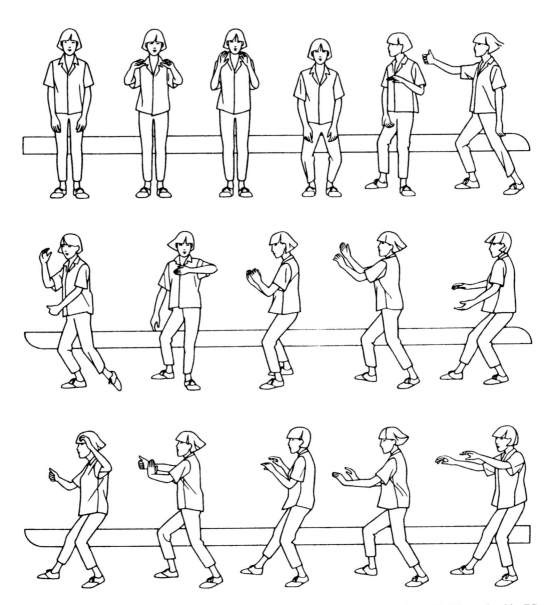

Figure 10–4   The first set of Tai Chi. *Source:* Reprinted from *Knocking at the Gate of Life* (pp. 37–39) translated by EC Chang with permission of Rodale Press, © 1985.

stand that it is all but impossible to learn Tai Chi from a book or picture.

Improving the Environment

The elderly patient may lose the ability to function when a musculoskeletal injury or the accumulation of age-related impairments combines with a hostile environment. The static en-

vironment may pose an insurmountable physical barrier (eg, a child-resistant safety cap), or the dynamic environment may be too complex (eg, a crowded shopping mall) for the patient to interact with safely.

The Static Environment

Some static environmental concerns relating to sensorimotor deficits have already been ad-

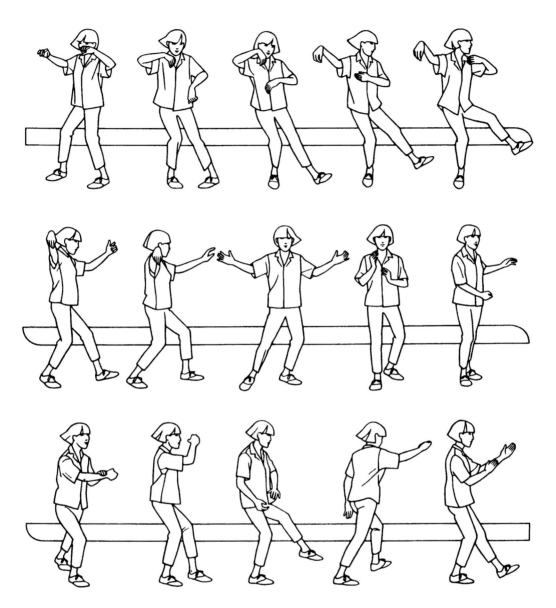

Figure 10–4   continued

dressed above. In addition, the clinician needs to assess other environmental barriers commonly found in the home, hospital, workplace, or recreational setting. Because the patient's last remaining domain is the home, the therapist should make the fewest alterations necessary to improve safety. The adaptations should be as esthetically pleasing as possible and affordable.[10] Contrasting grab bars can be installed near the toilet and tub. Safety frames can be bolted to the toilet to allow the patient to push off with the upper extremities instead of pulling up on grab bars. Slip-resistant adhesive strips or indoor-outdoor carpeting can be installed in front of the bathroom and kitchen sinks or bathtub to prevent sliding on a wet surface. Tub mats or decals can also be placed in the tub to prevent slipping.[10] Other changes could also include re-

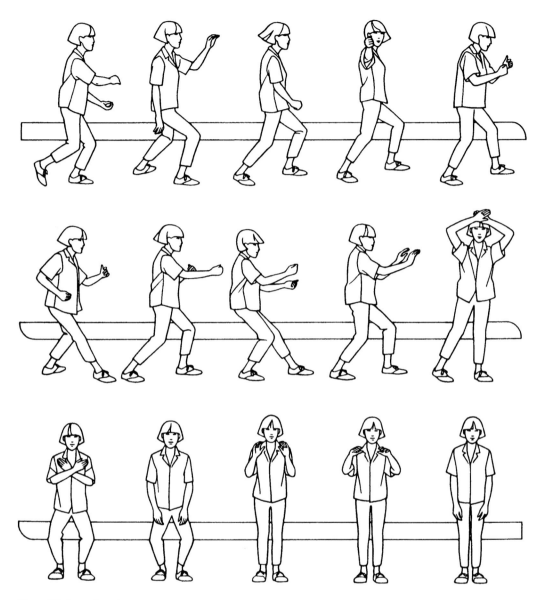

Figure 10–4   continued

moving clutter and electrical cords, placing double-sided tape on scatter rugs, and placing colored adhesive tape on changes in surface, such as steps or raised thresholds.

Other pieces of adaptive equipment are available to help the patient prepare foods, get dressed, perform personal hygiene, and so forth. For more information on environmental changes and designs see Chapter 6, and for more information about adaptive equipment, see Chapter 15.

The Dynamic Environment

With the demands imposed by declining sensorimotor abilities, the older adult has increased difficulty navigating in a dynamic environment. With reduced sensory input, the patient must visually track and time moving objects, such as people, cars, and escalators. Many problems arise during the functional activity of driving, especially at night. In some instances, the safety issues outweigh the benefits of independent transportation, forcing patients to reduce or give up their privilege to drive. In this automotive society, the inability to drive is a major handicap.

For most other functional activities, the patient can be taught to interact with the dynamic environment. Throwing, catching, and batting games can promote eye–hand coordination, and playing "bumper cars" (see Chapter 11) can teach patients to walk confidently in a crowd of people. Although certain adaptations may be needed, many elderly patients can learn to move safely about the home, shopping mall, restaurant, beach, or even the moving deck of a cruise ship.

The older patient also responds well to an alternative environment, such as the therapeutic pool. All the benefits of a buoyant medium combine with the soothing temperature of a heated pool to make the aquatic setting a delight for many achy bodies. Caution, of course, must be used in recommending a heated pool to elderly patients with cardiopulmonary diseases. For more information about the functional program in the aquatic environment, see Chapter 6.

THE FUNCTIONAL PROGRAM IN THE COMMUNITY SETTING

While working on improving the barriers to function, the patient simultaneously begins performing actual or modified functional tasks. The program can be done on an individual basis or in a group class (see Chapter 11). For patients with hearing loss, a one-to-one treatment session in a quiet space is probably of greater benefit than giving instructions in a group setting. The support offered by a peer group, however, can be beneficial to elderly patients who may be wondering how the young ("I wonder if she has graduated high school yet?") group leader can possibly understand what it means to be old.

The older patient does extremely well in a functional program compared with traditional therapy. Emphasis is on the patient's abilities (not inabilities) and how to optimize them to accomplish the patient's own goals. Immediate improvements in function are seen within weeks of initiating a function program. As the patient gains confidence in newfound abilities, more independence occurs. The patient and family often report an improved attitude and outlook on life.

The following two case studies illustrate the benefits of the functional program to community-dwelling elderly patients who, with growing loss of independence, faced the undesirable prospect of being institutionalized.

Case Study 1: Mr. J

August 20, visit 1

- *Diagnosis:* spinal stenosis and bulging disc
- *Age:* 74 years old
- *Past Medical History:* onset 1 year prior— progressive weakness left lower extremity

    onset 5 years prior—heart attack, on warfarin and nitroglycerin
- *Patient Goals:* walk 1 mile, climb stairs, play softball and bowl, garden, fix-it chores
- *Significant Findings on Evaluation*
  1. Abnormal ROM: bilateral ankle dorsiflexion 0°

      left knee extension –30°

      left hip flexion 93°
  2. One-legged standing balance test (OLSBT) eyes open: 2 seconds on right, 0 seconds on left
  3. Function Questionnaire: hard to rise from chair, unable to rise from floor

      unable to climb stairs unassisted

can walk in home, but reports falls of at least 10 times/week

unable to garden, do carpentry, play softball or bowl

independent in daily grooming, hygiene (not tub), driving

- *Social Information*: wife died 2 years prior, daughter died 6 months prior

  lives alone in two-story home, two sons in area

- *Assessment:* symptoms inconsistent with diagnosis, physician consulted

  patient requires functional program, approved by physician

- *Physical Therapy:*
  1. Eight visits over 1 month: ankle pumps, knee extension, hip flexion exercises in sitting

     standing balance in door jamb

     sit-to-stand transfer

     progress to Nautilus resistance training in sitting

     lower extremity locomotor (phase I) program

     step and stair training (4-in step-ups and step-downs)

     modified floor-to-stand transfer (floor raised 1 ft)

  2. September 21, reevaluation: independent chair-to-stand transfer, unable to rise from floor

     stairs with railing, one step at a time

     can walk 1 mile outdoors, reports decreased falls to 2 times /week

     unable to garden, do carpentry, play softball, or bowl

independent in daily grooming, hygiene (not tub), driving

reports improved attitude and hope for future

OLSBT (eyes open) increased to 5 seconds each leg

3. Four visits over 1 month: add Cybex training for left knee flexion and extension

   independent Nautilus program and home exercise program

   progress lunges, squats, and step-ups (7-in step)

   toe and heel walking, treadmill walking all directions

   balance training in door jamb

4. November 8, discharge status: bilateral ankle dorsiflexion 15°

   left knee extension −10°

   left hip flexion 115°

   OLSBT (eyes open) 30 seconds each leg

   independent chair-to-stand and floor-to-stand transfers

   can walk 2 miles, no reported falls over past month

   return to gardening and house chores, not sports

   independent in daily grooming, hygiene (including tub transfer)

   independent driving

   patient and son report improved outlook on life with patient stating he now "wants to live again"

- *Assessment:* patient independent in all desired functions (ADLs,

IADLs, and recreational activities)

independent in his rehabilitation program

safe to live alone

Case Study 2: Mrs. S

June 10, visit 1

- *Diagnosis:* undetermined cause of back pain and left lower extremity pain (hip to foot) for 7 years
- *Age:* 80 years old
- *Past Medical History:* extensive, including sleep disorder, angina, osteoarthritis
- *Patient Goals:* be able to go out to restaurants, play golf, visit friends, take care of cat, take in the mail, prepare light meals
- *Significant Findings on Evaluation:*
  1. Pain: complaint of severe (9/10) pain in left foot, calf, thigh, chest, neck on visual analog scale where 0/10 = no pain
  2. Posture: posterior pelvic tilt with posterior postural sway, thoracic kyphosis
  3. Two-legged standing balance test (eyes open): unsupported, 1 second
  4. Lower extremity strength: 2+/5
  5. Flexibility: moderate hip flexor tightness bilaterally
  6. Function Questionnaire: unable to eat, dress, or bathe by self

     unable to prepare meal

     unable to tolerate sitting for more than 10 minutes

     unable to tolerate supine for more than 5 minutes

     minimal assistance to transfer bed-to-chair, chair-to-stand

     house ambulator with rolling walker and supervision

     unable to shop, visit with friends, garden

     able to feed cat

     Function rating: 12 of 28 on clinic's scale (28 = independent)

- *Social Information:* husband died 3 years ago

  lives alone in two-story house with part-time attendant

- *Assessment:* diagnosis undetermined, past physical therapy palliative only, noneffective

  initiate functional program with focus on lower extremities

- *Physical Therapy:*
  1. Five visits over 1 month: two-legged balance training, postural correction

     modified sit-to-stand transfer with pillows (26-in high seat)

     question patient about chest and neck pain—reports past episodes of angina, recommend patient take her nitroglycerin

     begin stair climbing with railing and moderate assistance

     evaluate foot pain further: pressure sensitivity fifth metatarsal head

     —correct with padded doughnut (immediate pain relief)

—referral to podiatrist: no fracture, but fat pad deterioration

gait training forward and retro, small steps without walker

begin one-legged balance training in door jamb

gait training lateral motion with contact guard

2. June 29, reevaluation:

major decrease in chest and neck pain and foot pain (3/10)

left calf and thigh pain still present and severe (8/10)

independent sit-to-stand from regular height chair (no arm rests)

OLSBT: 2 seconds each leg

posture: neutral pelvis, decreased posterior postural sway

patient reports "I'm feeling much better. I feel like living again. Last night I went outside to look at Mercury. I feel more confident."

3. Four visits over 1 month:

gait training all directions, no device, larger steps

begin step training (4-in step)

begin floor-to-stand transfer with minimal assistance and table

begin standing hip exercises in door jamb

begin prone-lying (1 minute) to stretch out hip flexors

begin bilateral standing "putting" with golf club in house

begin bilateral standing while swinging small racquet

4. July 27, reevaluation:

major decrease in foot and calf pain (3/10), chest pain eliminated

hip and back pain decreased slightly (7/10)

OLSBT: 4 seconds each leg

dynamic standing balance improved with patient able to putt golf balls and swing small racquet without support or assist

house ambulator without device

sitting and supine tolerances unchanged and nonfunctional

5. Five visits over 2 months:

maneuvering through and over obstacle course

continue step-ups

continue chair-to-stand and floor-to-stand transfers (minimal assist)

throwing and catching balls, hitting balls with racquet in standing

begin light plyometrics, vertical leaps in door jamb (supported)

prone-lying up to 6 minutes with reduced back and thigh pain

stair climbing, full flight with railing

recommend railings be installed both sides of stairs in home

outdoor ambulation on uneven surfaces with minimal assistance

car transfers

6. September 28, discharge status:

foot and calf pain 2/10, chest and neck pain eliminated (nitroglycerin)

thigh and back pain reduced to 6/10

more erect standing posture with decreased posterior sway

OLSBT (eyes open): 5 seconds each leg

lower extremity strength 4/5

independent chair-to-stand transfer

independent floor-to-stand transfer with furniture for support

independent in eating, dressing, and bathing (sponge bath)

independent in stairs in own home with railings

can prepare light meal on stove

can walk one block with contact guard (no ambulation device)

can visit friends and go to restaurants with contact guard

Function rating: 24/28

• *Assessment:*   safe household ambulator without assistance

requires assistance of part-time helper for all IADLs and recreational activities

By participating in the function program, the two elderly patients in the above examples made remarkable gains in function. Both were intelligent, motivated, and without signs of dementia except for some short-term memory loss. Both had an excellent support system of caring relatives or helpers. Both had excellent senses of humor. The amount of actual therapy time was small: for Mr. J, 12 one-hour sessions over 2 months, and for Mrs. S, 11 one-hour sessions over 4 months. The bulk of the work was done independently by the patients in the comfort of their own homes or in the Nautilus gym. In other words, the actual performance of the phase II and III programs by the patients was the catalyst for the changes in functional ability.

Had these patients only attended therapy and not taken the initiative to help themselves, they would not have achieved such a high degree of success. Under these circumstances, the functional program is a cost-effective rehabilitation program with the potential to decrease the need for expensive and undesired institutionalization of the community elderly population.

THE FUNCTIONAL PROGRAM IN LONG-TERM CARE FACILITIES

There are many benefits to having nursing home residents improve their functional skills, even if there is no chance of their ever becoming fully independent or leaving the facility. For patients entering the long-term care facility with a medical diagnosis that can be helped through restorative services, physical therapy and/or occupational therapy is often ordered. These patients should engage in both a traditional and a functional rehabilitation program. Many other patients in the nursing home can also benefit from a functional program but are ineligible under Medicare guidelines. Glickstein and Neustadt[11] have developed a program for these elderly patients that works on optimizing their functional potential. The program is called functional maintenance therapy (FMT).

FMT is defined as the provision of services intended to enhance the residual functional abilities identified during an evaluation performed by rehabilitation professionals.[11] This is differentiated from the uncovered service of maintenance therapy, which keeps a patient at the same level and does not need the skills of a professional.

FMT comprises six interrelated steps:

1. screen: identify residents who qualify for short-term intervention
2. evaluate: perform functional assessment
3. program: implement FMT program
4. train: train staff and resident in performing program
5. document
6. ensure quality: assess effectiveness of program

Glickstein and Neustadt[11] have successfully implemented their FMT system to the benefit of hundreds of nursing home residents and staff without insurance denial through meticulous and accurate documentation. They have found a way to work within the present system to provide a better life for residents in nursing homes while being reimbursed for their professional time by Medicare. The FMT offers small but important gains in function to persons otherwise ignored by the system. One patient may wish or need to learn how to feed him- or herself, another might want to be able to get back into bed independently (and not have to wait for understaffed personnel to assist), and another might simply want to be able to water his or her plants.

THE OLDER PATIENT AND FUNCTIONAL REHABILITATION

The older patient, regardless of ability, can benefit from functional training. In fact, it is probably the most cost-effective treatment around to prevent the decline in independence that results in admission to expensive long-term care facilities. Even greatly debilitated patients can improve their condition through low-level restoration or FMT programs. This not only improves their own self-image but frees up assistive personnel to help other needy patients. Although this chapter primarily deals with musculoskeletal impairments and their effects on the geriatric patient's daily function, the reader can easily see that the same principles apply to the neurologically involved patient. Whether through restoration, compensation, or FMT, the elderly patient can improve the quality of his or her own life.

REFERENCES

1. Roach KE. The epidemiology of musculoskeletal disorders and their associated disability in the elderly. *Orthop Phys Ther Clin.* 1993;2:215–224.
2. Fiatrone MA, Evans WJ. Exercise in the oldest old. *Top Geriatr Rehabil.* 1990;5:63–77.
3. Kauffmann T. Posture and age. *Top Geriatr Rehabil.* 1987;2:13–18.
4. Lewis CB. *Improving Mobility in Older Persons.* Gaithersburg, Md: Aspen; 1989.
5. Neumann DA. Arthrokinesiologic considerations in the aged adult. In: Guccione AA, ed. *Geriatric Physical Therapy.* St. Louis, Mo: Mosby–Year Book; 1993: 51–54.
6. Daleiden S. *Aging, balance, and falling* (course notes). Burlington, Mass: Quality Educational Seminars for Therapists; 1989.
7. Johnson JH, Searles LB, McNamara S. In-home geriatric rehabilitation: improving strength and function. *Top Geriatr Rehabil.* 1993;8:51–64.
8. Judge JO. Resistance training. *Top Geriatr Rehabil.* 1993;8:38–50.
9. Craik RL. Sensorimotor changes and adaptation in the older adult. In: Guccione AA, ed. *Geriatric Physical Therapy.* St. Louis, Mo: Mosby–Year Book; 1993: 71–97.
10. Tideiksaar R. Environmental adaptations to preserve balance and prevent falls. *Top Geriatr Rehabil.* 1990;5: 78–84.
11. Glickstein JK, Neustadt GK. *Reimbursable Geriatric Service Delivery.* Gaithersburg, Md: Aspen; 1992.

ADDITIONAL READING

Carr JH, Shepherd RB. *A Motor Relearning Programme for Stroke.* Gaithersburg, Md: Aspen; 1987.

Felsenthal G, Garrison SJ, Steinberg FU. *Rehabilitation of the Aging and Elderly Patient.* Baltimore, Md: Williams & Wilkins; 1994.

Goldstein T. *Geriatric Orthopaedics.* Gaithersburg, Md: Aspen; 1991.

Guccione AA. *Geriatric Physical Therapy.* St Louis, Mo: Mosby–Year Book; 1993.

Hartke R. *Psychological Aspects of Geriatric Rehabilitation.* Gaithersburg, Md: Aspen; 1991.

Kane RA, Kane RL. *Assessing the Elderly.* Lexington, Mass: Lexington Books; 1981.

11

Group Treatment: Function Classes

As patients progress in their individual therapy sessions, oftentimes a group treatment program benefits them greatly. A function class works on normalizing entire body movement patterns as they relate to personal activities of daily living (ADLs) and instrumental ADLs (IADLs) rather than emphasizing the diagnosed physical impairment. Participants may enter the group with any diagnosis or skill level.

Most people respond positively to group therapy and progress faster than with one-on-one treatment. The mutual support provided by the group at the peer level is invaluable in helping each of the members achieve or exceed functional goals. Words of encouragement from a fellow patient encourage the group member better than the same words spoken by the therapist. Education classes on posture, body mechanics, warning signs, and the like teach the group important information needed to confront the everyday world. If the therapist urges active participation, the education classes abound with discussions about everyday functional problems and potential solutions devised by members of the group. The camaraderie that develops from group participation often flows over into daily life, with members socializing or performing activities together outside the formal class.

The group size should be small to maintain an instructor-to-student ratio of 1:3. A therapist with an assistant can successfully run a group of five or six members. The small group size encourages intimacy and interaction among all members. Because the therapist will be constantly evaluating the ability to perform a task as well as the quality of the performance, the number of patients must be kept reasonable. If the group is too large, supervision and safety may be compromised.

In general, function groups work best in four settings:

1. inpatient in a rehabilitation hospital
2. inpatient in a long-term care facility (nursing home)
3. outpatient clinic
4. community classes

In each of these different phases of rehabilitation, the treatment goals will address the most important aspects of functional recovery for the level of the facility. For example, the balance component of the community class would work on the task of balancing on one leg or on a balance board to improve community ambulation, whereas the nursing home class might address two-legged balance at a sink for hygiene and grooming. Yet each of the classes would still cover the same fundamental skills required to perform basic ADLs and IADLs:

- aerobic capacity
- static and dynamic posture (alignment of segments)
- flexibility
- strength
- balance
- speed (acceleration)
- stability (deceleration)
- motor control (coordination, efficiency, etc.)
- mobility, all levels (bed, chair, floor, transfers, etc.)
- ambulation (distance, velocity, assistance)
- advanced ambulation (maneuverability, uneven surfaces, thresholds, etc.)
- lifting
- reaching
- carrying
- pushing and pulling

In addition, the patient determines additional areas to work on to achieve a specific skill, such as golfing or painting.

THE INPATIENT CLASS IN A REHABILITATION HOSPITAL

Functional groups in rehabilitation hospitals work better if orthopaedic and neurological patients have separate groups. Because therapists already place major emphasis on the functional restoration of neurological patients, the following discussion focuses on the function group for orthopaedically involved patients, such as those with hip fractures, total knee replacements, amputations, osteoporosis of the spine, multitrauma from car accidents, and the like.

An occupational therapist and a physical therapist co-lead the group so as to blend the specialties and give equal emphasis to the ability to perform the task as well as to the quality of the movement in performing the task. In general, the orthopaedic condition is of such severity as to require protection during functional activities. Both therapists must be aware of any weight bearing or positional precautions as well as contraindications due to any physical impairment or pathology present. Many therapists, however, are overly cautious and retard functional achievements through unnecessary conservative treatment.

Such is often the case when a patient with an intertrochanteric fracture of the hip repaired with compression screw and plate tries to become independent in grooming and dressing. Although the patient may have partial weight-bearing (PWB) orders, the therapist warns the patient not to stand while washing or shaving and forces the patient to learn these ADL skills in a seated position. Bilateral standing causes a joint reaction force of one times the body weight, which is the equivalent of 50% weight bearing or a heavy PWB (PWB being defined as 25% to 50% weight bearing). Therefore, if the patient slightly unloads the affected side (which usually happens automatically to protect the hip), the patient will be protected while standing on two legs. This is a much more natural position in which to teach washing and grooming. Nothing irritates patients (and insurance carriers) more than paying professionals thousands of dollars to teach a skill, such as washing, in a position that the patient will never use at home.

If the same patient had a subcapital fracture of the hip repaired with Knowles' pins, the patient would probably require a longer healing time with weight precautions of a longer duration. This patient may only be able to ambulate at touch-down weight bearing and would require a seated position for most ADLs to protect the hip.

The group leaders require this level of detailed knowledge of orthopaedic and musculoskeletal impairments to run a function group safely and successfully. The function group provides the highest level of skilled rehabilitation and cannot be run by the aides or even by the licensed assistants without the presence of a licensed physical therapist or occupational therapist.

A patient is eligible to participate in the group if he or she is already oriented to both physical therapy and occupational therapy and will be able to attend the group for at least 1 week. The classes run daily for a minimum of 5 days and last 1.5 hours. They supplement, not replace, individual therapy. Complete evaluations of the individuals are available in the medical record.

Each class consists of the following general format:

- the warm-up
- general total body strengthening and flexibility
- low-level aerobics
- function skills
- education component

The Warm-Up

Patients should begin group by first sitting or standing in corrected postural alignment. If possible, group members should leave their wheelchairs and sit in more supportive chairs with arm rests. Any necessary additions, such as pillows or lumbar supports, should be placed so that the patient is sitting in a comfortable posture (ankles at 90° to the floor, knees at 90°, hips at 90°). The therapists teach the group the importance of good posture and its effect on breathing and movement at this time. The leaders should then instruct the group in deep breathing techniques (Figure 11–1) for 2 to 4 minutes. Depending on ability, group members can stand or sit for warm-up exercises consisting of ankle pumps or circles, marching (alternating hip flexion), kicking (knee extension), upper extremity proprioceptive neuromuscular facilitation (PNF) skill diagonals or straight-plane elevation, neck circles, and any other activities desired.

General Total Body Strengthening and Flexibility

The immobilization that normally accompanies severe orthopaedic insult results in atrophied muscle, loss of strength, and increased stiffness. For patients with an inactive premorbid life style, the problems of weakness and inflexibility are worse. The patients begin open- and closed-chain exercises for both the upper and the lower extremities. The supervising therapists

carefully evaluate the exercises to determine whether postural alignments are maintained and the correct muscles are firing. The leaders emphasize quality and pain-free motions over completion of repetition. Often during this portion of the program, old injuries are newly discovered. A patient with a fractured ankle cannot elevate the arms over shoulder height without pain or substituted motion. Another patient with a total knee replacement cannot lift a weight in the right hand, perhaps because of a Colles' fracture 23 years ago. Now is the time to address these ghosts of the past. The coleaders roam the room correcting movement patterns, adjusting resistance, providing manual techniques to restore range of motion (ROM), and encouraging the group to persevere or rest as indicated. After 15 minutes or so, the group is ready to move on to a short aerobics program.

Low-Level Aerobics

Generally patients in a rehabilitation facility are highly deconditioned and only require a low-level program of about 10 minutes to begin to rebuild the aerobic capacity and endurance necessary for community living. Ambulation, bicycle riding, or even light circuit training is highly effective at this stage. Patients should be taught to take their own pulses and to understand the exercise warning signs. The therapist, after consulting with the patients' physicians, should establish a light to moderate target heart rate of about 65% of maximal heart rate for each patient (the age-predicted maximal heart rate is 220 – age). All patients should be able to talk while exercising aerobically. Although it is highly unlikely that any patients will exceed their target heart rate in this mini–aerobics program, the cardiopulmonary information is invaluable for the group members in case they pursue an active life style after discharge.

Function Skills

The patients perform three or more functional activities per class. An example of a week's worth of function skills is as follows:

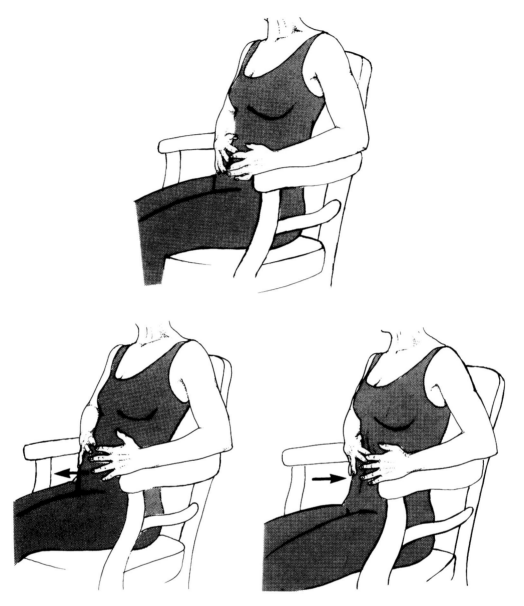

Figure 11–1 Diaphragmatic breathing. *Source:* Reprinted from *Health Promotion and Exercise for Older Adults* (p. 25) by CB Lewis and LC Campanelli, Aspen Publishers, Inc., © 1990.

- day 1: bed mobility, standing balance, car transfers, dressing skills

- day 2: ambulating all directions, lifting to waist height, sit-to-stand transfer

- day 3: toilet transfers, reaching, stair climbing, kitchen skills

- day 4: standing balance at sink, bed mobility, wheelchair transfers

- day 5: ambulating all directions, reaching, transfers, kitchen skills

- day 6: stair climbing, bed mobility, quadruped mobility

If a patient will be discharged shortly to home, he or she should begin floor-to-stand transfers by going through the developmental sequence.

The ability to get on and off the floor can be a life saver.

The therapist schedules sufficient rests for all patients because these functional skills are demanding both physically and mentally. Allowing patients to watch their fellow group members attempt the activities helps their own performance as well. Oftentimes, patients suggest excellent solutions to problems that arise in functional skills. The coleaders should ask the patients for other functional tasks that are important for them to be able to perform and should incorporate them into the functional part of the program.

Education Program

At the end of the daily session, a question-and-answer period or a more formal education program can be instituted. Some suggestions for possible educational topics are as follows:

- warning signs of exercise (perceived exertion)
- effects of aging
- effects of exercise
- body mechanics
- diabetes, osteoarthritis, rheumatoid arthritis, and similar diseases
- safety in the home

Patients may suggest topics about which they want to learn more. Each group will have its own unique needs. An ad lib format works equally well most of the time.

THE INPATIENT CLASS IN A LONG-TERM CARE FACILITY (NURSING HOME)

With the advent of diagnosis-related groups (DRGs) and stricter Medicare guidelines, many patients require discharge to a long-term care facility because they simply do not have the time to recover in the acute care and rehabilitation hospitals. With continued therapy, many of these patients can return home. Unfortunately, personnel shortages in nursing homes translate into a lower level of therapy than these patients need. Many times, occupational therapy services are not even provided. A well-run function group can help these patients acquire the skills necessary to return home in a cost-effective manner.

The Function Group for Temporary Residents

A physical therapist or occupational therapist leads the group with the help of a licensed assistant or rehabilitation aide. Group size should not exceed four patients to an instructor. In general, most of the patients with orthopaedic conditions have only minimal weight-bearing or positional precautions in effect at this time. The leader must possess an in-depth knowledge of musculoskeletal impairments and their relationship to functional loss. Although offered in a group format, this class provides extremely skilled rehabilitation care and cannot be run successfully by rehabilitation aides.

A patient is eligible to participate in the group if he or she expects (or hopes) to be discharged home within 6 months. The classes run two times a week for 2 months and last 1.5 hours. Complete physical therapy and occupational therapy evaluations should be performed for each individual.

Each class consists of the following general format:

- the warm-up
- general total body strengthening and flexibility
- low-level aerobics
- function skills
- safety in the home class

The Warm-Up

The warm-up is basically the same as in the rehabilitation hospital group. All participants must sit in supportive chairs with arm rests (not wheelchairs or cardiac chairs). Patients must learn to use pillows or lumbar supports to sit in the best posture possible. The leader should instruct the members in deep breathing (Figure 11–1) or Tai Chi (see Figure 10–3) for 5 to 7 minutes. The warm-up exercises may be performed in sitting or supported standing.

General Total Body Strengthening and Flexibility

The atmosphere of even the best long-term care facilities promotes passivity in many patients. Decreased activity levels in combination with normal aging and pathology cause major losses in strength, ROM, and function. The leader teaches both open- and closed-chain exercises with resistance as indicated. The therapist corrects movement patterns while ensuring efficient and pain-free exercising. Group members are encouraged to rest as needed. Exercises can include developmental sequence activities, minisquats, resisted pulley work, chair push-ups, PNF techniques, bench presses, biceps curls, Yoga stretches, and the like.

Low-Level Aerobics

Many nursing home patients are severely deconditioned and need to restore their aerobic capacity. Working at 40% to 60% of their maximum heart rate is usually sufficient to achieve an aerobic effect. Ambulation, bike riding, dance, and Tai Chi can all be used to build endurance. A 5-minute program the first day is progressed an additional 2 minutes per class. By the end of the first month, the group will be at a 20-minute workout in a safe manner. The leader teaches the participants to take their own pulses and explains the exercise warning signs and the need not to exceed the patient's own perceived exertion. The leader should engage the group in discussion to ensure that all members can speak while exercising. The aerobics workout can also be set to music with patients encouraged to sing along while exercising.

Function Skills

The patients learn four functional activities per week. An example of an 8-week program is as follows:

- week 1: bed mobility (including prone), sit-to-stand transfer, two-legged balance, reaching overhead
- week 2: toilet transfers, ambulation all directions, kitchen skills, car transfers
- week 3: stair climbing, lifting to waist height, pushing, pulling
- week 4: ambulation for speed, dressing skills, sit-to-stand transfer, bed mobility
- week 5: one-legged balance, floor-to-stand transfer, kitchen skills, dressing skills
- week 6: ambulation uneven surfaces, reaching overhead, pushing, car transfers
- week 7: one-legged balance, crawling, floor-to-stand transfer, bed mobility
- week 8: ambulation for speed, reaching to floor, kitchen skills, toilet transfers

The program, of course, is adjusted to fit the particular needs of the group members so that they will have the physical ability to return home. By attending the group, some members may achieve high physical function but remain so cognitively impaired that they cannot be discharged to home safely. These patients require an occupational therapy consult for specialized evaluation and treatment.

Safety in the Home Class

The education portion of the function group revolves around problem solving in the home. After being institutionalized, some members may forget the basics of how to be safe at home. Family members may be afraid that their loved one will get hurt living at home as a result of poor judgment or lack of safety. Discussions and simulations of problems that may arise can help the group members plan for potential trouble at home. An occupational therapist or social worker can offer valuable expertise in this area.

The Function Group for Permanent Residents

A similar group can be created for those residents of nursing homes who are not expected ever to have the capability of returning to a life style at home. The format of this group is similar, and its goal is to optimize the level of independence in personal ADLs for each member. This would serve not only to increase the patient's dignity and sense of self-worth but also to decrease the amount of assistance required of the nursing staff. Any resident with sufficient cognitive abilities could join after receiving medical clearance and evaluations from physical therapy and occupational therapy. The classes run two or three times a week for 1 hour as an ongoing service of the nursing home. A physical therapist or occupational therapist should attend at least one class per week to perform evaluations and to upgrade or adjust the program. The therapist should also teach the licensed physical therapist assistant or occupational therapist assistant how to run the group in his or her absence. The emphasis of this functional program is improving ambulation, transfers, balance, dressing, and grooming skills. Class size should not exceed six participants per instructor.

Each class consists of the following general format:

- the warm-up
- general conditioning and aerobics
- function skills

The Warm-Up

If possible, residents transfer from their wheelchairs to more supportive chairs. Deep breathing and postural awareness begin each class. These are followed by some light sitting exercises, beginning with ankle pumps and working up.

General Conditioning and Aerobics

Circuit training is the best way to run this part of the program. The therapist designs seven or eight exercise stations to create the circuit. The participants exercise at each station (nonstop if possible) for a specified amount of time, (eg, 2 to 3 minutes). If this exercise program for strengthening and flexibility continues at a con-

stant pace, an aerobic effect may be achieved. Any resident who is ambulatory may walk to the next station; others may have to propel their wheelchairs to the next station. Some suggested stations are as follows:

- station 1: rock board (wobble board): sitting ankle dorsiflexion, plantar flexion, inversion, eversion, circles
- station 2: resisted knee extension (open-chain) and hip flexion in sitting
- station 3: upper body station with dowel: wrist extension, biceps curls, bench press, military press in sitting, armchair push-ups (dips)
- station 4: sit-to-stand with 10-second bilateral standing balance
- station 5: supported standing, minisquats, marching
- station 6: bicycle riding (stationary)
- station 7: ambulation around exercise room
- station 8: prone-lying or prone press-ups on plinth

Many of these activities require close supervision or assistance for balance and safety as well as for helping group members in and out of positions or onto and off equipment. The leader of the group has to assess whether sufficient personnel are available for the particular function group to run safely or if modifications to the circuit stations need to be made. During a planned rest period, the leader should encourage group discussions on various topics of interest.

Function Skills

Each class should concentrate on one or two function skills. Because each participant will require close supervision, only one member at a time can perform a function skill. The other members watch and offer suggestions to improve the performance. Some important skills for this population to master are independent:

- bed mobility (including supine-to-sit)
- bed-to-chair transfer
- chair-to-toilet transfer

- unsupported standing balance
- standing balance at sink
- hygiene and grooming at sink
- ambulation to toilet
- ambulation in room
- ambulation in hallways

A short question-and-answer period is a good way to end the group. If a resident happens to make exceptional progress in this group, he or she can graduate to the other function group, which has more challenging activities.

THE OUTPATIENT CLASS IN A CLINIC OR HOSPITAL

Functional groups work well in the outpatient setting. If the group is run in a hospital, both a physical therapist and an occupational therapist can colead the class. In a private clinic one therapist can lead the group because patients have already attained a higher level of function. Quite often, patients have been fully rehabilitated from the original physical impairment only to find themselves still unable to function normally. A combination of old injuries or poor postural habits with the new diagnosis makes the patient function in an abnormal manner. The therapist in charge of the group must be knowledgeable about pathology as it relates to function as well as postural alignments and movement patterns.

A patient is eligible to participate in the group after attending at least 2 weeks' worth of one-on-one therapy. In general, the patient's therapist observes difficulty in restoring function or believes that the patient would benefit more from group treatment. The classes run twice weekly for 1.5 hours for 4 to 8 weeks. Participants can still attend one individual treatment session per week in addition to the group if needed. The therapist should perform a functional assessment on each patient before the class begins (see Chapter 13).

Each class consists of the following general format:

- the warm-up
- general total body strengthening and flexibility
- low-level to midlevel aerobics
- function skills
- education

The Warm-Up

The class begins with participants attaining proper posture in a supportive chair. The patients learn to place any necessary pillows, lumbar rolls, or cushions for good positioning (hips, knees, and ankles at 90°). In the beginning the leader teaches diaphragmatic breathing, with patients placing their hands over the lower ribs to feel each chest expansion. By the second or third week, a more complex breathing pattern, such as that used in Tai Chi, is introduced. If the leader does not know Tai Chi, upper extremity PNF diagonal patterns may be substituted. Warm-up exercises of ankle pumps, marching, kicking, shoulder circles, and so forth can be done in sitting or standing.

General Total Body Strengthening and Flexibility

Although this outpatient group is operating at a higher functional level than the groups mentioned previously, major strength and flexibility deficits remain. In the beginning, the exercise program is similar to the inpatient programs and consists of gentle open- and closed-chain exercises done first in sitting and progressing to standing. At this time, the therapist corrects any movement dysfunctions, such as loss of scapulohumeral rhythm during arm elevation or excessive hip internal rotation during minisquats (which will cause patella tracking problems). During the middle stages, the intensity of the exercise program increases, with patients doing isokinetic exercises or using resistive equipment such as cuff weights, plyoballs, rubber tubing, or Nautilus machines. Closed-chain work also intensifies, with patients performing low-level step-ups, deeper squats, and modified plyometrics. In addition, the leader works on improving the flexibility of the ankles, hips, and shoulders through the use of wobble boards (biomechanical ankle platform system [BAPS], rock board, Xerboard, etc.), developmental sequence, and manual techniques.

Low-Level to Midlevel Aerobics

Because the patients are already warmed up, the aerobics portion begins in either sitting or standing. Participants can follow a low-impact program, ride stationary bicycles, try a step class, or exercise continuously from a seated position. The leader teaches the patients to take their own pulses and also educates them about the exercise warning signs. In general, this group can safely exercise at 60% to 75% of maximal heart rate. All participants should be able to talk while exercising aerobically. Initially, the aerobics portion consists of about 5 minutes of exercising. The leader can add 3 minutes per class if tolerated by the attendees. A cool-down exercise period follows the aerobics program.

Function Skills

The community dwellers require a higher level of functional abilities. Being able to walk with an efficient, pain-free gait pattern is no longer good enough. They want the ability to cross streets, negotiate curbs and cracks on sidewalks, maneuver through shopping malls, get in and out of bathtubs, carry groceries, go banking, put away dishes, push grocery carts, pull golf carts, chop vegetables, lift children, drive a car, take public transportation, wash floors, vacuum rugs, make dinner, play softball, and go to work.

The group members work to master the basic mobility skills:

- bed mobility (including prone-lying and getting in and out of bed)
- sit-to-stand transfers
- floor-to-stand transfers
- ambulation (including pattern, distance, velocity, negotiating uneven terrain and stairs, maneuvering through crowds, etc.)

In addition to mobility, the participants need to accomplish the function skills of lifting to waist height and shoulder height, reaching (to the floor, across a counter, above head height), carrying, and pushing and pulling as well as ADLs and sport skills such as throwing, batting, cleaning, using tools, and the like.

The therapist makes the function portion of the class as fun and practical as possible. Patients can perform advanced gait activities such as side-stepping and retrowalking in a Conga line (this is especially good for patients with balance problems). They can also play another fun but extremely important game called bumper cars (Exhibit 11–1) to help alleviate the fear of walking in crowds, such as those found in a shopping mall or on a busy sidewalk. In addition, modified sports such as Nerf baseball, kickball, Frisbee tossing, basketball, balloon volleyball, etc., help with the total body coordination needed for everyday function.

Before each game, the therapist determines the position a group member can safely play while building important new skills. During the game, the therapist examines the movement patterns of the group members, correcting inefficient or harmful motions. Patients with known shoulder problems may need to pitch underhand initially, and batters with back problems must learn to swing with the spine stabilized and the lower extremities rotating. Fielders with knee problems must side-step carefully to track down the ball and must learn to squat with the patellae positioned properly over the feet. These fun activities promote normal motion and, it is hoped, will be carried over into everyday living activities.

Education Program

At the end of the daily session, the therapist can teach the patients about various topics of interest, such as:

Exhibit 11–1   Bumper Cars

- **Level 1:** One member stands still while the others walk past him or her, getting closer and closer without making contact.
- **Level 2:** The leader and other group members gently brush by so that their shoulders make small contact.
- **Level 3:** The rest of the group stands still as if frozen in a crowded walking space while the member maneuvers around or through the motionless crowd.
- **Level 4:** The member walks against the flow of traffic while the rest of the group walks past him or her without contact.
- **Level 5:** The member walks against the flow of traffic initiating small shoulder contact with other members.
- **Level 6:** The member walks against the flow of traffic while the rest of the group initiates contact with him or her as they walk by each other.
- **Level 7:** The member walks against the flow of traffic while trying to avoid (by changing speed or direction) other group members who are trying to make contact.

Additional advances in the program include having members carry shopping bags or boxes, push a cart, or drag (pull) a bag while advancing through the levels. Adjusting the weight carried, pushed, or pulled affects the difficulty of the task.

- effects of hypokinetics and exercise
- effects of aging
- body mechanics
- types of footwear
- warning signs of exercise
- safety during community activities (shopping, banking, sports, etc.)
- importance of body awareness

The group can also suggest topics about which they wish to learn more.

COMMUNITY CLASSES

Many community classes exist to promote the general health and fitness of its members. This class differs in that it exists only to promote functional abilities. Many adults with prior impairments (eg, weakness, stiffness, bursitis, degenerative changes, etc.) or old pathologies (eg, Parkinson's disease, rheumatoid arthritis, etc.) have been told simply to live with it. Thus begins a downward spiral of abilities, with one impairment promoting further impairments and disabilities.

The group operates on a format similar to that of the other function groups. The difference is that none of the attendees is an official patient. The group members have not been to therapy in

years or at all. They hear about the group through their internist, a newspaper advertisement, an elderly housing bulletin, or a local recreation department. The attendees pay out of pocket for the service, as they would if they joined a fitness center (alternatively, the therapist offers the group free of charge as a community service). Each participant must attend one individual therapy session for an evaluation. The therapist then recommends whether the participant needs a medical examination, individualized therapy, or the function group.

HOW TO SET UP FUNCTION CLASSES

This section describes how to organize and start a function class. Since most therapists already work in some type of facility, a written or oral proposal needs to be made to the administration promoting the need and benefits of such a group. (Generally speaking, most administrators favor therapy projects that require no major purchases nor time nor labor constraints, promote the patient's well being, and generate revenues for the facility.) The therapist usually has no problem getting reimbursement for a function group. This is one area in health care where all parties, the patient, physician, therapist, facility, and insurance carrier, agree: a function group is a cost-effective way to manage patients with disabilities.

Requirements

Beginning function classes in either an inpatient or an outpatient environment require minimal space, equipment, time, and effort expended for the benefits reaped.

Space

A small therapy gym or recreation room is needed for the general exercises, aerobics, and function skills. Ideally the space should be light, roomy, and quiet. The environment should be maintained at a comfortable temperature of about 68° to 70° F for adults and about 5° warmer for older adults. So that changes in ambulation can be reported objectively, a 100-ft track or corridor should be marked off. A stairway and bathroom need to be close by. The area should be handicapped accessible. If the facility already has ADL rooms set up, such as an occupational therapy kitchen or mock bedroom and bathroom, the therapist should reserve these rooms for function work as needed.

Equipment

Equipment requirements are modest and are found in most physical therapy and occupational therapy departments. The therapist might need to make a few modest purchases (total cost, about $300). The minimum equipment necessary (see Chapter 14) is as follows:

- a chair with arm rests for each group member
- pillows, lumbar support rolls, and foam wedges
- a mat, plinth, or bed
- a mercury manometer
- a stopwatch
- a full-length mirror
- a wobble board (rock board, BAPS board, etc.)
- cuff weights or pulley weights
- a goniometer

- an aerobic step or sturdy 4-in high platform
- a sturdy step stool
- a Gymnik ball (65 cm)
- a Nerf ball, Nerf turbo football, Wiffleball and bat, or foam ball and bat
- a soft flying disc (Frisbee)
- a 9-in children's plastic play ball
- a plastic milk crate
- plyoballs (4 and 8 lb)
- a small floor exercise mat
- a screwdriver and screws
- a hammer and nails
- a 2-in-thick piece of wood
- a wheeled cart on which to place equipment

Aside from the chairs, the group uses only selected pieces of equipment at each session.

Labor and Time

One skilled physical therapist or occupational therapist needs to be present for every three or four patients. An inexperienced therapist may only be able to handle two patients. In a long-term care facility, one leader can instruct no more than six participants safely. The leader should be certified in cardiopulmonary resuscitation and should be aware of all code procedures in the facility. Licensed physical therapy and occupational therapy assistants or rehabilitation aides may assist in the group at the discretion of the leader. The therapist should allot an additional half hour for every class for proper set-up, break-down, and documentation (ie, 30 minutes of nonreimbursable time).

Communication with Physicians

For outpatient clinics and inpatient long-term care facilities, form letters can be sent to covering physicians (and insurance carriers) to request referral to the group, to inform them that a patient has entered a group, or to inform them that a patient has completed the program (see Exhibits 11–2 through 11–5). The same information can be reported orally in a rehabilitation facility at team meetings.

Exhibit 11–2   Sample Physician's Referral Letter

Dear Dr. _____,

   Your patient, _____, has been evaluated and treated at this clinic for _____ weeks. I have

determined that he/she would benefit greatly from our Function Group. The Function Group consists of 16 1.5-hour

sessions of exercise to improve strength, flexibility, aerobic capacity, and functional skills in a small group setting.

   You will receive copies of your patient's functional assessment and 8-week reassessment. Please sign the enclosed

Physical (Occupational) Therapy Function Group Referral Form and indicate whether any problems or precautions ex-

ist for this patient. Thank you.

                                           Sincerely yours,

                                           Jamie E. Sandler, PT

Exhibit 11–3   Sample of Follow-Up Letter to Referring Physician

Dear Dr. _____,

   Thank you for referring _____ to the Function Group. A complete Functional Assessment was

performed by _____, PT (OT) on _____, 1996. A copy of the assessment is en-

closed for your records.

   Unless you indicate otherwise, your patient's heart rate will not be allowed to exceed _____ beat/min, and the pa-

tient's blood pressure will be maintained at _____ mm Hg during the exercise and aerobics sessions. Please advise us

immediately if these cardiac parameters are not safe for this patient!

   The Function Group began on _____, 1995, and consists of 8 weeks of progressive therapeutic exercise, aero-

bic training, balance training, functional training, and educational sessions. A follow-up assessment will be completed

at the end of the 16 sessions, and you will be apprised of the results.

   If you have any questions or recommendations, please feel free to call me. Your input is most welcome.

                                           Sincerely yours,

                                           Jamie E. Sandler, PT

Exhibit 11–4   Sample Letter to Referring Physician with Reassessment

Dear Dr. _____,

Your patient, _____, has successfully completed the Function Group 8-week program. Based on the enclosed results, I recommend that this patient:

___ repeat the program.

Although good gains have been made in _____,
severe deficits remain in _____,
requiring a supervised therapy program. Please authorize continued therapy (group or individualized) on the enclosed form.

___ be discharged from therapy and continue with an independent program.

___ return to you for medical consultation concerning _____.

Thank you for referring this patient to the Function Group.

Sincerely yours,

Jamie E. Sandler, PT

Exhibit 11–5   Sample Therapy Referral Form

PHYSICAL THERAPY GROUP REFERRAL

NAME _____   DATE _____

DIAGNOSIS _____

___ EVALUATE AND TREAT TWO TIMES/WEEK FOR 8 WEEKS

Active and Resistive Exercise
Neuromuscular Reeducation
Mobility Training
Nautilus Strengthening
Flexibility Training
Balance Training
Postural Awareness and Education
Body Mechanics
Activities of Daily Living (Basic and Instrumental)
Patient Education

___ This patient has no medical restrictions to participate in group class.

___ This patient has the following limitations: _____

Observe the following restrictions or precautions: _____

_____, MD
Signature

Setting Up Community Classes

Promoting a community class requires the additional work of finding both physical space and willing participants. The therapist searches for a suitable facility with sufficient space and handicapped accessibility. Many hospitals, fitness centers, senior centers, and private clinics may eagerly provide space as a community service. Finding participants means advertising or announcing the group in newspapers, posting flyers in the community, mailing brochures, and/or informing local physicians of the service. Local newspapers allow free announcements of community services. If the leader plans to charge only a nominal fee to cover costs or plans to run the group completely free of charge, the following sample announcement could be used:

RESTORING FUNCTION

Having difficulty getting out of bed? or chairs? A unique exercise workshop promoting strength and flexibility, gentle aerobics, and functional mobility skills such as walking, stair climbing, squatting, carrying bundles, and getting out of chairs will be offered free of charge to the public by Elyse J. Schultz, PT. Classes run twice a week for 2 months. For more information, call Schultz Physical Therapy at 555-0239.

The therapist can also inform local physicians of this service through the telephone or mail (see Exhibit 11–6). The physicians could then mention the function group to any interested patients.

Because the participants may not be official patients, the therapist may wish the attendees to sign a release of liability form (see Exhibit 11–7) or a consent form. It is important for the therapist to be aware that no one can legally sign away all their rights and that the therapist is still liable for any acts of negligence that may occur. A current liability policy is excellent protection in our society. The group leader may wish to consult an attorney for legal advice before running a community-based program.

CONCLUSION

The functional program runs well within a group format. The group leader has to be an extremely skilled and experienced clinician to observe the many members of the group and adjust their programs based on both their impairments and their functional goals. Suggestions for group formats have been presented in this chapter to give the reader some frameworks in which to create a group or groups within his or her own setting and needs. Little research has been done on the efficacy of group treatment. Clinical experience suggests that it is a cost-effective and pleasurable way to restore functional performance.

Exhibit 11–6   Sample Letter to Physician Introducing Function Group in Community

Dear Dr. _____,

I am pleased to introduce you to a novel fitness program run by the therapists of Schultz Physical Therapy. The Function Group is an 8-week wellness program designed to reverse gently the effects of hypokinetics and immobility that your middle-age or geriatric patients may experience as a result of injury, disease, or disuse.

After a comprehensive Physical Therapy Evaluation, your patient will participate in 16 1.5-hour sessions of cardiopulmonary, musculoskeletal, and functional activities training in a small group setting. Patients will be taught to monitor their own pulses while exercising in a safe range that you prescribe. The exercises will slowly progress from active total body work to resistive Nautilus training. Strengthening, flexibility, balance, and daily function will be emphasized. Patients with specific musculoskeletal impairments (eg, subdeltoid bursitis, arthritis of the knee, history of low back pain, etc.) will be given individual exercises in addition to the group program.

To ensure good communication, you will receive a copy of both the patient's initial evaluation and the 8-week reassessment. The therapist will recommend whether your patient is ready to continue with an independent exercise program, needs to repeat the program, or is not benefitting from the program.

If you would like to refer a patient to the Function Group, please send the enclosed Group Referral Form to us by _____.

If you have any questions about this new program, please call me at 555-0239.

Sincerely yours,

Elyse J. Schultz, PT

Exhibit 11–7   Release of Liability Form

I understand that I am voluntarily participating in an exercise group to increase my general fitness and functional capabilities.

Adequate opportunity has been given to me to ask any questions concerning the Function Group. I understand that I may at any time discontinue participation in the activities of the group if for any reason I see fit to do so.

I expressly agree that all instruction in and use of all facilities and equipment shall be undertaken at my own risk. In addition, I represent that I am physically and medically able to undertake any and all instruction provided.

_____
Signature

_____
Date

Please list all conditions, limitations, or sensitivities on the reverse side of this form. Also, please list any conditions for which you have seen a physician in the past year.

Please comment on any concerns that you may have about which you feel the group therapist should know.

12

Fitness and Function

A patient who attends therapy, completes the exercise and functional programs, becomes cured, and returns to a normal functional routine is considered a rehabilitation success. Yet if that patient comes back 2 months or 1 year later with the original complaint, how successful was the treatment? When asked at what point in time the problem returned, the patient invariably answers that after feeling "all better," he or she "got lazy" or "too busy" and stopped exercising. After 1 to 2 months of inactivity, the problem or pain seemed to return slowly.

A total body fitness program is essential to functional well-being. After reading the previous chapters, the clinician may get the impression that short-duration exercises and activities of daily living performed throughout the day will solve all the patient's functional problems. Although that is sometimes the case, the majority of people need to maintain an active life style, including some form of aerobic fitness routine. For some patients this means a return to a 45-minute step aerobic class performed three times a week, whereas for others it means a daily brisk walk of 30 to 60 minutes. In general, patients should exercise aerobically at 60% to 80% of their maximal heart rate for 20 to 30 minutes three times a week[1] (the reader is referred to the many texts about aerobic conditioning for complete details on creating a safe

cardiovascular training program for both healthy and unfit subjects).

Most rehabilitation and sports medicine clinicians agree about the many benefits of working out[1]:

- a reduction in pulse rate and blood pressure
- an increase in stroke volume and cardiac output
- an increase in maximum oxygen uptake
- an increase in pulmonary function
- an increased number of mitochondria
- an increase in muscle size
- a decrease in body fat and blood cholesterol level
- an increase in strength of bones, ligaments, and tendons

There is also an undeniable risk of further injury from the fitness program itself, however. Requa et al[2] found a moderate risk of musculoskeletal injury due to participating in an aerobic or weight-lifting fitness program. Sporadic exercising (the Weekend Warrior syndrome) can be worse than not exercising at all because sudden exertion by an unfit subject can easily cause physical harm.

Nevertheless, the benefits of improving the body's system reserves seem to far outweigh the potential damage. In fact, sufficient cardio-pulmonary endurance is a prerequisite for performing basic ADLs that are considered aerobic activities.[1] Therefore, while the patient is still attending therapy the clinician should recommend a suitable fitness program to complement the exercises and functional program. The benefits and risks should also be explained, so that the patient can make an informed decision. In addition, the patient should be taught to stop exercising if any of the following warning signs appear[3]:

- a decrease in pulse rate
- labored breathing or inability to speak while exercising
- pale or cool skin
- excessive fatigue
- any pain in the chest, jaw, or upper extremities
- incoordination or lightheadedness

There are many fitness options available today for home or club use. Together, the therapist and patient can choose the best program based on the patient's life style, desires, and any remaining physical limitations. This is important because the rate of injury from participating in a fitness program is doubled in the presence of a pre-existing injury.[2] Table 12–1 shows a list of fitness options and the skeletal structures potentially stressed by those activities. The patient should obviously avoid any fitness activities that place the injured site at higher risk than necessary.

Whatever the aerobic or strengthening program, the patient must use the information learned in therapy about skeletal alignment and muscle balance to customize the fitness program to diminish the risk of future injuries. For example, in an upper body weight-lifting program, many of the maneuvers force the glenohumeral joint into excessive abduction, extension, and external rotation, the so-called at-risk position for instability[4] (Figure 12–1). If a patient already has a shoulder or neck problem, the same activities can easily be modified to allow the activity to continue in a less stressful manner (Figure 12–2). This may not be the clas-

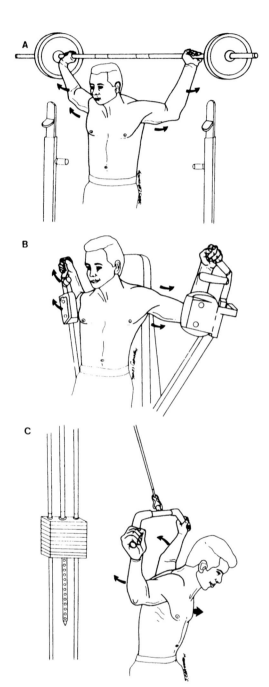

Figure 12–1 Weight-lifting maneuvers producing forced abduction, extension, and external rotation. (**A**) Military press. Note the behind-the-neck positioning. (**B**) Flys. Note the full stretch with elbows behind the plane of the body. (**C**) Pull-downs. Note the forward leaning position and wide grip. *Source:* Reprinted with permission from the *American Journal of Sports Medicine* (1993;21[4]:600), Copyright © 1993, American Orthopaedic Society for Sports Medicine.

Table 12-1 Common Fitness Exercises with Associated Areas of Skeletal Stress

Fitness Activity	*Structures at Risk*	*Avoid If This Acute Impairment Is Present*
Cross-country skiing Cross-country ski machine	Tibiofemoral joint Ankle/foot complex	Genu varum or valgum Pronated foot (uncorrected) Bunion Atrophied plantar fat pad Achilles tendinitis Plantar fasciitis Anterior compartment syndrome
Rowing (boat or machine)	Spine Patellofemoral joint Scapulothoracic "joint"	Low back pain Patellofemoral dysfunction Glenohumeral instability Glenohumeral impingement
Stair climbing Stair machine Step aerobics Hiking	Sacroiliac joint Hip joint Patellofemoral joint Tibiofemoral joint	Sacroiliac dysfunction Hip or knee osteoarthritis Patellofemoral dysfunction Tibiofemoral cartilage/bone defect Torn meniscus
Rock climbing VersaClimber	All extremity joints	Glenohumeral impingement Hip muscle imbalance Patellofemoral joint Achilles tendinitis Plantar fasciitis
Walking	Lower extremity weight-bearing joints	Acute lower extremity fracture, severe sprain or strain
Swimming	Shoulder complex Tibiofemoral joint	Impingement syndrome
Martial arts	All joints	Fractures
Jogging Running	All lower extremity weight-bearing joints	Iliotibial band syndrome Hip or knee osteoarthritis Anterior compartment syndrome Achilles tendinitis Plantar fasciitis Bunion
Bicycling	Spine Sacroiliac joint Ischium Patellofemoral joint	Low back pain Sacroiliac dysfunction Ischial bursitis Patellofemoral dysfunction
Ice skating In-line skating (roller blading) Glide board	Hip joint Patellofemoral joint Tibiofemoral joint Talocrural (ankle) joint Subtalar joint	Trochanteric bursitis Patellofemoral dysfunction Anterior cruciate ligament or meniscal tear Achilles tendinitis Plantar fasciitis Lateral ankle sprain

Note: Patients with the acute or uncorrected conditions listed in the last column should not choose the corresponding fitness exercise as part of a beginning fitness program. The patient may resume the fitness exercises initially avoided as the injury heals or corrections (tape, splint, orthotics, etc.) are made.

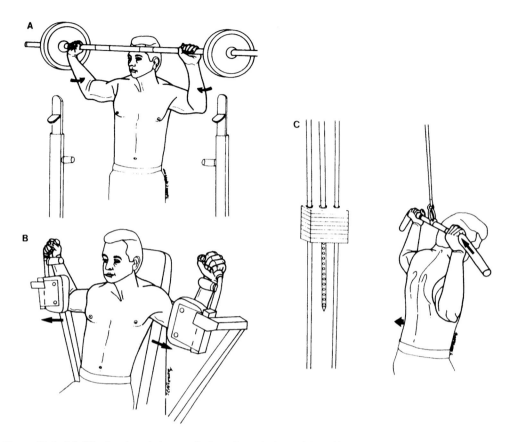

Figure 12–2   Modifications in technique to eliminate forces in the at-risk positions. (**A**) Military press done in front of the body. (**B**) Flys. Elbows do not go posterior to the plane of the body. (**C**) Pull-downs in erect position with narrow grip. *Source:* Reprinted with permission from the *American Journal of Sports Medicine* (1993;21[4]:601), Copyright © 1993, American Orthopaedic Society for Sports Medicine.

sic way to build strength in the upper body, but it allows safe continuation of a desired sport. Table 12–2 shows a list of fitness activities along with an accompanying list of postural reminders to maintain skeletal alignment and minimize potential injury.

As formal therapy sessions become less frequent, the patient should continue the independent fitness program about four times a week. After discharge from therapy, the patient should continue to perform both functional and fitness programs at the same (or higher) intensity for at least 2 months. For the next 4 to 8 months, both programs can continue on an every other day basis. As the patient approaches 1 year from onset of injury, the functional program should be completely automatic and require no further formal exercise. Efficient, pain-free movement should now be the patient's normal motor pattern. The fitness program should ideally continue two to three times a week for life, however.

Table 12–2 Fitness Activities and Postural Alignment

Fitness Activity	Postural Reminders To Minimize Injury
Cross-country skiing Cross-country ski machine	Keep knee over foot (hip in neutral rotation) Wear orthotics if feet are pronated
Rowing	Keep patella centrally tracked Make sure scapulae adduct during row and that not all movement (eg, shoulder extension) is coming from the glenohumeral joint
Stair climbing Step aerobics	Do not let spine forward bend excessively Do not let pelvis drop to each side excessively Keep hip in neutral rotation with patella centrally tracked
Rock climbing	Keep good scapulohumeral alignment Maintain hip muscle balance (especially for shorter people) Keep patella centrally tracked
Walking	Keep spine erect Maintain neutral hip rotation with patella centrally tracked
Swimming	Keep good scapulohumeral alignment If impingement present, keep humerus in neutral rotation (eg, middle finger, not thumb, enters water first during crawl stroke) If impingement present, avoid butterfly stroke
Martial arts	Maintain neutral hip position (knee over foot) especially in low stances
Jogging Running	Maintain hip muscle balance (hamstrings, iliopsoas, iliotibial band) Keep knee over foot Wear orthotics if feet pronated or supinated Maintain length of Achilles tendon (gastrocnemius and soleus)
Bicycling	Use padded seat or stand if ischial pain present Adjust seat height for comfort or injury protection Maintain pelvic alignment Keep patella centrally tracked
Skating Glide board	Do not let spine forward bend excessively Maintain hip muscle balance Keep patella centrally tracked

Note: When engaging in fitness activities, skeletal alignment must be maintained to prevent further injury. When posture is not optimally held, the joint centers of rotation are altered with forces transmitted to different soft and bony tissues. This can lead (over time) to musculoskeletal damage.

REFERENCES

1. Burnett CN. Principles of aerobic exercise. In: Kisner C, Colby LA, eds. *Therapeutic Exercise.* 2nd ed. Philadelphia, Pa: Davis; 1990: 637–666.

2. Requa RK, DeAvilla LN, Garrick JG. Injuries in recreational adult fitness activities. *Am J Sport Med.* 1993;21: 461–467.

3. Lewis CB. Effects of aging on the cardiovascular system. *Clin Manage.* 1984;4:24–29.

4. Gross ML, Brenner SL, Esformes I, Sonzogni JJ. Anterior shoulder instability in weight lifters. *Am J Sports Med.* 1993;21:599–603.

13

Measuring Function

In all medical practice, including rehabilitation, the effectiveness of treatment can only be assessed through outcome measures, such as measuring reductions in symptoms, improvements in daily functioning, or improvements in the patient's sense of well-being and quality of life.[1] In addition, there is recent evidence that a patient's ability level, not the severity of the disease present, dictates the quality of life and may predict the quantity of life in rheumatoid arthritis and other diseases.[2] Initial evaluations of function as well as outcome measures of function are imperative for better health care in our society.

ESTABLISHING A BASELINE

To treat any condition, a therapist must first be able to assess or identify the problems present. The therapist includes the observations and findings from clinical tests into a baseline data set, also called an evaluation. Based on this evaluation, the therapist develops a treatment plan. To determine whether this therapeutic plan in fact is working, the clinician needs to be able to reassess the problem and observe whether any change has occurred from the original data taken (ie, the baseline data set). If the patient's problems remain the same or worsen, the thera-

pist needs to design a new therapeutic plan. The evaluation includes an assessment of the patient's physiological systems, which determines the presence of physical impairments, and an assessment of the patient's functional abilities, which identifies any functional limitations present.

Assessing the Physiological Systems

Physical therapy and occupational therapy evaluations commonly include the following information about the patient's neuromuscular, musculoskeletal, and cardiopulmonary systems:

- inspection: a generalized statement of observation
- history: the patient's report of past medical information and current complaints
- vital signs: measures of heart rate, blood pressure, respiration rate, etc.
- posture: observation of musculoskeletal alignment
- palpation: observation by touch of the integrity of the soft and bony tissues
- strength: manual muscle test or isokinetic measure

- range of motion (ROM): goniometric measure of active or passive osteokinematics, accessory motion availability of arthrokinematics, end-feel determination of tissue tension at the end of ROM
- mobility: observation of ability to move in all positions
- balance: observation of ability to maintain postural control in sitting, standing, kneeling, and so forth
- motor control: observations of proprioception, timing, movement patterns, and the like
- pain: report of level of pain by description or visual analog scale

Other important areas assessed include:

- cognitive status: observation of orientation, memory, intelligence, judgment, impulsiveness, and ability to follow directions
- emotional status: observation of cooperation, motivation, coping skills, and fear
- social support: report of family or community resources, architectural layout, and so forth

A detailed discussion of evaluating the above areas is beyond the scope of this book, and the reader is referred to the many excellent assessment texts available in both physical therapy and occupational therapy. The information gathered during this portion of the evaluation will identify physical impairments that will correlate with the patient's ability to function.

Assessing Function

The standard method of assessing function is to address patient issues in activities of daily living (ADLs) and instrumental ADLs (IADLs). The therapist can assess disability or functional limitation or both.

Evaluating Disability

The term *disability* is not used here to identify permanent loss of function that requires

compensation but as discussed in Chapter 2. Disability, in this sense, is simply what the patient believes he or she cannot do that is meaningful in life. It is the patient's subjective determination of ability level. It takes into account what the patient can no longer accomplish due to both physical inability and psychological inability (eg, fear, anxiety, depression, etc.).

The easiest way to assess disability is to have the patient independently fill out a disability questionnaire (the therapist can also interview the patient instead). The patient is asked to determine how much difficulty is involved in accomplishing a selected list of functional tasks. Although not necessary, pain can be evaluated as well. An example of a disability questionnaire created for an outpatient physical therapy clinic is shown in Exhibit 13–1.

Assessing Functional Limitations

Another way to determine functional ability is for the therapist to test the patient for functional limitations. In this instance, the therapist asks the patient to perform selected tasks and observes the patient's ability to do so. The therapist might ask the patient to squat, kneel, reach onto a shelf, or pick up a milk crate in a simulated (ie, in the clinic) or real (ie, at home or work) setting. The therapist would then determine the limitation in functional performance. In a work-hardening center, this evaluation of function is called a functional capacity evaluation (FCE) and may take up to 8 hours or more to accomplish to simulate a work day. Such an extensive test often requires specialized equipment and dedicated space in the clinic (Figure 13–1).

SELECTING AN ASSESSMENT TOOL

Choosing the proper functional test or questionnaire may not be as easy as it first appears. At present, there is no all-encompassing instrument with which to measure all types of patients regardless of problem or clinical setting. Questions regarding reliability and validity abound. Should the clinician use one of the standard

Exhibit 13–1 Function Questionnaire for an Outpatient Clinic

Function Questionnaire

Name: _____   Date: _____

Please fill out the form below, indicating your level of ability and whether any pain is present during that activity. Fill in and rate any work, sports, hobbies, or other activities that are important to you.

Daily Functional Tasks	*Unable/ Need Help*	*Very Hard*	*Hard*	*Easy*	*Painful*
Getting in and out of bed					
Daily Grooming • brush teeth/make-up • bath or shower • dressing					
Sitting Tolerance (1 hour)					
Getting up/down from • chair • toilet • floor					
Driving Tolerance (1 hour)					
Riding Tolerance (1 hour)					
House Activities • cleaning • cooking • laundry • vacuuming/sweeping • wash/dry dishes					
Walking Distance (1 mile)					
Stairs or ladder (1 flight)					
Shopping (grocery)					
Child or Elder Care					
Work Activities 1. 2.					
Sports or Fitness Activities 1. 2.					
Hobbies or Other Activities 1. 2.					

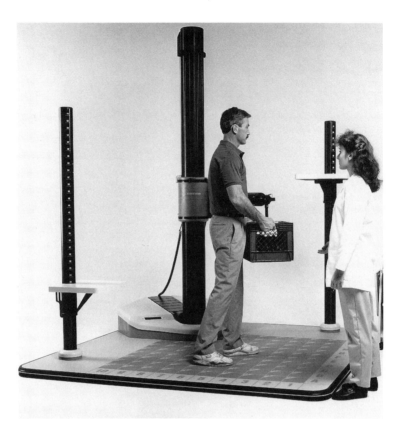

Figure 13–1   The LiftStation®. This device may be used in a work-hardening center to accurately assess three-dimensional functional lifting, including lifting, twisting, carrying, and lowering while carrying specified loads. *Source:* Photo courtesy of Isotechnologies Inc., Hillsborough, North Carolina.

tools or create one specific to the population the clinician sees? Kane and Kane[3] caution against simply picking an assessment tool cafeteria style from the menu of scientific literature because the measurement may not be suited to the population or problem at hand. The clinician does need some guidance in choosing or creating a proper measuring tool. Jette[4] proposes that therapists ask themselves the following questions before choosing a functional assessment tool:

- What is the purpose of the assessment?
- What items need to be assessed?
- Do the items need to be scaled?
- Is the assessment reliable?
- Is the assessment valid?
- Is the assessment responsive?

The Purpose of the Assessment

The purpose of this assessment is to evaluate change in the patient's functional status. Any assessment tool selected or created must be able to measure the magnitude of change occurring as a result of treatment (other assessment tools are created to classify a group or individual or to predict a particular outcome).

The Item Pool

The assessment tool must include functional activities or *items* that are important to the particular patient population. Determination of which items are appropriate can be based on the clinician's professional judgment and experience, information obtained from the literature, and the patients' opinions.[4]

For example, assessing the ability to transfer from bed to chair may be a crucial item to include for patients in nursing homes and rehabilitation facilities but not for those in outpatient clinics. Conversely, determining lower extremity skill level by measuring the ability to jump or run may be fine for an athlete but not for a bilateral above-knee amputee.

At some point, the therapist should review the item pool to determine whether all items are truly necessary or whether some can be eliminated (item reduction). Oftentimes, questionnaires or tests are longer than necessary and can be shortened without significant loss of important data or sensitivity.

The Scale

After choosing the items to be assessed, the clinician must decide how to judge those items. In other words, what are the criteria for successfully completing a functional assessment? First and foremost is the ability to perform. Can the patient accomplish the task? The remaining available options measure the quality with which the task is accomplished[4]:

- dependence: How much assistance (physical or equipment) is needed?

- pain: What level of pain occurs during the task?

- difficulty: How hard is it to accomplish the task?

- speed: How much time does it take to perform the task?

In some instances the measurement of the manner in which a task is accomplished is more important than just the measurement of the ability to perform the task. For example, the ability to walk is a major functional milestone, yet the ability to walk at a pace that is safe is imperative for the patient who needs to walk across a busy street.

Reliability

For obvious reasons, clinicians would like to use an assessment tool with the highest possible reliability. Reliability, in its simplest context, refers to the notion that a change or variation in a measurement occurs because of a true change in the patient's function and not because of an error in measurement. An instrument is considered reliable if it consistently measures similar values upon repeated application of the test in the same quantity. Sources of error exist throughout all measurement and cannot be totally eliminated. Because no assessment tool can ever be error free, the level of reliability can never reach 100% . In research terminology, this means that the correlation coefficient can never achieve 1. The closer the coefficient is to 1, the higher the reliability of the instrument. An instrument with a correlation coefficient of 0.94 may be considered highly reliable, whereas one with a coefficient of 0.69 may have only poor reliability.[5]

Validity

Simply put, an instrument is considered valid if it measures what it is supposed to measure. To be valid, an instrument must also be reliable. However, an instrument can be highly reliable but not measure the intended item (ie, not be valid). For example, a therapist wishes to measure the strength of the quadriceps femoris. Using a highly reliable tape measure and meticulous technique, the therapist measures the girth of the thigh exactly 10 cm above the patella. Although a measurement is taken, it is highly questionable whether strength is the only entity that is measured. In the same light, a function questionnaire that is filled out independently by a patient can only measure disability, or the patient's perception of his or her own functional capacity. To determine functional limitation or capacity more accurately, the clinician must observe the patient actually performing the activity. Even this method contains many sources of error. Observing the patient perform cannot take into account hard to measure qualities such as motivation, fear, or pain or how the patient would perform at home versus in the clinic.

Responsiveness

The responsiveness or sensitivity of an instrument refers to the power of the assessment tool to detect clinically relevant differences.[4] This quality is important for evaluating change in a patient's functional status.

Summary of Assessment Tool Qualities

The appropriate assessment tool changes for each patient population as well as for each clinical setting. The clinician must choose the best available instrument based on sound judgment. Whether one is measuring disability or functional limitations, the following qualities should be evident:

- the instrument measures change in functional status
- the instrument measures appropriate items for the clinical setting
- the instrument measures performance
- the instrument is reliable and valid
- the instrument is responsive enough to detect clinically relevant changes in functional status

STANDARD ASSESSMENT TOOLS

The major benefits of using standard assessment tools include time savings, established reliability and validity, and name recognition. Many of these tools were created under scientific conditions, however, and may not suit the particular needs of each clinical setting. A sampling of a few available impairment and disability tools is presented here. In general, there are two ways to evaluate function: observation of performance, and the use of questionnaires (interview or self-administered). The Functional

Independence Measure (FIM), the Physical Performance Test, the FCE, and the Athletic Functional Performance Test all have the patient performing selected tasks while being observed and graded by a clinician.

Performance tests allow for great objectivity, but the clinician can easily overestimate a patient's function by testing functional capacity in an artificial situation.[6] For example, a patient may be able to carry a 10-lb bag of groceries for 50 ft and pass a performance test but be unable to go shopping, a much more complicated activity. The remaining assessment tools are self-administered questionnaires. Although not objective at all, they may give more realistic measures of the patient's actual performances in his or her own environment.[6]

The FIM

In the fall of 1983, the American Congress of Rehabilitation Medicine and the American Academy of Physical Medicine and Rehabilitation recommended the establishment of a joint task force to develop a uniform national data system for medical rehabilitation. Supported by a grant from the National Institute on Disability and Rehabilitation, the task force created an instrument that would be reliable, valid, and precise in its measurement of impairment, disability, and other related functional outcomes. The FIM assesses self-care, sphincter management, mobility, locomotion, communication, and social cognition on a seven-level scale that is easily administered by any health care clinician or researcher. The FIM is a measure of disability, not impairment. Therefore, if a patient has different abilities when in therapy and when on the nursing floor, the lower score is recorded to reflect more accurately what the patient usually does. The tool has undergone revisions and will continue to change as needed. Facilities may add the FIM to their own data sets if appropriate, but they cannot change the FIM itself in any manner. Each of the 18 items on the FIM has a maximum score of 7 (highest possible total, 126) and a minimum score of 1 (lowest possible total, 18).[7]

Although the FIM is easy to use, therapists must learn how to assess function properly and reliably using the FIM and not simply start filling out forms in a haphazard manner. The guide for using the FIM (complete with instructions, blank FIMs, and sample cases) is reasonably priced at $20 and is readily available by contacting UDS Data Management Service at 82 Farber Hall, State University of New York South Campus, Buffalo, NY 14214 or by calling (716) 831-2076. The therapist or rehabilitation facility might also wish to subscribe to UDS Data Management Service and become part of the computer network. A new FIM has been developed for evaluating disability in children and is called WeeFIM. The guide for using WeeFIM is also available by contacting UDS Data Management Service.

A general description of the levels of function and their scores is provided in Exhibit 13–2 and the actual FIM is shown in Exhibit 13–3. Spe-

cial forms for inpatient coding of functional evaluation and discharge reassessment as well as a follow-up coding sheet come with the guide.

One of the best reasons for using the FIM over other functional assessment tools is its acceptance and use nationwide by all health care disciplines. Many facilities and home care agencies are using the FIM exclusively to ascertain functional level. In the March 1993 issue of *Topics in Geriatric Rehabilitation,* Johnson et al[8] show the relationship of rehabilitation to improving strength and function in the elderly. They present the case of Mrs. C, a frail, 90-year-old woman referred for home physical therapy after suffering a right hip fracture. They describe her functional status as follows[8(p52)]:

> Mrs. C scored 89 of 126 on the [FIM], which indicated modified independence in ADL. Mrs. C was dependent in bathing, dressing the lower extremity, and bladder management. She ambulated partial weight

Exhibit 13–2 Description of the Levels of Function and Their Scores

INDEPENDENT—Another person is not required for the activity (NO HELPER).

7 **Complete Independence**—All the tasks described as making up the activity are typically performed safely without modification, assistive devices, or aids and within reasonable time.
6 **Modified Independence**—Activity requires any one or more than one of the following: an assistive device, more than reasonable time, or there are safety (risk) considerations.

DEPENDENT—Another person is required for either supervision or physical assistance for the activity to be performed, or it is not performed (REQUIRES HELPER).

—**MODIFIED DEPENDENCE**—The subject expends half (50%) or more of the effort. The levels of assistance required are:

5 **Supervision or Set-Up**—Subject requires no more help than stand-by, cueing, or coaxing without physical contact. Or, helper sets up needed items or applies orthoses.
4 **Minimal Contact Assistance**—With physical contact the subject requires no more help than touching, and subject expends 75% or more of the effort.
3 **Moderate Assistance**— Subject requires more help than touching, or expends half (50%) or more (up to 75%) of the effort.

—**COMPLETE DEPENDENCE**—The subject expends *less* than half (*less* than 50%) of the effort. Maximal or total assistance is required, or the activity is not performed. The levels of assistance required are:

2 **Maximal Assistance**—Subject expends less than 50% of the effort but at least 25%.
1 **Total Assistance**—Subject expends less than 25% of the effort.

Source: From *Guide for Use of the Uniform Data Set for Medical Rehabilitation including the Functional Independence Measure (FIM),* Version 3.1 (p. 17) with permission of State University of New York at Buffalo, 14214 © March 1990.

Exhibit 13–3   The FIM

L E V E L S	7 Complete Independence (Timely, Safely) 6 Modified Independence (Device)	NO HELPER

	Modified Dependence
	   5 Supervision
	   4 Minimal Assist (Subject = 75%+)
	   3 Moderate Assist (Subject = 50%+)
	Complete Dependence
	   2 Maximal Assist (Subject = 25%+)
	   1 Total Assist (Subject = 0%+)
		HELPER

	ADMIT	DISCHG	FOL-UP
Self Care A. Eating B. Grooming C. Bathing D. Dressing-Upper Body E. Dressing-Lower Body F. Toileting	☐☐☐☐☐☐	☐☐☐☐☐☐	☐☐☐☐☐☐
Spincter Control G. Bladder Management H. Bowel Management	☐☐	☐☐	☐☐
Mobility Transfer: I. Bed, Chair, Wheelchair J. Toilet K. Tub, Shower	☐☐☐	☐☐☐	☐☐☐
Locomotion L. Walk/wheel Chair M. Stairs	wc☐☐	wc☐☐	wc☐☐
Communication N. Comprehension O. Expression	a v☐☐ v n☐☐	a v☐☐ v n☐☐	a v☐☐ v n☐☐
Social Cognition P. Social Interaction Q. Problem Solving R. Memory	☐☐☐	☐☐☐	☐☐☐
Total FIM	☐	☐	☐

NOTE: Leave no blanks; enter 1 if patient not testable due to risk.

Source: From *Guide for Use of the Uniform Data Set for Medical Rehabilitation including the Functional Independence Measure* (Version 3.1) Buffalo, NY: State University of New York at Buffalo, 14214, 1990.

Exhibit 13–4 Physical Performance Test Scoring Sheet

	Physical Performance Test		
	Time	*Scoring*	*Score*
1. Write a sentence *(Whales live in the blue ocean)*	_____ sec*	≤ 10 sec = 4 10.5–15 sec = 3 15.5–20 sec = 2 >20 sec = 1 unable = 0	_____
2. Simulate eating	_____ sec	≤ 10 sec = 4 10.5–15 sec = 3 15.5–20 sec = 2 >20 sec = 1 unable = 0	_____
3. Lift a book and put it on a shelf	_____ sec	≤ 2 sec = 4 2.5–4 sec = 3 4.5–6 sec = 2 >6 sec = 1 unable = 0	_____
4. Put on and remove a jacket	_____ sec	≤ 2 sec = 4 10.5–15 sec = 3 15.5–20 sec = 2 >20 sec = 1 unable = 0	_____
5. Pick up a penny from the floor	_____ sec	≤ 2sec = 4 2.5–4 sec = 3 4.5–6 sec = 2 >6 sec = 1 unable = 0	_____
6. Turn 360°	discontinuous steps continuous steps unsteady (grabs, staggers) steady	0 2 0 2	_____
7. 50-ft walk test	_____ sec	≤ 15sec = 4 15.5–20 sec = 3 20.5–25 sec = 2 >25 sec = 1 unable = 0	_____
8. Climb one flight of stairs[†]	_____ sec	≤ 5sec = 4 5.5–10 sec = 3 10.5–15 sec = 2 >15 sec = 1 unable = 0	_____
9. Climb stairs[†]	Number of flights of stairs up and down (maximum 4)		_____
TOTAL SCORE (maximum 36 for nine-item, 28 for seven-item)			_____ nine-item _____seven-item

*For timed measurements, round to nearest 0.5 second.
[†]Omit for seven-item scoring.

Source: Reprinted with permission from *Journal of the American Geriatrics Society* (1990;38[10]:1111), Copyright ©
1990, American Geriatrics Society.

bearing on the right leg (50%) with a standard walker. Mrs. C required moderate assistance of one person for bed, chair, and toilet transfers. Tub transfers were not tested at this time because of safety reasons. Memory loss was evident and was graded a four of seven on the FIM as Mrs. C required prompting and reminders 10%–25% of the time.

After describing the treatment protocols for 6 weeks of rehabilitation at home, the investigators report that Mrs. C's FIM score improved to 113 of 126, thereby establishing the link of improved function to their rehabilitation program.

The Physical Performance Test

Another all-around performance test created by Reuben and Siu[9] primarily for the geriatric patient is the Physical Performance Test. The therapist observes the patient perform seven or nine activities and times the performance to the nearest 0.5 second. The times are converted into

a numeric score ranging from 0, which means that the patient was unable to perform the task, to 4, meaning that the task was performed in a timely manner. The maximum score for the nine-item test (includes tests of stair-climbing ability) is 36 and for the seven-item test is 28. The scoring test sheet is shown in Exhibit 13–4.

The administration of the tasks and simulated activities of the Physical Performance Test are as follows:

1. While seated at a table or desk, the patient is asked to write the sentence *Whales live in the blue ocean.* Punctuation is not necessary, and the time is stopped when the pen is lifted from the page.
2. While seated at a table or desk, the patient simulates eating by picking up 5 kidney beans with a teaspoon (using the dominant hand) out of a dish placed 5 inches from the table edge and placing them into an empty coffee can located on the nondominant side. The time is stopped when the last bean hits the bottom of the can.

Exhibit 13–5 Sample FCE Chart

Name: Xavier Jones FCE TASK	UNABLE	0%–33% of Day Occasionally	34–66% of Day Frequently	67%–100% of Day Constantly
LIFTING: Floor to Waist Waist to Shoulder		40# 20#	20# 10#	10# 5#
CARRY: Right Hand Left Hand		30# 40#	15# 20#	10# 10#
PUSH:		80#	40#	20#
PULL:		60#	30#	15#
WALK		✔		
SIT			✔	
STAND			✔	
CROUCH			✔	
REACH				✔
CLIMB		✔		
BALANCE				✔
USE HANDS–MILD GRASPING				✔
USE HANDS–STRONG GRASPING			✔	

Source: Reprinted with permission from *Orthopaedic Physical Therapy Clinics of North America* (1992;1(1):95), Copyright © 1992, WB Saunders Co.

3. While standing, the patient lifts a heavy book from a table and places it on a shelf above shoulder height. The time is stopped when the book is freestanding on the shelf.

4. While standing, the patient puts on a jacket so that it hangs correctly and then completely removes it. The jacket does not have to be zippered or buttoned, and the time is stopped when the jacket is removed.

5. While standing, the patient picks up a penny that has been placed on the floor 1 ft from the dominant side and stands up erect. The time is stopped when the patient is standing up straight, penny in hand.

6. During this untimed test, the patient is asked to turn in a small circle (360°) while the therapist rates two scores: the continuity of the steps and the steadiness of the patient.

7. While standing, the patient is asked to walk forward for 25 ft, turn, and walk back 25 ft. The time is stopped when the patient completes the 50-ft walk.

This completes the seven-item test. The maximum score available is 28 points (4 × 7), and the lowest possible score is 0. If the therapist wishes to measure stair-climbing ability, the patient is asked to complete the next two activities (ie, the nine-item test).

8. The patient climbs up 9 to 12 steps and can use a railing or assistive device as needed. The clock is stopped after the last step is negotiated.

9. This untimed endurance test measures the number of flights of stairs a patient can negotiate both up and down. One point is given for each flight of stairs completed with a maximum of four.

Modified FCE

From the work-hardening arena comes the performance test related to vocations: the FCE. In its original form, the therapist assesses the worker's ability to perform the tasks of sitting, standing, walking, carrying, lifting, reaching, and grasping over the course of 5 hours of a full work day or a couple of work days.[10] The therapist determines how much time (by percentage)

of the work day the worker can safely perform the tasks. By convention, there are four grades of time[11]:

1. unable: the worker cannot safely perform the task at all
2. occasionally: the worker can perform the task from 0% to 33% of the work day
3. frequently: the worker can perform the task from 34% to 66% of the work day
4. constantly: the worker can perform the task 67% to 100% of the work day

The therapist further determines lifting and carrying capacities by weight. An example of an FCE form is shown in Exhibit 13–5.

Although this lengthy test of a worker's abilities and functional limitations is impractical in many instances, the functional tasks making up the FCE are needed often in everyday life. Therapists may wish to include these items in newly created functional assessment forms discussed later in this chapter.

Athletic Functional Performance Tests

Many sports medicine participation evaluations include functional performance tests. Items such as the 50-yard dash, standing long jump, 1.5-mile run, pull-ups, shuttle run, bench press, and the like are observed and measured to reveal any functional limitation that would not be found by conventional means (eg, tests of strength, flexibility, blood pressure, etc.). In addition, sports medicine rehabilitation evaluations are beginning to include functional performance tests before an athlete is allowed to return to sport. The reader should know that many functional performance tests have not been proved to be valid or reliable indicators of readiness to resume sports activities.

Lephart et al[12] describe one of the few functional performance tests proven to determine readiness (in combination with other assessments) for the patient with a deficient anterior cruciate ligament (ACL). The three tests are a cocontraction semicircular maneuver (with resisted tubing), a carioca maneuver (12 m in both

Exhibit 13–6 Functional Status Index

Activity	Assistance (1 to 5)	Pain (1 to 4)	Difficulty (1 to 5)	Comment
Mobility				
Walking inside	_____	_____	_____	
Climbing up stairs	_____	_____	_____	
Transferring to and from toilet	_____	_____	_____	
Getting in and out of bed	_____	_____	_____	
Driving a car	_____	_____	_____	
Personal care				
Combing hair	_____	_____	_____	
Putting on pants	_____	_____	_____	
Buttoning clothes	_____	_____	_____	
Washing all parts of the body	_____	_____	_____	
Putting on shoes/slippers	_____	_____	_____	
Home chores				
Vacuuming a rug	_____	_____	_____	
Reaching into high cupboards	_____	_____	_____	
Doing laundry	_____	_____	_____	
Washing windows	_____	_____	_____	
Doing yard work	_____	_____	_____	
Hand activities				
Writing	_____	_____	_____	
Opening containers	_____	_____	_____	
Turning faucets	_____	_____	_____	
Cutting food	_____	_____	_____	
Vocational				
Performing all job responsibilities	_____	_____	_____	
Avocational				
Performing hobbies requiring hand work	_____	_____	_____	
Attending church	_____	_____	_____	
Socializing with friends and relatives	_____	_____	_____	

Key Assistance: 1. independent; 2. uses devices; 3. uses human assistance; 4. uses devices and human assistance; 5. unable to do. Pain: 1 to 4 (1, no pain; 4, extremely severe pain). Difficulty: 1 to 5 (1, not difficult; 5 extremely difficult). Time frame: on the average, during the past 7 days.
Source: Reprinted with permission from the *Archives of Physical Medicine Rehabilitation* (1980;61:395), Copyright © WB Saunders Company.

directions, total 24 m), and a shuttle run (four lengths of 6.1 m, reversing direction every length).

The criterion for their three tests is elapsed time measured with a stopwatch. Lephart et al[12] discovered that, if the combined time scores of all functional tests together was around 31 seconds, the athletes successfully returned to sport. If the time scores were closer to 48 seconds, the athletes were unable to resume sport activities after ACL injury.

Research into functional performance testing continues in sports medicine. As the results become available, there will be carryover into the general population as well. Many aspects of the high-level maneuvers associated with sports apply to everyday activities. Quick starts and stops (accelerations and decelerations) as well as lateral motions are needed when one is walking in shopping malls or crossing a busy street.

The Functional Status Index

Jette[13] developed the Functional Status Index as an easy, quick, inexpensive clinical tool for assessing function in the elderly population. This tool evaluates the noninstitutionalized geriatric patient's perception of ability level concerning the degree of dependence, pain, and difficulty involved in performing ADL and IADL tasks. It is useful for describing and monitoring the patient's functional level but has no predictive validity. The ideal is to have the patient score a maximum of 1 on each category.[14] This tool has been proved reliable and valid in the rheumatoid arthritic and elderly populations.[6,13]

The patient fills out the Functional Status Index (Exhibit 13–6) using the following key:

- **list I:**
  1. no help
  2. use equipment
  3. use human assist
  4. use human assist and equipment
  5. unable to do
- **list II:**
  1. no pain
  2. mild pain
  3. moderate pain
  4. severe pain
- **list III:**
  1. extremely easy
  2. somewhat easy
  3. neither easy nor difficult
  4. somewhat difficult
  5. extremely difficult

The Arthritis Impact Measurement Scales 2

The revised Arthritis Impact Measurement Scales (AIMS 2) assess the health status of patients with rheumatoid arthritis or osteoarthritis. It was designed to measure improvements produced by therapeutic intervention for clinical research.[15] The entire AIMS 2 contains 78 items and takes approximately 20 minutes to fill out. Patients are simply asked to complete the questionnaire with no coaching. Of special interest are the first 28 items making up the six scales of the physical component:

1. Mobility Level
2. Walking and Bending
3. Hand and Finger Function
4. Arm Function
5. Self-Care Tasks
6. Household Tasks[16]

Other components include affect, pain, social interaction, satisfaction, health perceptions, arthritis impact, and work.

There are no established criteria for determining improvement with the AIMS 2. Users select the scales they deem appropriate and decide the percentage of change they think will indicate improvement. Exhibit 13–7 shows the first 28 items (the physical portion) of the AIMS 2. In general, low scores (1 or 2) indicate high ability, but special recoding needs to be done on selected items (4 through 10 and 21 through 24). For these items, the scoring is changed so that 1 = 5, 2 = 4, 3 = 3, 4 = 2, and 5 = 1. For more information about the AIMS 2 and the user's guide, or to use this copyrighted instrument for commercially sponsored research, please contact Robert Meenan, MD, MPH, Director, Boston University School of Public Health, 80 East Concord Street, Boston, MA 02118-2394.

Hip-Rating Questionnaire

Many functional tools exist to assess the outcomes of surgery or other therapeutic treatments at specific joints. One example of this kind of instrument is the Hip-Rating Questionnaire (Exhibit 13–8) developed by Johanson et al.[17] This tool was originally created to assess the arthritic hip and the effects of total hip replacement surgery on the patient's function.

The questionnaire is divided into four equally weighted sections with a maximum score of 25

Exhibit 13–7   Physical Scales of the AIMS 2

Please check (X) the most appropriate answer for each question.

These questions refer to MOBILITY LEVEL.

DURING THE PAST MONTH . . .	All Days (1)	Most Days (2)	Some Days (3)	Few Days (4)	No Days (5)
1. How often were you physically able to drive a car or use public transportation?	___	___	___	___	___
2. How often were you out of the house for at least part of the day?	___	___	___	___	___
3. How often were you able to do errands in the neighborhood?	___	___	___	___	___
4. How often did someone have to assist you to get around outside your home?	___	___	___	___	___
5. How often were you in a bed or chair for most or all of the day?	___	___	___	___	___

These questions refer to WALKING AND BENDING.

DURING THE PAST MONTH . . .	All Days (1)	Most Days (2)	Some Days (3)	Few Days (4)	No Days (5)
6. Did you have trouble doing vigorous activities such as running, lifting heavy objects, or participating in strenuous sports?	___	___	___	___	___
7. Did you have trouble either walking several blocks or climbing a few flights of stairs?	___	___	___	___	___
8. Did you have trouble bending, lifting, or stooping?	___	___	___	___	___
9. Did you have trouble either walking one block or climbing one flight of stairs?	___	___	___	___	___
10. Were you unable to walk unless assisted by another person or by a cane, crutches, or walker?	___	___	___	___	___

These questions refer to HAND AND FINGER FUNCTION.

DURING THE PAST MONTH . . .	All Days (1)	Most Days (2)	Some Days (3)	Few Days (4)	No Days (5)
11. Could you easily write with a pen or pencil?	___	___	___	___	___
12. Could you easily button a shirt or blouse?	___	___	___	___	___
13. Could you easily turn a key in a lock?	___	___	___	___	___
14. Could you easily tie a knot or a bow?	___	___	___	___	___
15. Could you easily open a new jar of food?	___	___	___	___	___

continues

Please check (X) the most appropriate answer for each question.

These questions refer to ARM FUNCTION.

DURING THE PAST MONTH . . .	All Days (1)	Most Days (2)	Some Days (3)	Few Days (4)	No Days (5)
16. Could you easily wipe your mouth with a napkin?	____	____	____	____	____
17. Could you easily put on a pullover sweater?	____	____	____	____	____
18. Could you easily comb or brush your hair?	____	____	____	____	____
19. Could you easily scratch your low back with your hand?	____	____	____	____	____
20. Could you easily reach shelves that were above your head?	____	____	____	____	____

These questions refer to SELF-CARE TASKS.

DURING THE PAST MONTH . . .	All Days (1)	Most Days (2)	Some Days (3)	Few Days (4)	No Days (5)
21. Did you need help to take a bath or shower?	____	____	____	____	____
22. Did you need help to get dressed?	____	____	____	____	____
23. Did you need help to use the toilet?	____	____	____	____	____
24. Did you need help to get in or out of bed?	____	____	____	____	____

These questions refer to HOUSEHOLD TASKS.

DURING THE PAST MONTH . . .	All Days (1)	Most Days (2)	Some Days (3)	Few Days (4)	No Days (5)
25. If you had the necessary transportation, could you go shopping for groceries without help?	____	____	____	____	____
26. If you had kitchen facilities, could you prepare your own meals without help?	____	____	____	____	____
27. If you had household tools and appliances, could you do your own housework without help?	____	____	____	____	____
28. If you had laundry facilities, could you do your own laundry without help?	____	____	____	____	____

Source: Reprinted with permission of the Boston University School of Public Health, © 1990.

Exhibit 13–8   Hip-Rating Questionnaire*

Which hip is affected by arthritis? (circle one)

Left   Right   Both

Please answer the following questions about the hip(s) you have just indicated.

1. **Considering all of the ways that your hip arthritis affects you, mark (X) on the scale for how well you are doing.**

0	25	50	75	100
very well	well	fair	poor	very poor

Circle one response for each question

(The score here is determined by subtraction of the number marked from 100, with the number being interpolated, if necessary, if the mark is between printed numbers. The result is divided by 4, and the answer then rounded off to the nearest integer. The maximum is 25 points.)

2. **During the past month, how would you describe the usual arthritis pain in your hip?** (maximum, 10 points)
   A) Very severe (2 points)
   B) Severe (4 points)
   C) Moderate (6 points)
   D) Mild (8 points)
   E) None (10 points)

3. **During the past month, how often have you had to take medication for your arthritis?** (maximum, 5 points)
   A) Always (1 point)
   B) Very often (2 points)
   C) Fairly often (3 points)
   D) Sometimes (4 points)
   E) Never (5 points)

4. **During the past month, how often have you had severe arthritis pain in your hip?** (maximum, 5 points)
   A) Every day (1 point)
   B) Several days per week (2 points)
   C) 1 day per week (3 points)
   D) One day per month (4 points)
   E) Never (5 points)

5. **How often have you had hip arthritis pain at rest, either sitting or lying down?** (maximum, 5 points)
   A) Every day (1 point)
   B) Several days per week (2 points)
   C) 1 day per week (3 points)
   D) One day per month (4 points)
   E) Never (5 points)

6. **How far can you walk without resting because of your hip arthritis pain?** (maximum, 15 points)
   A) Unable to walk (3 points)
   B) Less than one city block (6 points)
   C) 1 to <10 city blocks (9 points)
   D) 10 to 20 city blocks (12 points)
   E) Unlimited (15 points)

7. **How much assistance do you need for walking?** (maximum, 10 points)
   A) Unable to walk (1 point)
   B) Walk only with someone's help (2 points)
   C) Two crutches or walker every day (3 points)
   D) Two crutches or walker several days per week (4 points)
   E) Two crutches or walker once per week or less (5 points)
   F) Cane or one crutch every day (6 points)
   G) Cane or one crutch several days per week (7 points)
   H) Cane or one crutch once per week (8 points)
   I) Cane or one crutch once per month (9 points)
   J) No assistance (10 points)

8. **How much difficulty do you have going up or down one flight of stairs because of your hip arthritis?** (maximum, 5 points)
   A) Unable (1 point)
   B) Require someone's assistance (2 points)
   C) Require crutch or cane (3 points)
   D) Require banister (4 points)
   E) No difficulty (5 points)

9. **How much difficulty do you have putting on your shoes and socks because of your hip arthritis?** (maximum, 5 points)
   A) Unable (1 point)
   B) Require someone's assistance (2 points)
   C) Require long shoehorn and reacher (3 points)
   D) Some difficulty but no devices required (4 points)
   E) No difficulty (5 points)

10. **Are you able to use public transportation?** (maximum, 3 points)
    A) No, because of my hip arthritis (1 point)
    B) No, but for some other reason (2 points)
    C) Yes, able to use public transportation (3 points)

11. **When you bathe—either a sponge bath or in a tub or shower—how much help do you need?** (maximum, 3 points)
    A) No help at all (3 points)
    B) Help with bathing one part of your body, like back or leg (2 points)
    C) Help with bathing more than one part of your body (1 point)

12. **If you had the necessary transportation, could you go shopping for groceries or clothes?** (maximum, 3 points)
    A) Without help (taking care of all shopping needs yourself) (3 points)
    B) With some help (need someone to go with you to help on all shopping trips) (2 points)
    C) Completely unable to do any shopping (1 point)

13. **If you had household tools and appliances (vacuum, mops, and so on) could you do your own housework?** (maximum, 3 points)
    A) Without help (can clean floors, windows, refrigerator, and so on) (3 points)
    B) With some help (can do light housework, but need help with some heavy work) (2 points)
    C) Completely unable to do any housework (1 point)

14. **How well are you able to move around?** (maximum, 3 points)
    A) Able to get in and out of bed or chairs without the help of another person (3 points)
    B) Need the help of another person to get in and out of bed or chair (2 points)
    C) Not able to get out of bed (1 point)

This is the end of the Hip-Rating Questionnaire. Thank you for your cooperation.

*The maximum score is 100 points and the minimum is 16 points. The point values of the answers are not shown in the questionnaire that is administered to patients.

Source: Reprinted with permission from the *Journal of Bone and Joint Surgery* (1992;74-A[4]:589), Copyright © 1992, The Journal of Bone and Joint Surgery, Inc.

points per section (100 points maximum for the entire questionnaire): global or overall impact of arthritis, pain, ability to walk, and ability to perform daily functions. Johanson et al conclude that any difference of 12 points or more in total score reflects clinical change.

Other Standard Tests

Many other functional tests abound and have been used successfully in various rehabilitation settings to assess general function from an interdisciplinary point of view. Tools such as the Katz Index of ADL, the Barthel Index, the Older American Research and Service Center Instrument (OARS), and others are reliable and valid and are highly recommended in certain settings.[3] Discussion of all available functional assessment tools is beyond the scope of this book. The reader is referred to the texts on functional assessment referenced in this chapter for more information.

CUSTOMIZED ASSESSMENT TOOLS

Many facilities develop their own evaluation forms based on the particular needs of their clientele. In most instances, these forms are the result of clinical needs and insurance requirements. Often the forms include a myriad of assessment tools, some standard, some borrowed, some newly created. Some have not been tested in any fashion for reliability or validity. Although some investigators caution against using such tools,[3,18] these tools at least force the clinician to address the area of function and not simply ignore it because the perfect tool has not yet been developed to assess it.

The Functional Assessment Tool

The physical, occupational, and speech departments of Holmes Regional Medical Center in Melbourne, Florida, created the Functional Assessment Tool (FAT) to assess a patient's current level of function in an acute care hospital and to help design a rehabilitation program to return that patient to a normal life style. As such, the instrument was designed to meet three criteria in the acute care setting. The FAT focuses on attainment of therapy goals, assists in discharge planning, and provides an objective mechanism for assessing patient progress.[19]

The FAT (Exhibits 13–9 and 13–10) addresses the areas of bed mobility, transfers, ambulation, wheelchair mobility, dressing/bathing, and eating. The clinician awards points for the type of assistive device and amount of assistance required to perform the selected tasks. No points are awarded for independence, and a patient scores an 11 on any task that he or she is unable to perform. Therefore, the lower the score, the higher the function, with full independence in ADLs scoring a 0.

Group Class Functional Assessment (The Body Shop Evaluation)

The Body Shop Evaluation (Exhibit 13–11) is in development by the author for use in an outpatient clinic's group function class. The referring clinician fills out the majority of the four-page form during the patient's regular therapy session. The group leader then completes the evaluations of all the members of the group during the first group class. In addition to mobility and function skills, the therapist assesses general fitness, flexibility, and strength as well as balance and posture. Scales and target goals are included for ease of use by both practitioners and insurance reviewers. This form is used as both an initial evaluation and a discharge summary, thereby keeping paperwork to a minimum. The form has not been tested for reliability or validity. Flowsheets (Exhibits 13–12 through 13–14) are used to chart the patient's progress for the 6- to 8-week group program.

Rehabilitation Forum Documentation Forms

The Rehabilitation Forum and the Arizona Association for Home Care (AAHC) created

Exhibit 13–9 FAT for Acute Care Settings

Patient Name:_____ Age:_____ Date:_____

Diagnosis:_____ Physician:_____

PT Number:_____ MR Number:_____

PT Start Date:_____ PT D/C Date:_____ # of PT Sessions:_____

OT Start Date:_____ OT D/C Date:_____ # of OT Sessions:_____

Admission Date:_____ Discharge Date:_____ Length of Stay:_____

Insurance Code: ☐ Medicaid ☐ Medicare ☐ Group ☐ Self-Pay ☐ Workers Comp

Admit - PT Lag:_____ PT - D/C Lag:_____ Total PT $_____ # Days - PT:_____

Admit - OT Lag:_____ OT - D/C Lag:_____ Total OT $_____ # Days - OT:_____

Directions:
1. Award points for appropriate level of independence.
2. Multiply the amount of assistance needed by the number of persons required.
3. Total rows in column at right.
4. Total column for final score.

	Parallel Bars	Walker	Crutches	Cane	Maximal 51%+	Mod 26-50%	Minimal 1-25%	Contact Guard	Stand By Assist	Independent	# Persons	Unable	TOTAL
	4	3	2	1	5	4	3	2	1	0	#	11	
BED MOBILITY													
Rolling both sides													
Supine to sit													
Sit to supine													
TRANSFERS													
Sit to stand													
Stand to sit													
Stand - pivot													
Sliding board													
AMBULATION													
Level surfaces													
Curb													
Stairs													
WHEELCHAIRS													
Brakes													
Propulsion/Turns													
Ramps													
DRESSING/BATH													
Setup													
Upper body													
Lower body													
Footwear/Feet													
EATING													
Liquids (glassware)													
Solids (utensils)													

COMMENTS: Behavior/Mental Status/Safety Awareness/Ambulatory Distance)   TOTAL ☐

_____

D/C DISPOSITION:_____ THERAPIST:_____

Source: Reprinted with permission of *Physical Therapy Forum* (Midatlantic Edition–1992;11[2]:22–25) and Brimer MA, Schuneman G, and Allen B of the Holmes Regional Medical Center, Melbourne, Florida.

Exhibit 13–10   Example of a Completed FAT for a Patient with Total Hip Replacement

Patient Name: Anne Smith _____ Age: 69 _____ Date: 01-03-92 _____

Diagnosis: Severe DJD ® hip → ® THA _____ Physician: Orthopedist _____

PT Number: x _____ MR Number: y _____

PT Start Date: 01-03-92 _____ PT D/C Date: _____ # of PT Sessions: _____

OT Start Date: _____ OT D/C Date: _____ # of OT Sessions: _____

Admission Date: 01-02-92 _____ Discharge Date: _____ Length of Stay: _____

Insurance Code: ☐ Medicaid ☒ Medicare ☐ Group ☐ Self-Pay ☐ Workers Comp

Admit - PT Lag: _____ PT - D/C Lag: _____ Total PT $ _____ # Days - PT: _____

Admit - OT Lag: _____ OT - D/C Lag: _____ Total OT $ _____ # Days - OT: _____

Directions:
1. Award points for appropriate level of independence.
2. Multiply the amount of assistance needed by the number of persons required.
3. Total rows in column at right.
4. Total column for final score.

	Parallel Bars	Walker	Crutches	Cane	Maximal 51%+	Mod 26-50%	Minimal 1-25%	Contact Guard	Stand By Assist	Independent	# Persons	Unable	TOTAL
	4	3	2	1	5	4	3	2	1	0	#	11	
BED MOBILITY													
Rolling both sides							3				1		3
Supine to sit						4					1		4
Sit to supine							3				1		3
TRANSFERS													
Sit to stand							3				1		3
Stand to sit								2			1		2
Stand - pivot							3				1		3
Sliding board													N/A
AMBULATION													
Level surfaces						4					2		8
Curb												11	11
Stairs												11	11
WHEELCHAIRS													
Brakes													N/A
Propulsion/Turns													N/A
Ramps													N/A
DRESSING/BATH													
Setup										0			0
Upper body										0			0
Lower body					5						1		5
Footwear/Feet					5						1		5
EATING													
Liquids (glassware)										0			0
Solids (utensils)										0			0

COMMENTS: Behavior/Mental Status/Safety Awareness/Ambulatory Distance— **TOTAL 58**
Alert and oriented x3. Understands total hip precautions.

Gait 5' with walker, toe touch weight bearing.

Refer to OT for lower extremity dressing and bathing.

D/C DISPOSITION: _____ THERAPIST: _____

Source: Reprinted with permission of *Physical Therapy Forum* (Midatlantic Edition–1992;11[2]:22–25) and Brimer MA, Schuneman G, and Allen B of the Holmes Regional Medical Center, Melbourne, Florida.

Exhibit 13–11   The Body Shop Evaluation

ARLINGTON ORTHOPEDIC AND SPORTS PHYSICAL THERAPY

The Body Shop Evaluation

Initial Evaluation Date:_____   8 Wk Re-assessment Date:_____

Name:_____ DOB:_____ Age_____yrs

Occupation/Activities:_____

Medical Diagnosis:_____

Present Complaints:_____

_____

Medical History:_____

_____

Medications:_____

Personal/Functional Goals:_____

1. Weight (clothed without footwear):   Eval:_____lbs   8 Wk:_____lbs

2.   Cardiopulmonary Screen

	Vital Signs	Eval	8 Wk
RESTING	Pulse (bpm)		
(sitting)	BP (mm/Hg)		
	RR (rpm)		
EXERCISE (2 min)	Pulse (bpm)		

Max HR = 220 - age = _____bpm

Target Heart Rate:

    60% MHR = _____bpm

    80% MHR = _____bpm

3. Balance: one-legged standing balance (OLSB) test with eyes open

	L	R
Eval	sec	sec
8 Wk	sec	sec

Target OLSB:

Functional : 10 seconds

Normal   : 30-60 seconds

Note: This tool was developed for use by an outpatient clinic that runs group classes on functional restoration. The same form is used as both an initial and discharge summary for increased ease in comparing baseline data to progress made in the 6- or 8-week group session.

Source: Courtesy of Arlington Orthopedic and Sports Physical Therapy, Arlington, Massachusetts.

continues

4. Posture:

5. Flexibility Screen (aROM)

L		JOINT MOTION	R	
8 Wk	Eval		Eval	8 Wk
		NECK Rotation/SB		
		BACK Forward Bending		
		Backward Bending		
		SHLDR Flexion (180°)		
		Abduct (180°)		
		IR/ER (90°/90°)		
		ELBOW, WRIST, & HAND		
		HIP Flexion (120°)		
		Thomas Test (0°)		
		SLR (70°)		
		KNEE Ext-Flex (0-125°)		
		ANKLE Dorsiflex (10°)		

6. Strength Screen

L		Gross Strength at Joint	R	
8 Wk	Eval		Eval	8 Wk
		SHOULDER		
		HAND Grasp _____kg		
		TRUNK (# of curl-ups)		

continues

6. Strength Screen (cont'd)

L		CYBEX KNEE TEST (ft lbs)	R	
8 Wk	Eval	**60°/sec**	Eval	8 Wk
		Quadriceps		
		Hamstrings		
		H/Q ratio (60-70%)		
		MQT/BW_____ft lbs		
		180°/sec		
		Quadriceps		
		Hamstrings		
		H/Q ration (70-80%)		
		MQT/BW_____ft lbs		

7. Mobility Skills

	Eval		8 Wk	
	Assist	Quality	Assist	Quality
Bed Mobility				
Sit-to-stand				
Floor-to-stand				
Ambulation:				
Velocity	reg pace: fast pace:		reg pace: fast pace:	
Endurance				
Stairs:	# of steps	railing	step-over-step	# of steps	railing	step-over-step
Walk				
Run				

Target Gait: Community Ambulator: 100'/min. for 500'.   Normal velocity: ~262'/min.

> **Key:** 1/5 = Severely Limited or requires Maximal Assistance
> 2/5 = Moderately Limited or requires Moderate Assistance
> 3/5 = Minimally Limited or requires Minimal Assistance
> 4/5 = Slightly Limited or requires Contact Guard
> 5/5 = Normal or Independent

continues

8. Functional Skills

	Eval	8 Wk
Lifting: Waist Height		
Shoulder Height		
Reaching		
Carrying (lbs/distance)		
ADL		

Major Findings

Evaluation

1.

2.

3.

4.

Progress in 8 weeks

1.

2.

3.

4.

Initial Assessment: _____

_____

_____

8 Week Re-assessment: _____

_____

_____

Plan:

<u>Evaluation</u>

_____ Begin Group PT

_____ Requires Individual PT

_____ Refer to MD

<u>8 Week Re-assessment</u>

_____ Ready for Independent Program

_____ Repeat Group Program

_____ Refer to MD

_____   _____

Physical Therapist   Date

_____   _____

Physical Therapist   Date

Exhibit 13–12 Sample of Body Shop Flowsheet (Note Individualization of Flexibility, ADL & Sport Skills, Patient Comments, Assessment, and Plan of Treatment Sections)

Name: **PT NOTES**

CLASS	ONE	TWO	THREE	FOUR
Date				
RESPIRATION/WARMUP				
FLEXIBILITY				
1)				
2)				
3)				
STRENGTH/ENDURANCE				
Active ex (flowsheet)				
Nautilus (flowsheet)				
BALANCE (L/R)				
MOBILITY				
Rolling				
Floor-to-stand				
Amb vel. (reg/fast)				
Advanced gait				
Light job				
Stairs				
FUNCTIONAL SKILLS				
Lifting: waist height				
shoulder height				
Reaching				
Carrying (lb/distance)				
Push/pull activities				
ADL & SPORT SKILLS				
1)				
2)				
3)				
EDUCATION				
PT COMMENTS/PAIN				
PT ASSESSMENT				
PLAN OF TREATMENT				
PHYSICAL THERAPIST				

Source: Courtesy of Arlington Orthopedic and Sports Physical Therapy, Arlington, Massachusetts.

Exhibit 13–13 Body Shop Active Exercises Flowsheet (Number of Repetitions Is Recorded for the Group or Individual Exercises)

Body Shop Active Exercises																**Name:**
BODY SHOP CLASS	One	Two	Three	Four	Five	Six	Seven	Eight	Nine	Ten	Eleven	Twelve	Thirteen	Fourteen	Fifteen	Sixteen
1990 Date																
STANDING EXERCISES																
Neck Circles																
Shoulder Circles																
Shoulder Scissors																
Wall Push-Ups																
UE PNF Patterns																
Upper Trunk Rotation																
Backward Bends																
Yoga Forward Bend																
Marching																
Hip Abd/Sidestep																
Heel-Offs/Toe-Walk																
Toe-Offs/Heel-Walk																
Fencer's Lunge																
Squat																
Jump																
PRONE/QUADRUPED/KNEEL																
Press-Ups																
Rocking																
Angry Cat																
Sit onto Heels																
SUPINE																
Lateral Trunk Rotation																
3-Way Curl-Up																
Hamstring Stretch																
Piriformis Stretch																
INDIVIDUAL																
1)																
2)																
3)																

Source: Courtesy of Arlington Orthopedic and Sports Physical Therapy, Arlington, Massachusetts.

Exhibit 13–14   Fitness First Nautilus Exercise Flowsheet (Record Number of Plates under *P* and Number of Repetitions under R)

FITNESS FIRST
NAUTILUS TRAINING CENTER

P = PLATES R = REPETITIONS	DATE SETTING	/		/		/		/		/		/	
		P	R	P	R	P	R	P	R	P	R	P	R
1. HIP & BACK													
2. LEG EXTENSION													
3. LEG CURL													
4. PULLOVER													
5. TORSO ARM													
6. DOUBLE SHOULDER MACHINE													
A) LATERAL RAISE													
B) OVERHEAD PRESS													
7. DOUBLE CHEST MACHINE													
A) FLYS													
B) PRESS													
8. BICEP													
9. TRICEP													
OPTIONAL EXERCISES													
10. LOWER BACK													
11. ABDOMINAL													
12. ROTARY TORSO													
13. NECK & SHOULDERS													
14. ROWING													
15. MULTI-EXERCISER													
A) CALF RAISES													
B) DIPS													
C) WRIST CURLS													
D) CHIN-UPS													
16. FOUR WAY NECK													
17. ADDUCTOR													
18. ABDUCTOR													
19. SQUAT													

Source: Courtesy of Fitness First, Arlington, Massachusetts.

Exhibit 13–15   Physical Therapy Evaluation and Plan of Care for Home Care Setting

PHYSICAL THERAPY EVALUATION
and PLAN OF CARE

Agency _____   MR#_____

Date _____
Initial ☐   Recertification ☐

PATIENT	DX	ONSET	DATE OF BIRTH

SIGNIFICANT MEDICAL HISTORY / PERTINENT MEDICATIONS

PRIOR LEVEL OF FUNCTION:

PATIENT GOALS:

PROBLEMS

GOALS

Anticipated Completion Date

REHAB POTENTIAL:
☐ Good   ☐ Fair   ☐ Poor

DISCHARGE PLAN / LONG TERM GOALS:

PLAN OF CARE
_____ B1 Evaluation
_____ B2 Therapeutic Exercise: _____
_____ B3 Transfer Training
_____ B4 ☐ Establish ☐ Upgrade Home Program
_____ B5 Gait Training WB Status _____ Device____
_____ B6 Pulmonary Physical Therapy
_____ B7 Ultrasound _____

_____ Electrotherapy
_____ Prosthetic Training ☐ Preprosthetic
_____ B10 Fabrication of orthotic device
_____ B11 Muscle Reeducation
_____ B12 Management and evaluation of Patient Care Plan
_____ B15 Other _____

Frequency and Duration: _____

EVALUATION
Strength   ROM

Cervical

Trunk

Extremities

ENDURANCE / OUT OF BED TIME   BP:_____   HR:_____

POSTURE
SITTING   STANDING

PAIN / EDEMA

GAIT

BALANCE
SITTING   STANDING

SENSORY / TONE / NEURO

COGNITION / COMMUNICATION

FUNCTIONAL LIMITATIONS
specify level of assistance

Rolls _____
Assumes sitting over edge of bed _____
In and out of bed _____
Toilet independence _____
Feeds self_____
In and out of chair _____
Down and up from floor _____
In and out of shower / tub_____
Bathes / grooms self _____
Dresses self_____
Wheelchair independence indoors_____
Walks all directions / surfaces _____
Climbs stairs_____
Car transfers _____

EQUIPMENT IN HOME / ARCHITECTURAL BARRIERS

COMMENTS / NOTES / REHAB ENVIRONMENT

Plan of Care Established with:
☐ Patient   ☐ Family   ☐ Other _____

Therapist	Physician
Signature _____ Date _____	Signature _____ Date _____
PHYSICIAN PHONE	ADDRESS

Source: Reprinted with permission of Arizona Association for Home Care and Rehabilitation Forum, 1991.

Exhibit 13–16   Occupational Therapy Evaluation and Plan of Care for Home Care Settings

OCCUPATIONAL THERAPY EVALUATION
and PLAN OF CARE

Date _____

Agency _____   MR#_____   Initial ❑   Recertification ❑

PATIENT	DX	ONSET	DATE OF BIRTH

SIGNIFICANT MEDICAL HISTORY / PERTINENT MEDICATIONS   PRIOR LEVEL OF FUNCTION

PATIENT GOALS

PROBLEMS: GOALS:

Anticipated Comp. ___ Date:

PLAN OF CARE   FREQUENCY / DURATION

_____ D1 Eval   _____ D8 Sensory Treatm.

_____ D2 ADL Instruction   _____ D9 O___ ___linting

_____ D3 Muscle Reeducation   _____ ___daptive ___ Fabric./trn.   DC PLAN / LONG TERM GOAL

_____ D5 Perceptual Motor Training   _____ D1___

_____ D6 Fine Motor Development

_____ D7 Neuro Developmental Rx   REHAB POTENTIAL   ❑ Good ❑ Fair ❑ Poor

RUE	LUE
STRENGTH	STRENGTH
ROM	ROM
MENTAL STATUS: ORIENTATION, MOTIVATION, ATTENTION SPAN	ORAL MOTOR
SAFETY / ARCHITECTURAL BARRIERS	BALANCE/TRUNK CONTROL SITTING STANDING
CO-ORDINATION / FINE MOTOR	COMMUNICATION
TONE	PAIN/EDEMA
ENDURANCE BP:_____ HR:_____	SENSATION
VISION/HEARING	ADAPTIVE EQUIP/ORTHOTIC NEEDS
CARETAKER NEEDS	PERCEPTION

FUNCTIONAL LIMITATIONS   (specify level of assistance)

_____ U.E Dressing	_____ Transfers	_____ Bed Mobility	_____ Ambulation
_____ L.E. Dressing	_____ Grooming	_____ W. C. Mobility	_____ Homemaking
_____ Self Bathing	_____ Toileting	_____ Eating / Feeding	_____ Play / Leisure Skills

Plan of Care Reviewed with: ❑ Patient   ❑ Family   ❑ Other _____

Therapist Signature _____   Date _____

Physician Signature _____   Date _____

PHYSICIAN	ADDRESS	PHONE

Sample

Source: Reprinted with permission of Arizona Association for Home Care and Rehabilitation Forum, 1991.

Exhibit 13–17   Total Hip Arthoplasty Functional Milestones: Sample Flowsheet for Documenting Functional Progress in Patients after This Surgery.

Source: Sample courtesy of The Hospital for Special Surgery Rehabilitation Services Department, New York, NY, © The Hospital for Special Surgery.

Exhibit 13–18   Total Knee Arthoplasty Functional Milestones: Sample Flowsheet for Documenting Functional Progress in Patients after This Surgery.

TOTAL KNEE ARTHROPLASTY - FUNCTIONAL MILESTONES

DEPARTMENT OF REHABILITATION SERVICES
PHYSICAL THERAPY

DIAGNOSIS_____ PT_____

RIGHT/LEFT/BILAT   EPI/SPIN/GEN   ♀ ♂

HT(in.)_____WT(lbs.)_____

MANIP/R/L   COMPRESSION BOOTS   Y/N

VENOGRAM   L +/- R +/-

COMPLICATIONS/CO-MORBIDITY/COMMENTS _____

	RR	1	2	3	4	5	6	7	8	9	10	11	12	13	14	15	16	17	18	19	20
DISCHARGE																					
STAIRS UNASSISTED*																					
STAIRS ASSISTED																					
CANE UNASSISTED*																					
CANE ASSISTED																					
WALKER UNASSISTED*																					
WALKER ASSISTED																					
TRANSFER UNASSISTED*																					
TRANSFER ASSISTED																					
DANGLE UNSUPPORTED																					
DANGLE SUP																					
CPM (R/L)																					
ACTIVE EXT R																					
ACTIVE FLEX R																					
ACTIVE EXT L																					
ACTIVE FLEX L																					

DATE OF
SURGERY:_____   P.O.D.

COMMENTS:_____
_____
_____
_____
_____
_____
_____

*UNASSISTED = Not requiring the presence of another person to perform the activity

Source: Sample courtesy of The Hospital for Special Surgery Rehabilitation Services Department, New York, NY,
© The Hospital for Special Surgery.

physical and occupational therapy evaluation forms in 1991 to be used in home care. The forms incorporate essential documentation required for Medicare and other third party payers, Arizona state licensure, and the Joint Commission on Accreditation of Healthcare Organizations and standards of practice for home health therapists being developed by the forum and the AAHC.[20] The evaluations include functional limitations sections corresponding to the increased emphasis currently placed on functional restoration (see Exhibits 13–15 and 13–16). For more information or to purchase these forms (already printed in carbonless triplicate), contact the AAHC/Rehabilitation Forum, 20 East Main Street, Suite 710, Mesa, AZ 85201.

OutPatient Clinic Function Questionnaire

The functional needs of patients in outpatient settings exceed the basic self-care requirements of patients in institutional settings. The function questionnaire shown in Exhibit 13–1 attempts to address the issues that are important to the patient and even considers the patient's pain level during the activities. Blank spaces under work, sports, hobbies, and other allow the patient's goals and desires to be customized on the questionnaire. The patient fills out the questionnaire without being coached while sitting in the waiting room. If desired, the therapist can convert the patient's check marks under the ability category to a numeric scale (eg, easy = 0, hard = 1, very hard = 2, unable/needs help = 3). The lower the score, the higher the function, with 0 indicating complete independence.

DOCUMENTING PROGRESS

After the desired assessment tool is selected, the clinician needs to continue documenting functional changes that occur during treatment sessions. To keep within Medicare guidelines, the therapist must show that skilled services were provided and that progress occurred in

therapy. This means that it is no longer acceptable to document a patient's gait as simply "50' × 2 with a cane and close supervision." Lingering questions remain as to the presence of inefficient gait deviations and balance problems and whether the velocity of the gait is safe enough for the patient to perform tasks. In other words, simply reporting the facts in physical therapy jargon does not indicate the functionality of the patient's walking ability.

Although therapists are now documenting better the patient's progress in functional terms, there is still much room for improvement. In the above example, additional information as to the patient's ability or inability to maneuver around obstacles, the distances required to reach the bathroom in the home or hospital, the patient's steadiness and balance, and so forth should be included in the assessment portion of the progress note. This allows the reader of the medical record (eg, other team members or insurance reviewers) to get a better picture of the patient's functional ability. Good documentation takes both knowledge and time. Although many therapists know how to document properly, they simply do not have enough time to do it. (Documentation Catch-22: Many employers do not like to pay for nonreimbursable documentation time, commonly referred to as down-time, implying that the therapist is doing nothing rather than writing good progress notes.)

Nevertheless, because the problem is real, creative therapists continue to attempt to streamline the lengthy documentation note by using flowcharts. These handy devices allow the clinician to chart daily progress of strength, ROM, or gait by quickly filling in a daily box. (Documentation Catch 22: Sometimes flowsheets are disallowed as improper documentation by insurance reviewers, to the great dismay of the creative therapists who designed them.) In any event, now there are flowsheets that chart functional progress for quicker documentation.

Functional Milestones

The physical therapists at the Hospital for Special Surgery in New York have developed the

Functional Milestone form for their patients recovering from either total hip (Exhibit 13–17) or total knee (Exhibit 13–18) arthroplasties; these have proved to be both valid and reliable. The therapist records the postoperative day on the X axis and checks the appropriate functional milestone (eg, transfer unassisted) on the Y axis (Cioppa-Mosca J. Personal communication. July 1993).

These copyrighted forms are available in packages of 50 for a small fee by contacting JeMe Cioppa-Mosca, PT, Hospital for Special Surgery Rehabilitation Services Department, 535 East 70th Street, New York, NY 10021.

The Body Shop Evaluation Flowsheets

Based on the parameters assessed using the Body Shop Evaluation form (see Exhibit 13–11), the author has also developed documentation flowsheets to be used by the group leader. The therapist/group leader jots down objective data on each date the group meets. Some areas, such as flexibility and ADL/sport skills, are left blank to be individualized to each patient's needs. A sample flowsheet is shown in Exhibit 13–12. In addition, separate flowsheets for the active (Exhibit 13–13) and resistive (Exhibit 13–14) exercise portions of the program are included in the chart. During the function group, not all patients perform the same exercises, and many areas of the flowsheet may be left blank. Improvement is charted daily in number of repetitions completed or amount of time elapsed. For more information about functional programs for groups, please see Chapter 12.

DISCHARGE SUMMARIES

The discharge summary reports the patient's physical and functional status at the time of formal discharge from therapy. A quick way to assess the functional status at discharge is to simply readminister the original functional evaluation. The patient can fill out a discharge questionnaire, or the therapist can observe the patient performing selected tasks. Either on a specific discharge form or in narrative style, the therapist must report the patient's level of physical and functional ability (it is hoped that these will correlate).

In general, most patients do not fully recover while attending therapy and must continue with an independent home program before attaining prior functional status. This, too, should be noted in the discharge summary. Athletes seem to be the exception to this rule because they are often allowed to achieve the necessary skills before returning to their sport. On the other hand, therapists working with debilitated or geriatric patients usually need to fight tooth and nail with excellent documentation to eke out a few more treatments.

(Author's personal note: It is a sad reflection on our society that we think little of the expense of returning an athlete to a game but become miserly when faced with the expense of returning an elderly patient home instead of to a nursing home.)

DOCUMENTATION ALTERNATIVES

Documentation does not require a facility to choose or create specific tools to chart the patient's functional progress. The clinician need only take the time to write a specific, concise, but informative note in terms that all will understand. Some facilities use computer documentation, with therapists scanning bar codes that correlate with treatments provided. Some of these are for all types of therapy; others are only based on function. As our society becomes more computer oriented, the number-crunching ability of the computer will be used to measure the outcomes of different treatment approaches in the clinical (and not just the research) sector. If detailed diagnoses are input (eg, not just low back pain, which is too general an entity), these computer programs should aid the therapist and the insurance provider in determining the most efficacious treatments for our patients.

REFERENCES

1. Greenfield S. The state of outcome research: are we on target? *N Engl J Med.* 1989;320:1142–1143.

2. Pincus T, Callahan LF. Early mortality in RA predicted by poor clinical status. *Bull Rheum Dis.* 1992;41:1–4.

3. Kane RA, Kane RL. *Assessing the Elderly: A Practical Guide to Measurement.* Lexington, Mass: Lexington Books; 1981.

4. Jette AM. Disability assessment in clinical practice. Presented at the American Physical Therapy Association Annual Conference: June 1991; Boston, Mass.

5. Currier DP. Confidence in research and instruments. In: *Elements of Research in Physical Therapy.* Baltimore, Md: Williams & Wilkins; 1979: 143–180.

6. Harris BA, Jette AM, Campion EW, Cleary PD. Validity of self-report measures of functional disability. *Top Geriatr Rehabil.* 1986;1:31–41.

7. Research Foundation, State University of New York. *Guide for Use of the Uniform Data Set for Medical Rehabilitation Including the Functional Independence Measure (FIM)* (version 3.1). Buffalo, NY: Research Foundation, State University of New York; 1990.

8. Johnson JH, Searles LB, McNamara S. In-home geriatric rehabilitation: improving strength and function. *Top Geriatr Rehabil.* 1993;8:51–64.

9. Reuben DB, Siu AL. An objective measure of physical function of elderly outpatients. The physical performance test. *J Am Ger Soc* 1990;38(10):1105–1112.

10. Isernhagen SJ. Return to work testing. *Orthop Phys Ther Clin.* 1992;1:83–98.

11. US Department of Labor. *Dictionary of Occupational Titles.* 4th ed. Indianapolis, Ind: JIST Works;1991;2.

12. Lephart SM, Perrin OH, Fu FH. Relationship between selected physical characteristics and functional capacity in the anterior cructiate ligament-insufficient athlete. *J Orthop Sports Phys Ther.* 1992;16:174–181.

13. Jette A. The Functional Status Index: reliability of a chronic disease evaluation instrument. *Arch Phys Med Rehabil.* 1980;61:395–401.

14. Lewis CB. *Documentation and functional assessment* (course notes). Sarasota, Fla: Advanced Educational Seminars, Inc. 1992.

15. Meenan RF, Mason JH, Anderson JJ, et al. AIMS 2: the content and properties of a revised and expanded Arthritis Impact Measurement Scales health status questionnaire. *Arthritis Rheum.* 1992;25:1–10.

16. Boston University Arthritis Center. *AIMS 2 Users Guide.* Boston, Mass: Boston University Arthritis Center; 1990.

17. Johanson NA, Charlson ME, Szatrowski TP. A self-administered hip-rating questionnaire for the assessment of outcome after total hip replacement. *J Bone Joint Surg Am.* 1992;74:587–597.

18. Chamberlain A. The rehabilitation team and functional assessment. In: Goodwill CJ, Chamberlain MA, eds. *Rehabilitation of the Physically Disabled Adult.* London, England: Croom Helm; 1988:59–82.

19. Brimer MA, Shuneman G, Allen BR. Guidelines for developing a functional assessment for an acute care facility. *Phys Ther Forum.* 1993;12:22–25.

20. Feige M. Rehabilitation Forum documentation forms. *Inside Ariz.* Summer 1991.

ADDITIONAL READING

Gallo JJ, Reichel W, Andersen L. *Handbook of Geriatric Assessment.* Gaithersburg, Md: Aspen; 1988.

14

Functional Exercise Equipment

One of the nicer features of the functional exercise program is the lack of equipment needed to get a good result. In reality, the creative therapist can use any available pieces of existing equipment or any number of things found within the environment to promote functional return (this is no news to community therapists, who have been doing just that in the resource-starved setting of home care). Some excellent exercise equipment, however, has recently been designed that promotes strength, proprioception, coordination, flexibility, and motor control at extremely affordable prices.

This chapter discusses the functional exercise equipment needs of different rehabilitation settings and explores the various pieces of equipment themselves. This discussion can never be complete because new equipment is being created and marketed as this chapter is being written. At the end of the chapter, an equally incomplete list of vendors is provided to allow the clinician the ability to try out or purchase equipment if desired.

FUNCTIONAL EXERCISE EQUIPMENT NEEDS BY REHABILITATION SETTING

It is perhaps important to point out once again that no additional equipment need ever be bought to achieve good results from the functional exercise program. Even modest purchases of small but highly challenging pieces of exercise equipment, however, will greatly enhance the effectiveness of the exercise program. Because the equipment provides difficult motor problems for the patient to overcome, an element of risk is involved in using it. As mentioned previously, the degree of risk can be minimized by altering the exercise parameters (eg, widening the base of support, holding onto a table for balance, etc.). The therapist must carefully weigh the benefits of using the equipment against the potential harm caused by an accident. In general, a skilled physical therapist or occupational therapist can evaluate the situation quickly and easily.

The Home Care Setting

In some ways, the home care setting is the ideal environment to perform the functional exercise program. The patient can easily transfer the motor-solving skills from the phase I and II exercises to the phase III portion by actually solving real functional problems in the home environment (see Chapters 4 and 7). The home provides a ready-made challenging environment with which to interact. The therapist does not possess the resources of a fully equipped therapeutic gym to correct the patient's impairments, however (eg, strength, flexibility, stability, balance, etc.). To augment the functional exercise program, the traveling clinician needs the least amount of equipment that will provide the greatest results. The minimal functional equipment needed in this setting is:

- wobble boards (beginner or intermediate level)
- surgical tubing
- 8-in-diameter ball

The entire cost of this equipment package is less than $100 and is affordable by most home care agencies. Because the equipment accompanies the therapist while he or she is traveling, it is subject to great fluctuations in weather conditions. The therapist must frequently check the integrity of the rubber in the surgical tubing and check for any warping of the wobble board or playing ball.

Nursing Homes and Long-Term Care Facilities

Most of the skilled nursing facilities for the geriatric patient possess a small therapeutic gym. The facilities vary from being a fully equipped rehabilitation center to a small room with a plinth, cuff weights, ultrasound machine, full-length mirror, and some ambulation devices. The minimal functional exercise equipment needed in this setting is:

- wobble boards (beginner and intermediate levels)
- surgical tubing
- 8-in-diameter ball
- 65-cm (26-in) therapeutic ball
- 4-in aerobic step
- milk crate
- dowel
- full-length mirror

Aside from the mirror, which is usually standard in the therapy gym, the approximate cost of this equipment is $250 and can be shared among all therapists and patients. The frail elderly who generally reside in these facilities tend to enjoy the challenges of using the above equipment, but almost all require contact guard or minimal assistance when exercising.

The Acute Care Hospital

Patients are being discharged so quickly from the acute care hospital that little functional exercise actually occurs there. Yet most hospitals are still fully equipped with complete lines of exercise machines, weights, modalities, parallel bars, and so forth as well as all manner of functional exercise equipment. The acute care therapist is similar to the home care therapist, however, in that he or she often travels to the patient's room to provide therapy. The minimal amount of functional exercise equipment needed for bedside rehabilitation in this setting is:

- wobble board with a piece of Dycem for traction on slippery hospital room floors
- surgical tubing
- dowel
- cuff weights

If these are not already available in the facility, the cost of the above equipment is approximately $125. For patients attending therapy in the rehabilitation gym(s), the equipment requirements are similar for the outpatient setting (described below).

The Outpatient Clinic

Almost all patients attending therapy in an outpatient clinic can participate fully in the functional exercise program. A small facility with space or monetary constraints requires the same functional exercise equipment as the nursing home setting:

- wobble boards (beginner and intermediate levels)
- surgical tubing
- 8-in-diameter ball
- 65-cm (26-in) therapeutic ball
- 4-in aerobic step
- milk crate
- dowel
- full-length mirror

In addition to the equipment mentioned above, a larger facility can select from the following:

- glide board and/or Fitter™
- treadmill
- stair climber
- stationary bicycle
- Ethafoam™ rollers
- plyoballs
- Shuttle® or Plyo-Plus™
- Total Gym®
- miniature therapeutic pools

Because prices and quality vary, the therapist must call different vendors for price estimates. The rollers and balls cost less than $100; the larger pieces of equipment begin at $500.

The hand, sports medicine, and work-hardening clinics represent highly specialized variants of the outpatient setting. Much of the equipment previously mentioned is frequently used in these settings. Additional specialized equipment has also been designed to get the hand-injured patient, the athlete, and the injured worker back to function. For the patient with an injured hand, many assistive and resistive exercise devices are available. Some of the more basic pieces of hand equipment include:

- therapy putty
- hand grippers
- Eggsercizer™
- Exer-Stik™
- PowerWeb™

- Grip-Master®
- dexterity boards

Because of the intricacy of hand rehabilitation, the reader is referred to the many texts on hand rehabilitation for more information about exercise equipment and functional rehabilitation of the hand. In general, patients with a hand injury require the services of a certified hand specialist, and appropriate referrals should be made in all but the most basic cases.

For sports medicine rehabilitation, additional equipment is needed to stress the athlete above and beyond so-called normal parameters. This may include:

- sprinter's sleds
- weighted vests
- hurdles
- minitrampoline
- plyometric boxes
- parachutes
- plyoballs and rebounders

For work hardening, entire workstations are built to simulate the many types of injured workers encountered: secretaries, manual laborers, truck drivers, and so forth. Many texts are devoted exclusively to the injured athlete and worker, and the reader is referred to these sources for further information about equipment needs for these patients.

The Rehabilitation Hospital

The rehabilitation hospital has increased resources to possess a complete line of therapeutic and functional restoration equipment. Oftentimes, the therapist has the luxury of using a full-sized therapeutic pool as well as the latest exercise equipment used in sports and industrial medicine. Generally, the main focus of rehabilitation hospitals is the adult and geriatric patient who has become so severely disabled or debilitated that a complete rehabilitation team approach is required to restore function. The therapist with an interest in functional rehabilitation can find a plethora of equipment in the physical, occupational, and recreational therapy gyms. At minimum, this setting should provide the same equipment for its patients as is found in a medium-size outpatient clinic.

FUNCTIONAL EXERCISE EQUIPMENT

This section discusses the uses of the various pieces of functional exercise equipment presently available on the market today. Table 14–1 summarizes which common vendors sell specific pieces of equipment. Once again, the list is by necessity incomplete. Omission from this discussion does not indicate that a specific type of equipment lacks quality or worth. No gifts or donations were accepted in return for including a piece of equipment in this chapter, although many manufacturers kindly provided requested pictures of their products.

In addition, little documentation exists to support the premise that using a certain type of equipment actually benefits the patient. This chapter, however, describes gains attributed to

pieces of equipment that have been observed through clinical experience. Because this is by no means scientific, the reader must determine the equipment's worth based on the incomplete information available and his or her own experience. The reader is further cautioned not to accept vendors' (biased) claims for their own equipment. Remember: *Caveat emptor*—Let the buyer beware!

Aerobic Step

The aerobic step (Figure 14–1) is a sturdy 4-in-high platform that can be used to train in climbing and descending curbs and stairs. Postural faults of the hip rotators or patellar stabilizers can be assessed and trained without the patient becoming overly stressed from a high-rise platform. In addition, the patient can perform beginning plyometric jumps on and off this sturdy surface. The steps come in different widths and lengths. This piece of equipment ranges in cost from approximately $30 to $100 and can be purchased through mail-order catalogs or off the shelf in sports stores and department stores.

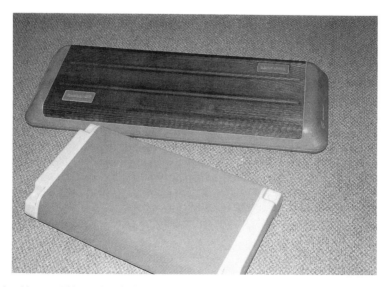

Figure 14–1   Aerobic step. This sturdy 4-in-high platform comes in standard or personal size. Platforms can stack for higher-intensity workouts (not recommended for patients with patellofemoral disorders).

Table 14–1 Functional Exercise Equipment Vendors

Functional Exercise Equipment	*Vendors (Incomplete Listing in Alphabetical Order)*
Aerobic steps	Flaghouse Rehab LL Bean
Aquatic equipment	Authentic Fitness Flaghouse Physical Education & Recreation LL Bean Perform Better (M-F Athletic Co) Sprint (Rothammer International, Inc) SwimEx Systems
Balls	Back Designs Ball Dynamics Flaghouse Rehab Perform Better (M-F Athletic Co) Sammons Saunders Group Sportime Abilitations Wolverine Sports
Bicycles (upper and lower body stationary) and RangeMaker®	Biodex Medical Cybex® Flaghouse Rehab Rainbow Rehabilitation & Fitness (RangeMaker®) Sammons Saunders Group Universal®
Cross-country ski machines	NordicTrack
Ethafoam™ rollers	Back Designs Dow Chemical
Fitter™ (Pro Fitter)	Fitter International Flaghouse Rehab Perform Better (M-F Athletic Co)
Games	Flaghouse Physical Education & Recreation
Glide boards	Flaghouse Rehab Improve Human Performance (Ultima Glide) Perform Better (M-F Athletic Co) Saunders Group Speed City
Hand equipment	Baltimore Therapeutic Equipment (BTE®) Fitter International Flaghouse Rehab North Coast Medical Sammons Sportime Abilitations

Table 14–1 Functional Exercise Equipment Vendors (continued)

Functional Exercise Equipment	*Vendors (Incomplete Listing in Alphabetical Order)*
Milk crates	Sammons
Sports rehabilitation equipment	Flaghouse Physical Education & Recreation Perform Better (M-F Athletic Co) Speed City Wolverine Sports
Stair-climbing machines	Flaghouse Rehab Sammons StairMaster™ Sports/Medical Products Universal® Gym Equipment
Surgical tubing	Innovation Sports (Body Lines) Lifeline-USA® Perform Better (M-F Athletic Co) PRO (Unit 10) Saunders Group SPRI Performance Systems TheraBand® Tubing (Hygienic Corporation)
Total Gym®	Engineering Fitness International (EFI/Total Gym) Perform Better (M-F Athletic Co) Saunders Group
Treadmills	Biodex Medical Cybex® Flaghouse Rehab Sammons
Wobble boards	CAMP® International (biomechanical ankle platform system, BAPS) Fitter International Flaghouse Rehab Orthopedic Physical Therapy Products Sammons SPRI Performance Systems
Work-hardening equipment	Advanced Therapy Products BTE® Flaghouse Rehab North Coast Medical Isotechnologies Sammons Smith & Nephew Rolyan

Note: This incomplete listing is provided as a service for those readers who do not know whom to contact to try out or purchase different pieces of equipment. Wherever possible, a selection of vendors has been provided. Many other excellent pieces of equipment and reputable vendors exist. Neither the specific products nor the vendors are endorsed or recommended over other products or vendors. The reader is referred to the annual buyer's guides for both physical therapy and occupational therapy published by the professional associations (American Physical Therapy Association and American Occupational Therapy Association) for more comprehensive listings of vendors. In addition, many pieces of equipment are available at local sports stores, department stores, and toy stores.

Aquatic Equipment

All sorts of aquatic exercise equipment are now available for functional training. For resistive exercise, the therapist can choose from:

- hand paddles
- buoyancy cuffs
- buoyant dumbbells
- aqua gloves (Figure 14–2)
- swim fins
- water boards

For more functional exercise, the patient can use similar but waterproof exercise equipment, such as:

- small step platform (Figure 14–3)
- treadmill
- water leash (like surgical tubing)
- games (volleyball, badminton, dive rings, basketball, etc.)

Many of the items are available in sports stores and through aquatics and therapeutic catalogs. Prices vary greatly. With the increase in popularity of aquatic therapy, many companies now offer miniature therapeutic pool environments (Figure 14–4), which can fit in a medium to large clinic. These are available through the manufacturers. Clinicians should examine and carefully try out this high-ticket item before purchasing.

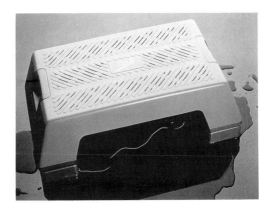

Figure 14–3 Speedo aquatic exercise step. *Source:* Photo courtesy of Authentic Fitness Corporation, Van Nuys, California.

Balls

Nothing brings a smile faster to more patients than an approaching therapist with any type of ball in hand. Balls somehow evoke happy memories in just about everyone, even patients who have never enjoyed sports. Balls come in so many shapes and sizes (Figure 14–5) that some companies specialize in therapeutic ball equipment. Unless the facility is large and has no breakable items nearby, baseball-size throwing balls should be made of foam rubber (eg, Nerf balls) to protect mirrors and other patients from errant throws or catches. Larger playing balls (8-in diameter) can be used for eye-foot or eye-hand coordination activities (eg, kicking or throwing). In addition, this size ball can be held between a patient's knees to promote hip adduction and activation of the vastus medialis obliques for patellofemoral retraining. The ball can also be placed between a patient's spine and a wall to decrease the friction of a wall slide (a squat performed against a wall). The ball can be used for dribbling, shooting baskets, or any other number of games. These items can be purchased in any toy store, department store, or sports store for less than $5.

Large Therapeutic Ball

The large therapeutic ball offers a large area of support, but on an unstable base. This provides an excellent challenge in balance, stabili-

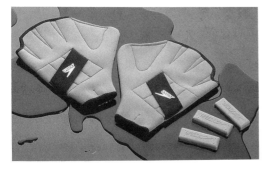

Figure 14–2 Speedo aqua gloves. Webbing increases resistance in water for a higher-intensity workout. *Source:* Photo courtesy of Authentic Fitness Corporation, Van Nuys, California.

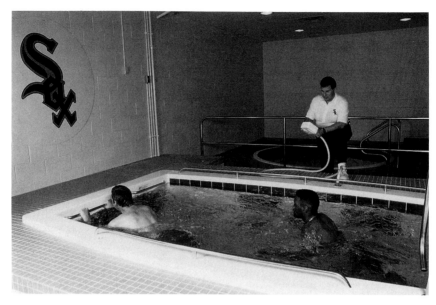

Figure 14–4   Miniature therapeutic pool environment. *Source:* Photo courtesy of SwimEx Systems, Warren, Rhode Island.

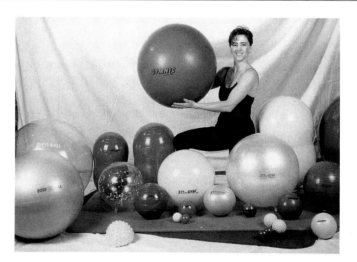

Figure 14–5   Therapeutic balls in all shapes and sizes, including Gymnic balls, sensory balls, plyoballs, and foam balls. *Source:* Photo courtesy of Ball Dynamics International, Denver, Colorado.

zation, and motor control. Greater stability can be gained by underinflating the ball. The balls are surprisingly comfortable to sit upon and may be helpful for the patient with pressure sensitivity. The patient can exercise in some of the following positions:

- sitting upon the ball
- prone over the ball
- quadruped over the ball
- standing with the ball between the patient and a wall
- supine (bridging) with feet flat upon the ball
- supine on the ball with feet on the floor
- standing while lifting or carrying the ball
- kneeling against the ball

The balls come sized for both children and adults. Persons ranging from 5 ft to 5 ft 10 in usually can use the 65-cm (26-in) ball; taller adults usually require the 85-cm (34-in) ball. Colors identify the ball size within companies but vary from manufacturer to manufacturer (therefore, ordering a green ball without specifying the exact size is not a good idea). The balls are readily available through the ball companies, many of the therapy catalogs, and even children's toy and adult mail-order catalogs for less than $40.

Plyoballs

Plyoballs or weighted balls (once called medicine balls) are used to challenge further the patient who can easily perform regular ball activities. Catching the plyoball requires a full-body response and can be used to improve total-body balance, stability, and coordination as well as to improve trunk and upper quarter strength. Some plyoballs are constructed so that they can bounce, providing additional activities, such as dribbling, for the patient. The patient can juggle a plyoball from one hand to the other or play catch with the therapist. If desired, the patient can use a Rebounder to throw and catch independent of the therapist.

Bicycle

The stationary bicycle is a common piece of rehabilitation and recreation equipment. It allows lower extremity closed-chain exercise while limiting weight bearing on the legs. By adjustment of the seat height, range of motion (ROM) can be promoted or assisted at various joints. For example, a high seat is recommended for the patient with patellofemoral joint dysfunction to avoid excessive knee flexion. Conversely a lower seat would benefit a patient with an anterior cruciate ligament reconstruction to avoid terminal knee extension. Patients with total joint replacements can use pedals to self-assist in gaining ROM. To avoid unnecessary torque, total knee replacement patients and those with genu varus or valgum should not use the toe clips but should instead place their feet

on top of the pedals. The bike can also be used for strengthening and aerobic fitness. The seat can be removed for the patient who must avoid hip or trunk flexion, allowing the patient to stand while pedaling. In addition, elderly or deconditioned patients or patients with low back pain can enjoy the benefits of cycling on a recumbent bicycle (Figure 14–6). Many rehabilitation bicycles have adaptors for upper extremity use, and some are designed specifically for upper extremity training (Figure 14–7). Stationary bicycles are available at all sports stores, department stores, and (of course) bicycle stores. The cost of a good quality bike for department use begins at $1000; a personal stationary bicycle retails for less than $500.

Because some patients lack sufficient knee ROM to attempt cycling, an adapter that changes the lever arm length can be attached to the pedals. The RangeMaker™ (Figure 14–8) allows the patient to gain the benefits of cycling

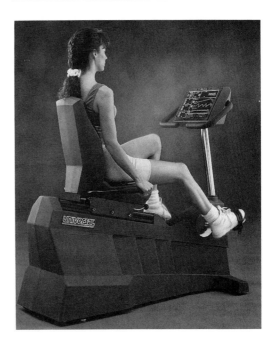

Figure 14–6 Universal® recumbent bicycle. Many patients find the seating on the recumbent bicycles more comfortable. In addition, it is generally easier to get on and off this type of unit than a regular stationary bike. *Source:* Photo courtesy of Universal Gym Equipment, Inc., Cedar Rapids, Iowa.

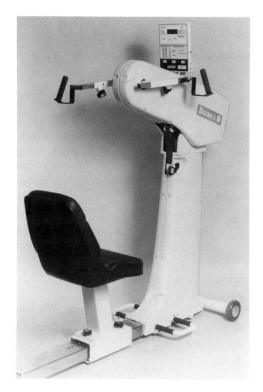

Figure 14–7   Upper body cycle. *Source:* Photo courtesy of Biodex Medical Systems, Inc., Shirley, New York.

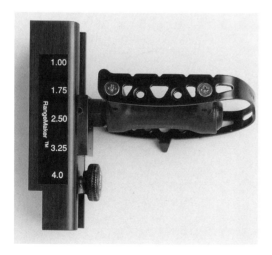

Figure 14–8   RangeMaker™. By attachment of this unit to a standard stationary bicycle, the lever arm can be adjusted to make cycling easier. The patient reaps the benefits of bicycling within tolerable ranges of knee motion. *Source:* Photo courtesy of Rainbow Rehabilitation & Fitness, Grayling, Michigan.

while simultaneously gaining the ROM needed to use the bicycle without adaptations. This product is especially useful in the geriatric population or specifically for the patient with an injured knee. The adapter is available through Rainbow Rehabilitation & Fitness Company and therapy mail order catalogs at a cost of about $250.

Dowel

Any sturdy wooden stick, even a yardstick or cane, can serve as a functional exercise tool. The dowel is an indispensable piece of equipment. The patient can use it to gain upper extremity ROM or can hang cuff weights on it to act as a miniature barbell. The therapist can place it along the patient's back or pelvis to provide additional sensory feedback to help with postural alignment. The patient can also play stickball with it (and a foam ball or balloon) or simulate a golf swing. This batting activity helps promote new problem-solving strategies for the patient. The dowel should be approximately 2 to 3 ft long and be sturdy enough to support 10 lb of cuff weights. This item can be purchased at any craft or garden store for about $1.

Cross-Country Ski Machine

Although obviously an aerobic exercise machine, the cross-country ski machine is valuable in promoting closed-chain exercise for the lower extremities while avoiding impact loading. Patients with varus or valgus knees should avoid this machine because excessive torque can occur when the patient's foot is locked into the toe clips. The machine does not have to be used in the standard fashion at all. Alternative exercises include having a patient face the side of the machine and place one foot on the ground and the other foot onto the ski but perpendicular to it. This allows the motions of hip abduction and adduction to be performed in a smooth gliding fashion but against resistance.

Ethafoam™ Rollers

Ethafoam™ rollers provide another exercise surface that has a supportive but unstable base of support. Exercising with the rollers may help promote varied motor recruitment patterns while self-mobilizing soft tissue and joint structures.[1] A patient can stand or assume quadruped position on the roller (Figure 14–9) to promote balance and proprioception (similar to standing on a wobble board). In addition, the roller can be used in many ways like the large therapeutic ball, with the patient lying supine or bridging on the roller as part of a lumbar stabilization program. The rollers come in various sizes of either 4 or 6 inches in diameter and either 1 or 3 ft in length. Ethafoam™ rollers can be purchased through mail order only. Prices vary greatly among vendors, ranging from $8 apiece to upwards of $90 per set.

Fitter™

The Fitter™ (sometimes called Pro Fitter) is a closed-chain exercise machine that simulates downhill skiing. Accessories for the machine include ski poles for balance. The Fitter™ can also be used in a variety of ways for upper extremity closed-chain exercise, however, as well as for seated lower extremity work (Figure 14–10). It provides a different and challenging workout for the high-level patient, promoting proprioception, coordination, and strength. It places large acceleration and deceleration forces on the joints and is therefore excellent in retraining joint stability. The whole body tends to be involved in Fitter™ exercising, and the device also provides an aerobic workout in a fun and stimulating way. The Fitter™ is available through therapy catalogs and through the manufacturer, Fitter International, at a cost of approximately $500.

Games and Sports Equipment

Many games and pieces of sports equipment can be used as functional exercise equipment. Perusing the clearance aisle in sports and toy stores can yield many rehabilitation tools. In ad-

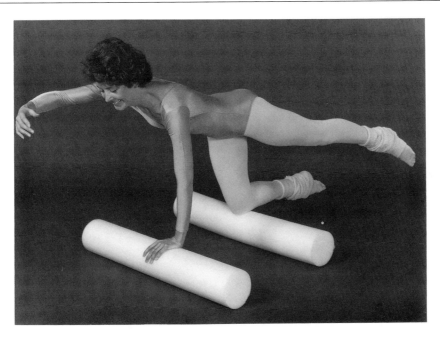

Figure 14–9 Ethafoam™ roller used in quadruped position to promote joint stability, proprioception, and improved motor control. *Source:* Photo courtesy of Back Designs, Inc., Berkeley, California.

A

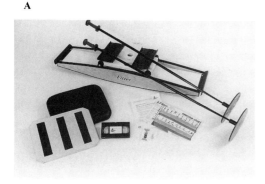

B

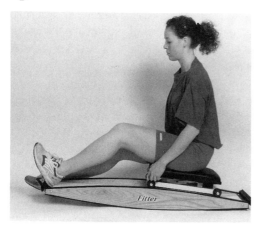

Figure 14–10 (**A**) The Fitter™ and accessories. (**B**) Closed-chain lower extremity work done in sitting position. *Source:* Photos courtesy of Fitter International, Inc., Calgary, Alberta, Canada.

dition, some rehabilitation-oriented companies have recreation subdivisions as well. Creative clinicians find unlimited opportunities for equipment ideas from the recreational arena.

Glide Board

The glide board (Figure 14–11) simulates speed skating; the original design is attributed to Eric Heiden, an Olympic speed skating champion (some of these boards are called Heiden boards). By pushing off the side bumpers, the patient accelerates and decelerates the entire lower quarter in a flowing type of movement. The patient can also stand in the middle of the board and control hip abduction

and adduction by scissoring the legs apart and together. When the patient masters the movement pattern needed to glide back and forth, the therapist can throw balls to the patient in midglide. Patients enjoy exercising on the glide board, likening it to the fun they had as children when sliding across the kitchen floor in socks. Great balance and control are needed to glide successfully, and many elderly patients may wish to forego this high-level and somewhat dangerous exercise.

Many companies make both large, adjustable glide boards and portable boards. Special booties are worn over sneakers to decrease friction and allow smooth gliding. The portable boards are available in sports stores and department stores; the full-size rehabilitation boards are available through the manufacturers and therapy mail-order catalogs. The portable boards begin at $50, and the full-size boards begin around $300.

Milk Crate

A sturdy milk crate is another one of those low-technology pieces of functional exercise equipment that comes in handy. The crate can be used while empty or weighted to allow the patient to practice the functional activities of lifting, carrying, pushing, and pulling. (A word of caution: Milk crates are not designed for climbing or jumping on and off. If the facility has a large population of patients requiring plyometrics, Plyoboxes or aerobic steps should be used instead.) Laundry baskets, cardboard boxes, or storage totes can be substituted for milk crates in the clinic or home. After being used for exercising, the milk crate can be used to store some of the other pieces of functional exercise equipment. This item is available in most office stores or from a local milk company for less than $10.

Sports Rehabilitation Equipment

It is beyond the scope of this book to discuss sport-specific rehabilitation equipment. Many tools exist to promote speed, agility, and power.

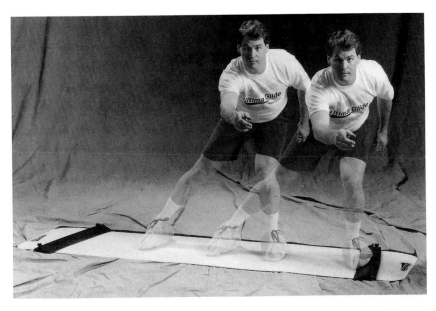

Figure 14–11 Ultima glide board: Adjustable length board for clinic use. *Source:* Photo courtesy of Improve Human Performance, Inc., Abingdon, Maryland.

Aside from the items mentioned in this section, the reader is referred to sports medicine books and catalogs for more information about sports medicine equipment.

Stair-Climbing Machines

Stair-climbing machines fall into one of two categories: those for complete closed-chain exercising (as found in the StairMaster™ 4000 PT® exercise system, Figure 14–12), and those for simulated stair climbing with both open- and closed-chain work (as found in the StairMaster™ Stepmill™ exercise system, Figure 14–13). Clinics should purchase models that have guard rails, which allow protective weight bearing or assisted balance for the patients. Machines with adjustable step heights are also helpful. All stair climbers promote lower extremity strengthening and proprioceptive retraining. Aerobic training can also be achieved with this device. The machines are available in sports stores and through therapy mail-order catalogs. Quality and pricing vary greatly, and the clinician should examine and try out several models of this expensive equipment before purchasing.

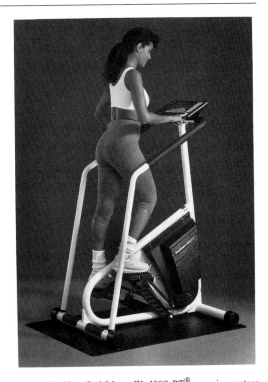

Figure 14–12 StairMaster™ 4000 PT® exercise system for complete closed-chain work in which the feet stay in contact with the pedals for the duration of exercise. *Source:* Photo courtesy of StairMaster™ Sports/Medical Products, Inc., Kirkland, Washington.

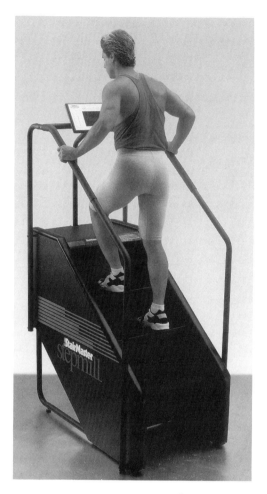

Figure 14–13   StairMaster™ Stepmill® exercise system, which more closely simulates actual stair climbing, including both open- and closed-chain work. *Source:* Photo courtesy of StairMaster™ Sports/Medical Products, Inc., Kirkland, Washington.

Surgical Tubing

Before companies sold complete kits of resistive exercise equipment based on surgical tubing, therapists were sneaking into the nurses' supply closet for catheter tubing. From such an inauspicious start came a line of variable resistive exercise equipment. Surgical tubing can be used to promote strength, stability, and motor control of the extremities and can as act as a miniature treadmill by providing resistance to ambulation activities. Although the clinician can easily construct individual exercise kits by

purchasing separately an entire box of surgical tubing, ready-made exercise units possess superior quality for a slight increase in cost. Some units, such as the PRO Stretch or Body Lines (Figure 14–14), have built-in handles that are soft and flexible, which are an advantage for patients with arthritis. Some handles are made of strong, hard plastic, which may be preferred in an athletic setting (Lifeline-USA®, Figure 14–15). Most have foot/ankle straps for lower extremity exercising. The ready-made kits come in different strengths of tubing, which must be specified when one is ordering. Portable surgical tubing kits can be purchased from the manufacturers, through therapy catalogs, and even in

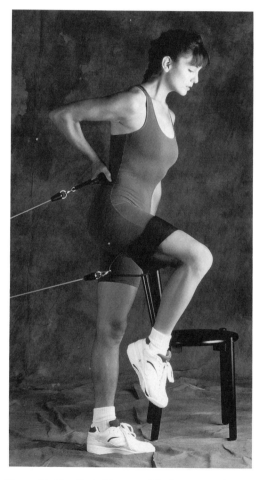

Figure 14–14   Body Lines conditioning system. *Source:* Photo courtesy of Innovation Sports, Inc., Irvine, California.

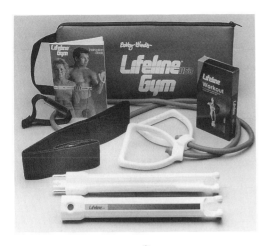

Figure 14–15   Lifeline-USA® portable exercise system. This system comes with a sturdy bar and carrying case. *Source:* Photo courtesy of Lifeline-USA®, Madison, Wisconsin.

some sports stores. The prices vary between $30 and $60. Wall units (Figure 14–16) based on tubing can replace standard pulleys and are available through Lifeline® for less than $400.

Total Gym®

The Total Gym® (Figure 14–17) is a versatile total body exerciser that can strengthen, stretch, and increase proprioceptive input while also protecting the joints from excessive weight-bearing forces. The patient can exercise in both open- and closed-chain patterns. New movement patterns emerge as the patient attempts to solve the challenging motor problems provided by this unique piece of exercise equipment. The Total Gym® can also be used in conjunction with other functional equipment, such as surgical tubing or the biomechanical ankle platform system (BAPS) board (Figure 14–18). This equipment is available through therapy catalogs and the manufacturer, Engineering Fitness International, at a cost of about $1200.

Treadmill

Treadmills provide a moveable surface for all aspects of gait training. Patients who have diffi-

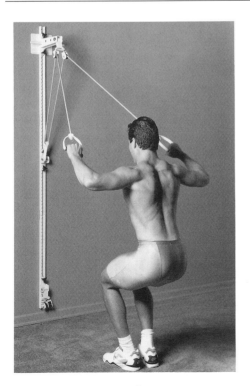

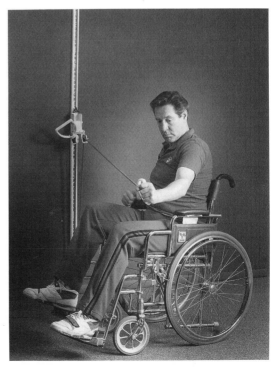

Figure 14–16   Lifeline-USA® wall unit. This unit allows flexibility of resistance cord placement and therefore multiple angles of pull. It also provides a safe and stable surface from which to exercise. *Source:* Photo courtesy of Lifeline-USA®, Madison, Wisconsin.

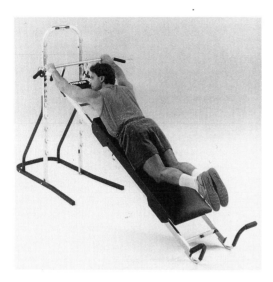

Figure 14–17   The Total Gym®, shown being used for upper body exercise. *Source:* Photo courtesy of Engineering Fitness International/Total Gym®, San Diego, California.

culty with a dynamic environment may find the treadmill useful for improving the timing of the gait pattern. Without using a lot of space, patients can work on side-stepping, carioca stepping, Groucho walking, regular forward walking, retro-walking (Figure 14–19), and running on the treadmill. Some treadmills have the abil-

ity to raise on an incline, simulating hill climbing. For the clinic, a wide and extra long treadmill with guard rails is preferred. Since treadmills seem to break down with incredible frequency compared with other types of exercise machinery, the clinician needs to examine both the equipment and the service contract carefully before purchasing. Although personal treadmills are available in department and sports stores, clinics should only consider heavy-duty professional units for purchase. Prices begin at approximately $3500.

Wobble Boards

Wobble boards or balance boards are flat discs or rectangles with some sort of a beveled bottom to reduce the base of support. Exercising on the boards strengthens the ankle and knee musculature and can improved balance in sedentary subjects.[2] The boards also promote proprioceptive input into the entire lower or upper quarter. The patient can work on individual joint motions (eg, ankle dorsiflexion/plantar flexion or inversion/eversion) or simply try to balance on the board without letting the board rim touch the ground (Figure 14–20). For upper extremity use, patients can place either their hands or their

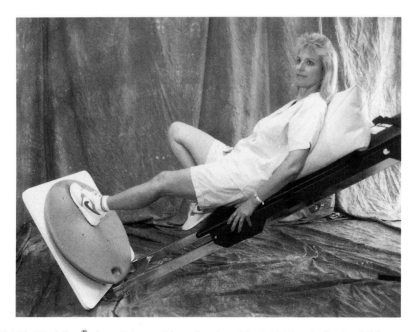

Figure 14–18   The Total Gym®, shown being used in conjunction with a BAPS board, allowing full foot contact with protected weight bearing. *Source:* Photo courtesy of Engineering Fitness International/Total Gym®, San Diego, California.

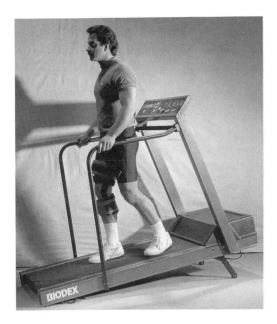

Figure 14–19 Biodex treadmill used for retro-walking. Note the guard rails for protected weight bearing and the ability of the treadmill to incline, increasing the intensity of the exercise. *Source:* Photo courtesy of Biodex Medical Systems Inc., Shirley, New York.

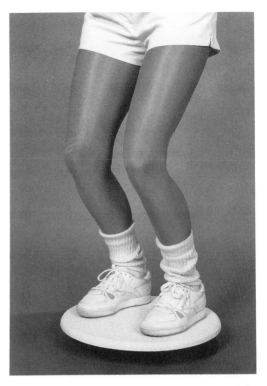

Figure 14–20 SPRI intermediate wobble board used for promoting bilateral standing balance and proprioception. *Source:* Photo courtesy of SPRI Performance Systems, Deerfield, Illinois.

forearms on the board (which is on a table or plinth) for proprioceptive retraining.

The boards come in a variety of materials, shapes, and sizes (Figure 14–21). Beginner and intermediate boards are suitable for most patients (including geriatric patients); advanced boards are reserved for the high-level patient or athlete. The wobble board usually has a slippery bottom surface, which needs to be placed on a carpet or a piece of Dycem for safety reasons (if the same area of the gym or clinic is to be used for wobble board training, an additional piece of carpet should be placed between the board and the floor to prevent wearing away of the carpet fibers). The wobble boards are available through therapy catalogs and from the manufacturers at a cost of about $30 to $60.

No discussion of wobble boards would be complete without mentioning the BAPS board. Although heavier and larger than the other wobble boards, the BAPS board (Figure 14–22) was designed to match more accurately the ankle axis of rotation for improved performance. In addition, the size of the hemiball base can be

adjusted by screwing in one of five standard modular components (Figure 14–23). The user also has the ability to adjust resistance by either adding plates or hooking up to surgical tubing. The BAPS board is available through therapy catalogs and the manufacturer, Camp International, for approximately $500.

Work-Hardening (Conditioning) Equipment

A discussion of industrial rehabilitation equipment is beyond the scope of this book. For basic work conditioning in the outpatient clinic, the therapist can choose from a variety of small but sturdy workstations (Figure 14–24). The clinician is referred to the plethora of work-hardening texts and equipment catalogs for more information concerning this type of equipment.

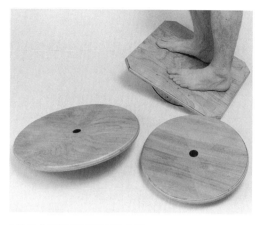

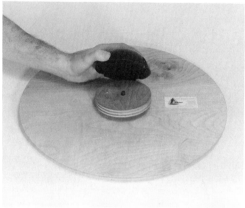

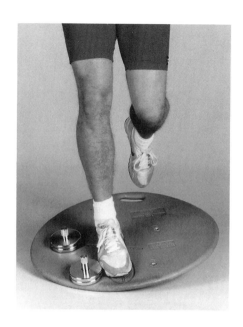

Figure 14–23 BAPS board with plates added to assist or resist desired ankle motion. *Source:* Photo courtesy of CAMP® International, BISSELL Healthcare Company Inc., Jackson, Michigan.

Figure 14–21 Wobble boards in a variety of shapes, materials, and levels. *Source:* Photo courtesy of Fitter International, Inc., Calgary, Alberta, Canada.

VENDOR LISTING

The following alphabetical listing of some vendors of exercise equipment is provided to help the clinician begin to find needed pieces of equipment. None of the vendors is recommended over others in this list or over other vendors nationwide or in the community. As mentioned several times previously, this list is incomplete. With the information provided here, however, the clinician can begin to obtain various catalogs and promotional materials for desired items.

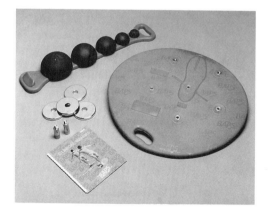

Figure 14–22 BAPS board with adjustable hemiballs. *Source:* Photo courtesy of CAMP® International, Inc., BISSELL Healthcare Company, Jackson, Michigan.

Advanced Therapy Products, Inc
PO Box 3420
Glen Allen, VA 23058-3420
(804) 747-8574

Authentic Fitness Corp
PO Box 10156
Van Nuys, CA 91410
(818) 376-0300

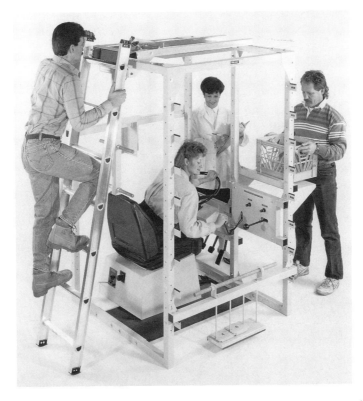

Figure 14–24 Work-hardening stations to simulate multiple occupations. *Source:* Photo courtesy of Advanced Therapy Products, Inc., Glen Allen, Virginia

Back Designs, Inc
1045 Ashby Avenue
Berkeley, CA 94710
(510) 849-1923

Ball Dynamics International, Inc
1616 Glenarm Place
Suite 1900
Denver, CO 80202
(800) 752-2255

Baltimore Therapeutic Equipment Company (BTE®)
7455-L New Ridge Road
Hanover, MD 21076-3105
(800) 331-8845

Biodex Medical Systems, Inc
Brookhaven R&D Plaza
20 Ramsay Road, Box 702
Shirley, NY 11967-0702
(800) 224-6339

CAMP® International, Inc (BAPS board)
PO Box 89
Jackson, MI 49204-0089
(800) 492-1088

CYBEX®, a division of Lumex
2100 Smithtown Avenue
Ronkonkoma, NY 11779
(800) 645-5392

Dow Chemical, Inc (Ethafoam™)
2040 Dow Center
Midland, MI 48674

Engineering Fitness International, Inc
(EFI/Total Gym®)
7766 Arjons Drive, Suite B
San Diego, CA 92126
(800) 541-4900

Flaghouse (Rehab and Physical Education
& Recreation)
150 N MacQuesten Parkway
Mt Vernon, NY 10550
(800) 793-7900

Fitter International, Inc (Pro-Fitter,
PowerWeb)
4515 1st Street SE
Calgary, Alberta, T2G 2L2, Canada
(403) 243-6830
(800) FITTER-1

Hygienic Corp (Thera-Band®)
1245 Home Avenue
Akron, OH 44310-2575
(800) 321-2135

Improve Human Performance, Inc
(Ultima glide board)
PO Box 506
Abingdon, MD 21009-0506
(800) 388-2666

Innovation Sports, Inc (Body Lines)
7 Chrysler
Irvine, CA 92718
(800) 222-4284

Isotechnologies, Inc
PO Box 1239
328 Elizabeth Brady Road
Hillsborough, NC 27278
(800) 487-5438

Lifeline-USA®
1421 S Park Street
Madison, WI 53715
(800) 553-6633

NordicTrack
104 Peavey Road
Chaska, MN 55318
(800) 468-4485

North Coast Medical, Inc
187 Stauffer Boulevard
San Jose, CA 95125-1042
(800) 821-9319

Orthopedic Physical Therapy Products
(rock board)
PO Box 47009
Minneapolis, MN 55447-0009
(800) 367-7393

Perform Better (M-F Athletic Co)
PO Box 8090
Cranston, RI 02920-0090
(800) 556-7464

PRO
PO Box 27525
Tucson, AZ 85726
(800) 523-5611

Rainbow Rehabilitation and Fitness
(RangeMaker®)
PO Box 49
100 Ottawa Street
Grayling, MI 49738
(517) 348-5220

Sammons
145 Tower Drive, Dept 966
Burr Ridge, IL 60521
(800) 323-5547

Saunders Group, Inc
7750 W 78th Street
Minneapolis, MN 55439
(800) 654-8357

Smith & Nephew Rolyan, Inc
PO Box 578
Germantown, WI 53022
(800) 558-8633

Speed City, Inc
PO Box 25690
Portland, OR 97225
(800) 255-9930

Sportime® Abilitations
1 Sportime Way
Atlanta, GA 30340-1402
(800) 283-5700

SPRI Performance Systems
111 Pfingsten Road, Suite 311
Deerfield, IL 60015
(800) 488-7774

Sprint (Rothammer International, Inc)
PO Box 5579
Santa Maria, CA 93456
(800) 235-2156

StairMaster™ Sports/Medical Products, Inc
12421 Willows Road NE
Suite 100
Kirkland, WA 98034
(800) 635-2936

SwimEx Systems
PO Box 328
Warren, RI 02885-0328
(800) 877-7946

Universal Gym Equipment, Inc
PO Box 1270
Cedar Rapids, IA 52406
(800) 843-3906

Wolverine Sports
PO Box 1941
Ann Arbor, MI 48106-1941
(800) 521-2832

For more information about equipment and vendors, the reader can also reference the following books and journals:

Aquatics: The Complete Reference Guide for Aquatic Fitness Professionals
Jones and Bartlett Publishers
20 Park Plaza
Boston, MA 02116

buyers guide issue of *PT Magazine*
American Physical Therapy Association
1111 N Fairfax Street
Alexandria, VA 22314-1488
(703) 684-2782

buyers guide issue of *OT Magazine*
American Occupational Therapy Association
1383 Piccard Drive
Rockville, MD 20850
(301) 948-9626

Physical Therapy Products™ Magazine
Novicom, Inc
3510 Torrance Boulevard, Suite 315
Torrance, CA 90503
(310) 316-8112

REFERENCES

1. Hauswirth B, Keyser K. Ethafoam roller. *PT Mag.* 1993; 1:93–94.
2. *Physiother Can.* 1992;44:23–30.

15

Adaptive Equipment

To create an environment that allows efficient movement patterns to emerge, the clinician often must alter the patient's surroundings or equipment. In many instances, the adaptations are only temporary until the patient's physical impairments are corrected through exercise. For example, a patient with low back pain complains of an increase in symptoms when rising from the toilet. The evaluation determines that insufficient lower extremity strength is preventing the patient from getting up without undulating the lumbosacral region. The patient needs to use a raised toilet seat until adequate strength is restored to the lower extremity through exercises, such as squats and the modified sit-to-stand functional exercise.

Some patients will require the adaptations for much longer periods of time if the insufficiency cannot be corrected. A patient with a total hip replacement will need a raised toilet seat to prevent the artificial joint from dislocating. Similarly, a patient with rheumatoid arthritis may need more permanent adaptations to perform many activities of daily living (ADLs) to protect the joints from further damage.

This chapter provides the rehabilitation specialist with a brief description of the types of adaptive equipment available for home and recreational use. The health care professional most qualified to prescribe adaptive equipment is the occupational therapist. When an occupational therapist is unavailable, other clinicians can find the necessary equipment through the (incomplete) list of vendors provided at the end of the chapter.

MAJOR TYPES OF ADAPTIVE EQUIPMENT

In general, patients resist the use of adaptive equipment. Some people cannot accept the social stigma of looking different. Other people cannot accept that their present physical condition (versus how they remember themselves) requires an alternative way of doing things. The therapist should recommend the use of adaptive equipment only when necessary, explaining the rationale carefully to the patient. The following general types of adaptive equipment are available for patient use at home.

Clothing and Shoes

Fashion has never been a friend of the human body until recently. The worst offenders were, of course, the dresses with 30 tiny buttons in the back (only Houdini could have managed them). Even able-bodied women could not fasten those kinds of dresses without assistance. Fortunately, some companies have attempted to design pleasant-looking clothing that is easier to don.

These clothes are mostly bought through mail-order companies and can mean the difference between being independent in dressing or requiring help, especially for people with arthritis. Many other types of clothing, such as pants with elastic waistbands and wraparound skirts, are available in clothing and department stores. Even bras that snap in the front can now be bought off the shelf. Existing clothing and footwear can be adapted easily by replacing buttons with Velcro closures or using elastic shoe laces.

The best thing to happen to feet was the acceptance of athletic shoes (sneakers) as fashionable. This footwear provides good heel counters, arch supports, and padded innersoles and can even accept prescription orthotics. Many patients with foot and ankle problems not only can look normal but can benefit from wearing supportive athletic shoes. Many of the elderly have also discovered the joys of wearing sneakers. Athletic shoes provide good traction and shock absorption for aging feet with diminished metatarsal fat pads.

If trunk flexion is a problem, patients can easily slip into loafers and pumps. They do not have to rely only on slippers (which can be dangerous) for wear around the house. Women's fashion shoes have also benefitted from advances in technology with companies such as Naturalizer, Easy Stride, and Cobbie Cobbler providing a full line of casual and dress shoes with good support, padded inner soles, shock absorption, and arch supports.

Communication

The patient can choose from both low- and high-technology adaptive equipment for assisting with communications. Writing can be made easier with special grippers for pens and adjustable table tops and desks. Telephones now come with large push buttons and amplification dials built into the handset. A phone holder allows the patient with arthritis to hold the handset without grasping it. Patients with neck or shoulder pain can purchase headsets to replace the handset, allowing hands-free phone operation.

Computers can also be used for communication, and some (eg, Apple computers) come with disability software built into the system. Voice recognition programs are allowing patients greater ability to input into the computer without the need for keyboard entries. For those with hand impairments, wrist pads and ergonomic keyboards are available to decrease the repetitive stress of keying in entries. The ability to access on-line information systems via modem and built-in facsimile machines increase the patient's ability to communicate even with high levels of physical impairment.

Dressing Aids

Despite the advancements in clothing, many problems can remain. For this reason, the following dressing aids may be helpful:

- button helper (Figure 15–1)
- sock starter (Figure 15–2)
- long-handled shoe horn
- zipper pull

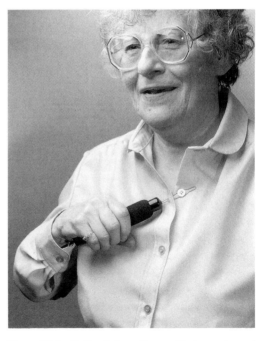

Figure 15–1 Button helper. *Source:* Photo courtesy of S&S Worldwide (AdaptAbility®), Colchester, Connecticut.

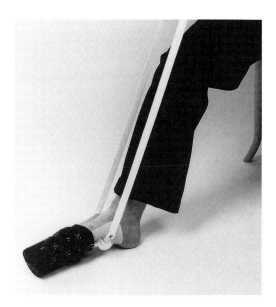

Figure 15–2   Sock starter. *Source:* Photo courtesy of S&S Worldwide (AdaptAbility®), Colchester, Connecticut.

These items can be purchased through mail order or in some pharmacies and department stores (eg, Sears, Bradlees, etc.).

Driving Adaptations

Because of the immense safety issues, automobile adaptations should be left to trained professionals in this area. The leading American automakers can provide information and the actual equipment to adapt cars for disabled drivers. In addition, many occupational therapy departments provide driving education programs for people with disabilities.

Minor adaptations regarding seat comfort and positioning can be handled easily by physical therapists and occupational therapists. Lumbar supports and wedge cushions can be prescribed as needed and can be used on regular chairs as well (Figure 15–3). These are available through mail order as well as in most drug stores.

Food Preparation

Pitfalls can arise in many areas of food preparation. The patient may be unable to reach or carry a required utensil, an oven door may be too difficult to open, a jar may be too tightly sealed, and so forth. After the clinician has evaluated the entire task, some of the following equipment may help the patient prepare meals more easily:

- modified cutting boards
- jar openers
- step-stools
- large-gripped utensils (Figure 15–4)
- adapted knives and parers (Figure 15–5)
- Dycem

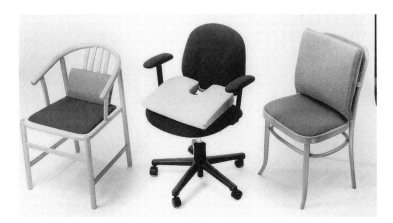

Figure 15–3   Lumbar supports and wedge cushions can promote improved seating when used on regular chairs (as shown above) or on car seats. *Source:* Photo courtesy of S&S Worldwide (AdaptAbility®), Colchester, Connecticut.

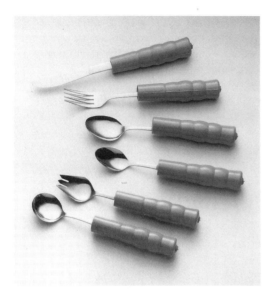

Figure 15–4   Large-gripped utensils. *Source:* Photo courtesy of Fred Sammons Incorporated, Burr Ridge, Illinois.

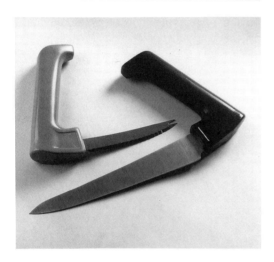

Figure 15–5   Adapted knives. *Source:* Photo courtesy of Fred Sammons Incorporated, Burr Ridge, Illinois.

Many of these adapted tools are readily available in department stores; others can be purchased through mail order.

Grippers

Many tools for everyday or recreational use need to be enlarged with padding for patients

with hand problems, especially arthritis. Some are designed specifically for tableware, pens and pencils, or utensils (Figure 15–6). For other tools, such as crochet hooks, toothbrushes, knitting needles, screwdrivers, and paintbrushes, generic foam tubing or thermoplastic tubing (eg, My-Grip®, Figure 15–7) can be custom-fitted for each patient's needs. These items are available through mail-order catalogs.

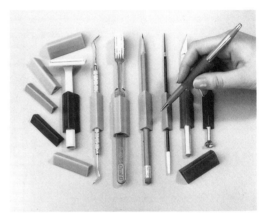

Figure 15–6   Grippers for assorted utensils. *Source:* Photo courtesy of Fred Sammons Incorporated, Burr Ridge, Illinois.

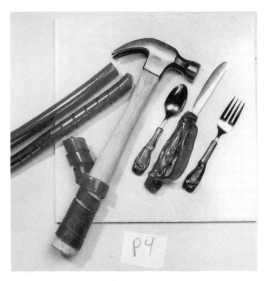

Figure 15–7   My-Grip® thermoplastic tubing to customize grips for other tools. *Source:* Photo courtesy of S&S Worldwide (AdaptAbility®), Colchester, Connecticut.

Hygiene (Personal)

Many patients have difficulty bending over to clean themselves properly. Long-handled sponges can help with washing of the lower extremity and even in applying body lotion. Long-handled sponge dishwashers can substitute nicely for the medical equipment and can be found in all food and department stores.

For washing the face, brushing teeth, shaving, or putting on make-up, the person with a painful low back can benefit from a make-up mirror attached to the wall with an accordian arm. This prevents the need to bend over the sink.

Many different types of tub seats are available for patients who are unsafe to shower and cannot sit into a bathtub. Another convenient washing item is a hand-held shower system (Figure 15–8). In addition, grab bars can greatly enhance patient safety and confidence and should be standard in all showers and tubs (considering the number of bathtub falls that occur annually). Most of these items can be purchased in hardware, drug, or even department stores as well as through mail-order companies.

Reachers

Reachers (Figure 15–9) come in handy to pick up things from the floor or to grab things from hard to reach places. They come in differ-

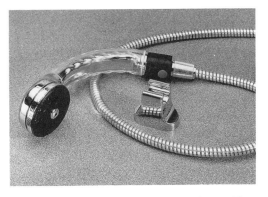

Figure 15–8 Hand-held shower system. *Source:* Photo courtesy of S&S Worldwide (AdaptAbility®), Colchester, Connecticut.

ent lengths (18 to 36 in) and weights. Most employ a pistol grip. They are wonderful for patients with back and shoulder problems, but they also work well for people who are less than the average height. These items can be purchased in drug and department stores and through mail-order catalogs.

Recreational Aids

Patients sometimes have to sacrifice enjoyable activities, such as sports and hobbies, because of physical impairments. Adaptive equipment is now available to return patients to avocational skills. Some of these include:

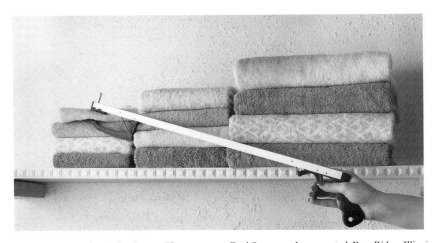

Figure 15–9   Reachers with pistol grip. *Source:* Photo courtesy Fred Sammons Incorporated, Burr Ridge, Illinois.

- playing card holders (Figure 15–10)
- adapted tenpin bowling balls and ramps (Figure 15–11)
- swimming aids
- modified exercise machines
- modified bats and balls

In addition, the padded grippers mentioned earlier can assist the patient with hand problems in doing other hobbies, such as painting, knitting, gardening, and woodworking. These items are mostly available through mail-order companies.

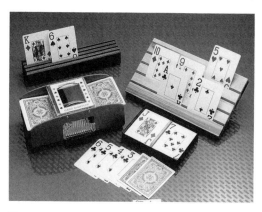

Figure 15–10 Playing card holder. *Source:* Photo courtesy of S&S Worldwide (AdaptAbility®), Colchester, Connecticut.

Instrumental Activities of Daily Living Simulator

Unlike the other adaptive aids described in this chapter, the Easy Street Environment helps patients learn to perform different instrumental ADLs (IADLs) such as shopping (Figure 15–12), getting on public buses (Figure 15–13) or into a car (Figure 15–14), going to a restaurant (Figure 15–15) or store, or doing laundry or kitchen work while in the protective environment of the rehabilitation clinic. Facilities can custom design which IADL modules they wish to provide for patients, but the minimum space requirement is 900 ft^2. In some ways, the Easy Street Environment is the ultimate in functional rehabilitation. Patients can attempt various solutions to the problems presented in the environment without external pressures. The simulator is only available through the HSM Group/Easy Street Environments.

Toileting

Different types of raised toilet seats now exist; some can clamp onto the toilet for stability and safety, and others are made of plastic and just fit into the normal seat (Figure 15–16). Although raised toilet seats are standard issue for

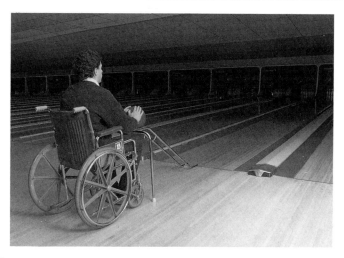

Figure 15–11 Bowling ramp. *Source:* Photo courtesy of Fred Sammons Incorporated, Burr Ridge, Illinois.

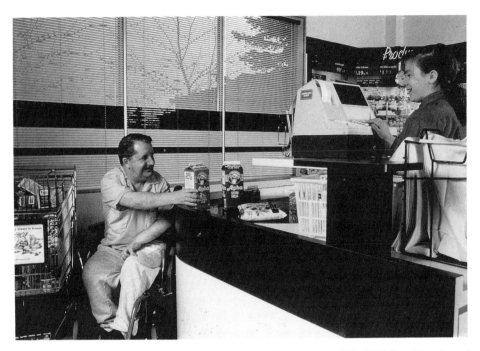

Figure 15–12   Easy Street Environment: shopping module. *Source:* Photo courtesy of The HSM Group/Easy Street Environment, Scottsdale, Arizona.

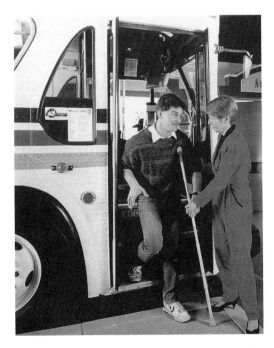

Figure 15–13 Easy Street Environment: transportation module—public transportation. *Source:* Photo courtesy of The HSM Group/Easy Street Environment, Scottsdale, Arizona.

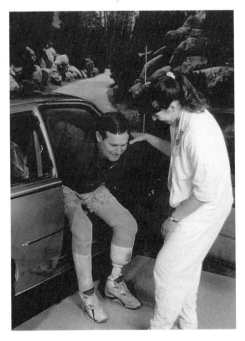

Figure 15–14 Easy Street Environment: transportation module—car transfers. *Source:* Photo courtesy of The HSM Group/Easy Street Environment, Scottsdale, Arizona.

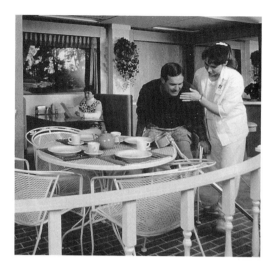

Figure 15–15 Easy Street Environment: restaurant module. *Source:* Photo courtesy of The HSM Group/Easy Street Environment, Scottsdale, Arizona.

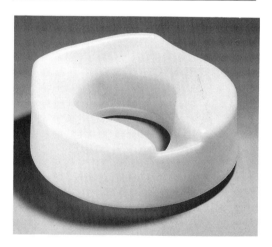

Figure 15–16 Raised toilet seat of molded plastic, which press-fits into a standard toilet seat. (Not recommended for patients with balance problems who require raised seats that are bolted to the toilet.) *Source:* Photo courtesy of Fred Sammons Incorporated, Burr Ridge, Illinois.

Other toilet equipment is available depending on the patient's needs. Safety frames (Figure 15–17) can be placed around the toilet to provide arm rests to assist the patient in getting on and off. For the patient with a hand or wrist injury, there is even an aid to help grip and use toilet paper (Figure 15–18).

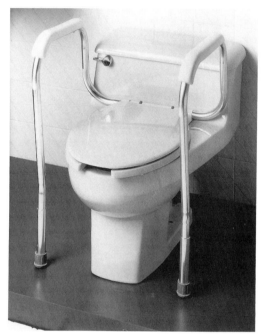

Figure 15–17 Safety frames for toilet. *Source:* Photo courtesy of S&S Worldwide (AdaptAbility®), Colchester, Connecticut.

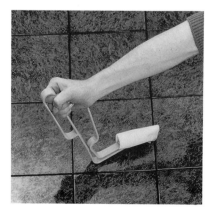

Figure 15–18 Toilet paper tongs. *Source:* Photo courtesy of S&S Worldwide (AdaptAbility®), Colchester, Connecticut.

patients recuperating from total hip replacement surgery, the therapist must remember to evaluate the size of the toilet in relation to the size of the patient to make sure that the patient is tall enough to need a raised seat. Raised toilet seats are available through mail-order catalogs, pharmacies, and even some chain stores (eg, Service Merchandise) for less than $100.

VENDOR LISTING

This alphabetical listing of some vendors of adaptive equipment is provided to help the clinician begin to find needed pieces of adaptive equipment. Each provides adaptive equipment for dressing, grooming, food preparation, hygiene, toileting, and recreation. None of the vendors is recommended over others in this list or over other vendors nationwide or in the community. As mentioned several times previously, this list is incomplete. With the information provided here, however, the clinician can begin to obtain various catalogs and promotional materials on desired items.

AdaptAbility®
PO Box 515
Colchester, CT 06415–0515
(800) 288-9941

AliMed, Inc
297 High Street
Dedham, MA 02026-9135
(800) 225-2610

Enrichments® **for Better Living**
145 Tower Drive
PO Box 579
Hinsdale, IL 60521
(800) 323-5547

Flaghouse
150 N MacQuesten Parkway
Mt Vernon, NY 10550
(800) 793-7900

HSM Group/Easy Street Environments®
6908 E Thomas Road, Suite 201
Scottsdale, AZ 85251
(800) 776-8078

Orthopedic Physical Therapy Products
PO Box 47009
Minneapolis, MN 55447-0009
(800) 367-7393

Sammons
145 Tower Drive, Dept 966
Burr Ridge, IL 60521
(800) 323-5547

Sportime® **Abilitations**
1 Sportime Way
Atlanta, GA 30340-1402
(800) 283-5700

Wheel-Chair Carrier, Inc
PO Box 79
Waterville, OH 43566-0079
(800) 541-3213

Appendix A _____

Six Phases of Gait as Described by Perry

The reader can use the detailed information presented here about the different phases of gait and the anatomic structures involved to initiate and control the lower extremities to customize the gait portion of the functional program for each patient.

Source: The following six plates are reprinted from _Principles of Lower-Extremity Bracing,_ (pp. 17, 21, 23, 25, 27, 29) edited by J. Perry and H. Hislop with permission of the American Physical Therapy Association, © 1967.

Plate 1. WEIGHT ACCEPTANCE

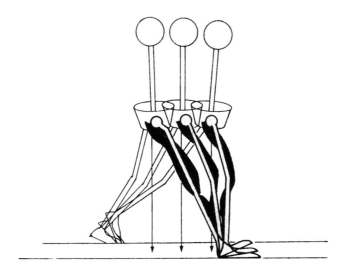

TASK: WEIGHT ACCEPTANCE (INTERVAL:.HEEL–STRIKE)
Heel–Strike to Foot–Flat: 0 to 15% of Walking Cycle.

DEMANDS:
1. Shock absorption
2. Limb stabilization
3. Forward travel without interruption
4. Balance on one limb

SITUATION:
1. Strong forward momentum just before heel strike
   a. Body traveling 2 mph (force from push of opposite limb)
   b. Swing limb traveling 5 mph (force from own push plus active hip and knee flexion)
2. Extremity reaching ahead of body
3. Heel strike abruptly stops forward travel of foot; momentum now concentrated on lower leg (tibia)

RESPONSE:

Events	Anatomical Activity
FORWARD PROGRESSION	
1. Immediate plantar flexion (due to ground contact of heel, body weight along tibia).	1. Restraint by ankle dorsiflexors: anterior tibialis, great and common toe extensors.
2. Rapid knee flexion to 15° (due to tibial advancement with thigh and trunk aligned behind foot).	2. Knee flexion restrained by: a. Tibial advancement restrained by soleus and posterior tibialis b. Quadriceps activity c. Thigh stabilization through hip extensor activity by semitendinosis, biceps (long head), gluteus maximus.
3. Hip flexion tendency (due to body weight being behind weight bearing foot).	3. Reversed by hip extensors and forward momentum.
SINGLE LIMB BALANCE:	
1. Tendency to fall away from support limb.	1. Lateral shift of body. Pelvis stabilization by hip abductors: Gluteus medius, gluteus minimus, tensor fascia femoris.
2. Valgus thrust on knee secondary to lateral shift.	2. Restrained by medial knee muscles: vastus medialis, semitendinosis, gracilis.
3. Valgus thrust on ankle.	3. Restrained by posterior tibialis and medial insertion of soleus.

Plate 2. TRUNK GLIDE

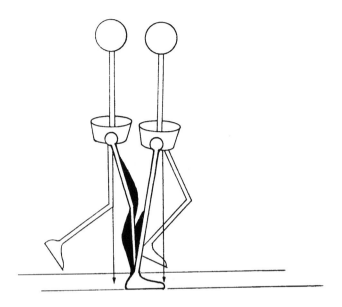

TASK: TRUNK GLIDE (INTERVAL: MID–STANCE)
Foot–Flat Period to Maximum Dorsiflexion: 15 to 40% of Walking Cycle

DEMAND:

Continue forward travel of body over flat foot.

SITUATION:

Complete single limb support has been attained.
Foot flat on the ground.
Extremity stable.
Momentum still active but lessening.
Rate of forward travel slowing a bit.

RESPONSE:

Events	Anatomical Activity
FORWARD PROGRESSION	
1. Momentum carries trunk and limb segments forward over stationary foot.	1. Rate of advancement controlled by tibial restraint: soleus and posterior tibialis activity.
a) Knee extended as thigh advancement over stable tibia.	a) Quadriceps quiet.
b) Hip extended by thigh advancement.	b) Hip extensors quiet.
2. Body weight passes from behind heel to over forefoot.	2. Ankle advances from 5 degrees plantar flexion to 10 degrees dorsiflexion.
SINGLE LIMB BALANCE:	
1. Total single limb support.	1. Continued hip abductor activity.
2. Lateral shift maximum at 20% point, then starts to decrease.	2. Knee stress relieved and protector muscles relaxed.
LIMB LENGTH ADJUSTMENT:	
Other limb swinging forward.	Simultaneous abduction, internal rotation, and extension demand on weight-bearing hip joint.

Plate 3. PUSH

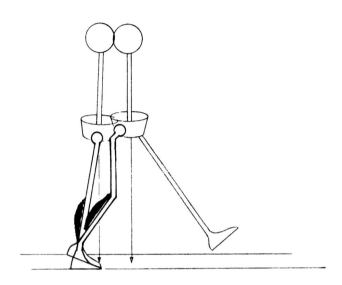

TASK: PUSH (INTERVAL: FIRST HALF OF PUSH–OFF)
Heel–Rise to Maximum Push Force: 40 to 50% of Walking Cycle

DEMAND:
Renew forward propelling force.

SITUATION:
Body slightly ahead of foot.
Knee fully extended.
Heel just starting to rise.
Ankle in 10 degrees dorsiflexion.

RESPONSE:

Events	Anatomical Activity
FORWARD PROGRESSION	
1. Body weight tends to pull:	
a. Hip into more extension	1. a. Hip extension restrained by iliacus.
b. Knee into more extension	b. Knee extension restrained by gastrocnemius to 10 degrees flexion.
c. Ankle into more dorsiflexion	c. All seven plantar flexors active: gastrocnemius, peroneus longus and brevis, great and common long toe flexors join soleus, and posterior tibialis which continue activity.
2. Create push force.	2 Increased activity of all seven plantar flexor muscles.
SINGLE LIMB BALANCE:	
1. Trunk returns to midline in preparation for weight transfer to other limb.	1. Hip abductors relaxed by middle of period.
2. This creates passive abduction of hip.	2. Shift controlled by hip adductors longus and magnus.

Plate 4. BALANCE ASSISTANCE

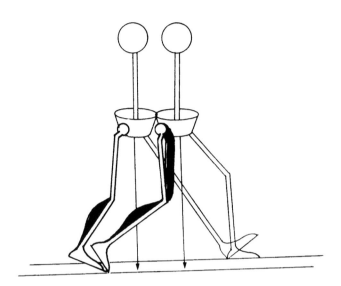

TASK: BALANCE–ASSIST (INTERVAL: LAST HALF OF PUSH–OFF)
Maximum Push Force to Toe–Off: 50 to 60% of Walking Cycle

DEMAND:
  Assist body balance as other limb "struggles" to accept weight.

SITUATION:
  Period of double limb support.
  Weight rapidly transferred to other limb.
  Primary limb maintains floor contact for balance while it prepares for swing.
  Body well ahead of limb.

RESPONSE:

Events	Anatomical Activity
FORWARD PROGRESSION:	
1. Rapid weight transfer removes resistance at knee and ankle.	1. Rapid and marked passive knee flexion (0 to 50°). No knee flexor muscle activity evident.
2. Floor contact maintained.	2. a. Postural equinus due to forward tipping of tibia by the knee flexion with the hip extended. b. Active plantar flexion: only gastrocnemius and posterior tibialis silent.
	3. Hip extension lessens (—10° to 0°). Adductor longus and magnus active (let's not quibble whether this is hip joint or pelvis motion).
SINGLE LIMB BALANCE (lateral alignment)	
Period of double limb support. Weight shifting rapidly across midline to other foot.	Adductors (magnus and longus) restrain lateral shift, hence add stability.

Plate 5. PICK-UP

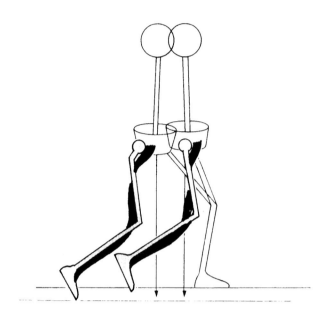

TASK: PICK–UP (INTERVAL: EARLY SWING)
      Toe–Off to End of Knee Flexion: 60 to 75% of Walking Cycle

DEMAND:
    Lift foot from ground in preparation for forward reach.

SITUATION:
    Weight entirely on other limb
    Extremity far behind body axis
    Toe extended down toward ground as a result of:
        1) the marked knee flexion
        2) the length of foot that protrudes beyond the line of the leg
        3) ankle in maximum equinis from assisting balance

RESPONSE:

Events	Anatomical Activity
FORWARD PROGRESSION:	
1. Entire extremity lifted to overcome postural and true equinus.	1. a. Active hip flexion (0° to 5°) by: iliacus, sartorius, tensor fascia femoris.
	b. Active knee flexion (50° to 70°) by: biceps femoris (short head), sartorius.
2. At toe-off, foot posterior and lateral to axis of body.	2. Extremity brought toward midline by adductor magnus.
LIMB LENGTH ADJUSTMENT:	
1. Limb shortened to aid toe clearance.	1. Pelvis rotates forward from its maximum posterior position.

Plate 6. REACH

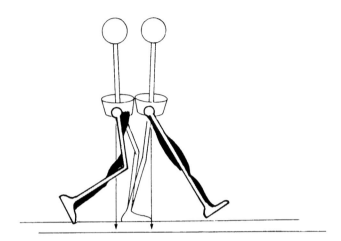

TASK: REACH (INTERVAL: LATE SWING)
   Period of Knee Extension During Swing: 75 to 100% of Walking Cycle

DEMAND:
   Advance foot for next step in forward progression.
   Be ready to receive the advancing body weight.

SITUATION:
   Body traveling forward as a result of previous push and stance activity of other limb.
   Extremity suspended in a flexed posture at every joint.
   Foot still behind axis of body.
   Toe clear.

RESPONSE:

Events	Anatomical Activity
FORWARD PROGRESSION:	
1. Limb advances rapidly to reach weight acceptance position before body weight is too far ahead for stability.	1. Knee extends rapidly from its 70 degrees flexed posture by relaxation of flexors and pendulum effect. Extensors (Vasti) become active at end of period to maintain full knee extension. Hip flexion increased slightly (to 30°) and maintained by adductors.
2. Toe kept clear of ground.	2. Active dorsiflexion.
LIMB LENGTH ADJUSTMENT:	
1. Limb lengthened.	1. Pelvis continues to rotate with advancing limb. Also drops into further adduction.

Index